Diabetes and Vascular Disease

Diabetes and Vascular Disease

Edited by

Morris D. Kerstein, M.D.

Professor, Department of Surgery
Associate Dean for Academic Affairs
Director, Graduate and Postgraduate Medical Education
Louis and Helen Sizelar Chair in Vascular Surgery
Tulane University School of Medicine
New Orleans, Louisiana

With 22 Contributors

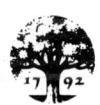

J. B. LIPPINCOTT COMPANY   Philadelphia
Grand Rapids   New York   St. Louis   San Francisco
London   Sydney   Tokyo

Acquisitions Editor: Lisa McAllister
Coordinating Editorial Assistant: Paula M. Callaghan
Project Editor: Lorraine D. Smith
Copy Editor: Mary Frawley
Indexer: Alberta Morrison
Design Coordinator: Doug Smock
Production Manager: Carol Florence
Compositor: TSI Graphics
Printer/Binder: R. R. Donnelley & Sons Company

Copyright © 1990, by J. B. Lippincott Company. All rights reserved. No part of this book may be used or reproduced in any manner whatsoever without written permission except for brief quotations embodied in critical articles and reviews. Printed in the United States of America. For information write J. B. Lippincott Company, East Washington Square, Philadelphia, Pennsylvania 19105.

1 3 5 6 4 2

Library of Congress Cataloging in Publication Data

Diabetes and vascular disease / edited by Morris D. Kerstein : with 22 contributors.
    p. cm.
Includes bibliographies and index.
ISBN 0-397-50985-5
1. Diabetic angiopathies.   I. Kerstein, Morris D.
[DNLM: 1. Diabetes Mellitus—complications.   2. Diabetes Mellitus—therapy.   3. Diabetic Angiopathies—complications.   WK 835 D5342]
RC700.D5D53 1990
616.4′62—dc20
DNLM/DLC   89-8177
for Library of Congress   CIP

The authors and publisher have exerted every effort to ensure that drug selection and dosage set forth in this text are in accord with current recommendations and practice at the time of publication. However, in view of ongoing research, changes in government regulations, and the constant flow of information relating to drug therapy and drug reactions, the reader is urged to check the package insert for each drug for any change in indications and dosage and for added warnings and precautions. This is particularly important when the recommended agent is a new or infrequently used drug.

To Margaret, Lars, and Minnie, without whose love and support I could not achieve.

To my students and residents, who reward me with the joy of teaching.

Contributors

Donald L. Akers, M.D.
Fellow, Vascular Surgery
University of Cincinnati
Cincinnati, Ohio
Chapter 15

Julian L. Ambrus, M.D., Ph.D.
Resident Professor of Internal Medicine and Experimental Pathology
State University of New York at Buffalo
Director of Cancer Research (Pathophysiology)
Roswell Park Memorial Institute
Buffalo, New York
Chapter 2

Prabhakar K. Baliga, M.D.
Chief Resident, Department of Surgery
Tulane University School of Medicine
New Orleans, Louisiana
Chapter 1

William T. Cefalu, M.D.
Assistant Professor of Medicine
Section on Endocrinology and Metabolism
The Bowman Gray School of Medicine
Wake Forest University
Winston-Salem, North Carolina
Chapter 10

Rex S. Clements, Jr., M.D.
Vice-President of Medical Affairs
Squibb Novo
Princeton, New Jersey
Chapter 10

Gordon Cohen, M.D.
Resident, Department of Surgery
University of California at Los Angeles
Los Angeles, California
Chapter 15

James M. Falko, M.D.
Professor of Medicine and Physiological Chemistry
Division of Endocrinology and Metabolism
Department of Internal Medicine
Ohio State University College of Medicine
Columbus, Ohio
Chapter 9

Eric I. Friedman, M.D.
Resident in Surgery
Oregon Health Sciences University
Portland, Oregon
Chapter 13

Morris D. Kerstein, M. D.
Professor, Department of Surgery
Associate Dean for Academic Affairs
Director, Graduate and Postgraduate Medical Education
Louis and Helen Sizelar Chair in Vascular Surgery
Tulane University School of Medicine
New Orleans, Louisiana
Chapter 1, Chapter 15

Charles Kilo, M. D.
Associate Professor in Clinical Medicine
Washington University School of Medicine
Attending Physician, Barnes Hospital
Chairman, Kilo Diabetes and Vascular Research Foundation
St. Louis, Missouri
Chapter 6

Brian W. King, Ph.D.
Assistant Director, Scientific Communications
Hoechst–Roussel Pharmaceuticals, Inc.
Somerville, New Jersey
Chapter 11

CONTRIBUTORS

John S. Kirkland, M.D., Ph.D.
Clinical Instructor in Surgery
Emory University; Section of Vascular Surgery
Harbin Clinic
Rome, Georgia
Chapter 14

Leo P. Krall, M.D., D.Sc. (Hon.)
Education, Joslin Diabetes Center
Lecturer on Medicine
Harvard Medical School
Senior Staff, New England Deaconess Hospital
Boston, Massachusetts
Chapter 7

Kevin J. Lafferty, Ph.D.
Director of Research, Barbara Davis Center for Childhood Diabetes
University of Colorado Health Sciences Center
Department of Microbiology/Immunology
University Hospital
Denver, Colorado
Chapter 16

Steven B. Leichter, M.D.
Professor of Medicine
Eastern Virginia Medical School
Director of Clinical Programs
Diabetes Center of Eastern Virginia
Norfolk, Virginia
Chapter 5

Marvin E. Levin, M.D.
Professor of Clinical Medicine
Associate Director, Diabetes and Metabolism Clinic
Washington University School of Medicine
Associate Physician, Barnes Hospital
St. Louis, Missouri
Chapter 12

Lyndee Paris, B.S.
    University of Colorado Medical School
    Denver, Colorado
Chapter 16

John M. Porter, M.D.
    Professor of Surgery
    Head, Division of Vascular Surgery
    Oregan Health Sciences University
    Portland, Oregon
Chapter 13

Philip Raskin, M.D.
    Professor, Department of Internal Medicine
    University of Texas Southwestern Medical Center
    Dallas, Texas
Chapter 4

Alan M. Reich, M.D.
    Clinical Assistant Professor of Medicine
    University of Illinois at Chicago
    Chicago, Illinois
    Lutheran General Hospital
    Park Ridge, Illinois
Chapter 8

D. Eugene Strandness, Jr., M.D.
    Professor of Surgery
    University of Washington
    Seattle, Washington
Chapter 3

Joseph R. Williamson, M.D.
    Professor of Pathology
    Washington University School of Medicine
    Pathologist, Barnes Hospital
    St. Louis, Missouri
Chapter 6

Foreword

The relationship between diabetes mellitus and vascular disease has long been recognized. With the discovery of insulin in 1921, our understanding of diabetes and its treatment has expanded rapidly, and sophisticated and precise control of blood glucose levels is now possible. Control of blood glucose levels, however, has not prevented the cardiovascular complications of diabetes, which continue to be the major source of morbidity and mortality in diabetic patients. Diabetes is associated with adverse effects throughout the cardiovascular system, including large elastic arteries, medium and small muscular arteries, arterioles, and capillaries. In addition to disturbances of flow in the microcirculation, abnormalities exist in the circulating blood itself. Our knowledge and level of understanding in these areas is increasing, but remains imprecise. The clinical cardiovascular manifestations of diabetes include myocardial infarction, stroke, peripheral occlusive disease, retinopathy, renal failure, and peripheral neuropathy. These diverse manifestations are incompletely understood and demand continuing close investigation by the research scientist and clinician. In this monograph, the relationship between vascular disease and diabetes mellitus is reviewed. Basic concepts of hemorrheology and microcirculation associated with metabolic alterations and glycemic control are carefully outlined and are related to the natural history and risk factors of vascular disease. Important considerations of clinical management of diabetes, including an understanding of peripheral neuropathy and considerations of nonsurgical hemorrheologic pharmacologic manipulations in the management of diabetic microvascular disease, are reviewed. The medical and surgical management of patients with diabetes and vascular disease is clearly presented. This is an important book because it compiles in one volume the current concepts related to both large and small vessel diabetic vascular disease, including pathophysiology, clinical assessment, medical management, and operative and nonoperative strategies of treatment. It provides a sound data base and background for clinicians managing patients with diabetic vascular disease and serves as a useful reference. Further investigation and focus on the problems, as outlined in this volume, should lead to new information that will help us to better treat and manage our diabetic patients in the future.

Christopher K. Zarins, M.D.
Professor of Surgery
Chief, Section of Vascular Surgery
The University of Chicago
Chicago, Illinois

Preface

"There are men too gentle to live among wolves."*
James Kavanaugh

Diabetes and the problems of associated vascular disease have plagued patients for centuries.

Multiple informational forces impact on the physician, yet basic science is the foundation of clinical knowledge. The authors have tried to present a clinical correlation of the problem of diabetes and vascular disease supported by some of the historic and current knowledge on progression of vascular disease from the chemistry of cellular change to intervention of transplantation.

To what doctrines should we cling? If the correct answers all were known, it would be easy. This monograph, "Diabetes and Vascular Disease," wishes to stimulate others by its simplicity and directness; avenues unexplored can be filled by the reader seeking more complete answers.

Many patients with diabetes suffer various disabilities, including amputation or death. Only through a better understanding of the pathology and methods of clinical assessment can the continuance of care culminate in a well patient.

Morris D. Kerstein, M.D.

*E. P. Dutton & Co., Inc., New York, 1970

Acknowledgments

I wish to express my appreciation to Laura Miller for her understanding, cooperation, and patience—for the hours in the library, for typing, and for support.

To the contributors who gave time from their already overcrowded schedules—a sincere expression of appreciation.

A special expression of gratitude is extended to Brian W. King and Hoechst–Roussel Pharmaceuticals for their cooperation, patience, and indulgence.

To Gae O. Decker–Garrad, editorial associate, friend—your help, support, and encouragement are the perfect blend of knowledge, reliability, perceptiveness, and patience.

Contents

Chapter 1
HEMORRHEOLOGY AND MICROCIRCULATION 1
Prabhakar K. Baliga and *Morris D. Kerstein*
Red Blood Cell Concentration and Aggregation 4
Red Blood Cell Deformability 5
Plasma Viscosity 6

Chapter 2
MICROVASCULAR CHANGES IN DIABETES 9
Julian L. Ambrus
Red Blood Cell Deformability 11
Stiff Cell Syndrome 21
Biochemical Mechanism of Pentoxifylline Action 27
Role of Cyclo-Oxygenase Inhibitors as Agents to Improve Blood Flow 30
Pentoxifylline to Facilitate Perfusion 31

Chapter 3
NATURAL HISTORY AND RISK FACTORS IN PERIPHERAL VASCULAR DISEASE 41
D. Eugene Strandness, Jr.
Historical Perspective 41
Prevalence 42
Risk Factors 43
Natural History—Progression of Disease 45

Chapter 4
ROLE OF HYPERGLYCEMIA IN DEVELOPMENT OF DIABETES COMPLICATIONS   49
Philip Raskin

Natural History of Diabetes	49
Diabetic Complications: Genetic Influences	53
Diabetic Complications: Metabolic Influences	56
Clinical Trials	64
Controlled Prospective Trials	68
Conclusions	80

Chapter 5
ASSOCIATION BETWEEN GLYCEMIC CONTROL AND DEGENERATIVE COMPLICATIONS OF DIABETES MELLITUS: A BRIEF REVIEW OF CURRENT CONCEPTS   87
Steven B. Leichter

Classification of Diabetic Complications	88
Metabolic Factors and Microvascular Complications	88
In Vivo Evidence About Metabolic Control and Diabetic Microvascular Complications	90
Questions About Strict Glycemic Control and Microvascular Complications	91
Diabetes Control and Complications Trial	92
Metabolic Control and Macrovascular Complications	92

Chapter 6
HORMONES, SUGAR ALCOHOLS, AND DIABETIC COMPLICATIONS   97
Joseph R. Williamson and *Charles Kilo*

Historic Commentary	97
Basic Studies in Diabetic Animal Model	98

Chapter 7
MODERN TREATMENT OF TYPE II DIABETES — 109
Leo P. Krall
Management	111
Short-Term (Acute) Effects of "Control"	111
Control	112
Treatment	113
Classification of Diabetes	114
Treatment of Type II Diabetes	116

Chapter 8
NEWER MODES OF TREATING TYPE II DIABETES — 123
Alan M. Reich
Pathophysiology	124
Therapeutic Modalities	125
Sulfonylurea Agents	130
Insulin	137

Chapter 9
NEW STRATEGIES IN THE TREATMENT OF TYPE II DIABETES — 143
James M. Falko
Impaired Insulin Secretion	143
Increased Hepatic Production of Glucose	145
Insulin Resistance	146
Management Strategies	146
C-Peptide	156

Chapter 10
DIABETIC NEUROPATHY — 163
William T. Cefalu and Rex Clements, Jr.
Prevalence	164
Clinical Presentation	164
Treatment	173

Chapter 11
DRUGS THAT AFFECT THE HEMORRHEOLOGIC PROPERTIES OF BLOOD — 181
Brian W. King
Hemorrheology in Diabetics — 181
Drugs Affecting Hemorrheology — 182

Chapter 12
MEDICAL MANAGEMENT OF THE DIABETIC FOOT — 193
Marvin E. Levin
Diabetic Peripheral Vascular Disease — 194
Diabetic Peripheral Neuropathy — 199
Saving the Diabetic Foot — 204

Chapter 13
NONOPERATIVE TREATMENT OF INTERMITTENT CLAUDICATION — 215
John M. Porter and *Eric I. Friedman*
Perspective — 215
Lack of Exercise and Smoking as Limiting Factors — 216
Pharmacologic Manipulation — 216

Chapter 14
MEDICAL AND SURGICAL MANAGEMENT OF PERIPHERAL VASCULAR DISEASE IN THE DIABETIC PATIENT — 229
John S. Kirkland
Pathophysiology of Atherosclerosis — 229
Diagnosis of Peripheral Vascular Occlusive Disease — 231
Medical Management — 233
Surgical Management — 235
Reconstructive Techniques — 235

Chapter 15
PERIPHERAL VASCULAR DISEASE AND THE DIABETIC PATIENT 241
Donald L. Akers, Gordon Cohen, and *Morris D. Kerstein*
Pathophysiology 241
Diagnosis 246
Clinical Investigation 249
Management 256

Chapter 16
ISLET TRANSPLANTATION IN ANIMALS AND HUMANS 267
Kevin J. Lafferty and *Lyndee Paris*
Allograft Response 267
Disease Recurrence 272

INDEX 279

Diabetes and Vascular Disease

CHAPTER ONE

Hemorrheology and Microcirculation

Prabhakar K. Baliga
Morris D. Kerstein

Hemorrheology is the study of the interaction of blood and its components and the vascular system with added foreign materials, such as drugs, plasma expanders, or prosthetic devices. It is also the study of deformation behavior, including flow of blood and those materials of blood vessels and surrounding tissues with which blood or its components come into direct contact.

The capillary bed forms the functional unit of nutrient exchange and consists of arterioles, which control flow into the capillaries, and venules, which drain the capillary bed. Lymphatics also form an integral part of this unit. The flow of blood through the capillary bed depends largely on the hemodynamic forces and pressure gradient between arterial and venous ends. In the smaller vessels, flow is inversely related to the diameter of the channels and viscosity of the fluid. The latter, in turn, is determined by four factors: red blood cell concentration, red blood cell aggregation, red blood cell deformability, and plasma viscosity.[2] The fluidity of blood in the microcirculation is dependent on adequate flow forces. High shear stress at the microcirculatory level can overcome deficiencies in the rheologic properties of blood. With the presence of stenosis, a reduction of shear stress may lead to increased red blood cell aggregation, decreased ability of red blood cells to deform, increased viscosity of blood, and impedance of fluid motion.

Hemodynamic compensatory changes follow arteriolar dilatation; these changes cause increased vascular conductance, with a local increase in driving pressures and shear stress. Because this mechanism is limited, fluidity depends largely on the fluid properties of blood. Axial migration of red blood cells results in aggregation and plasma marginates against the vessel wall.

Because red blood cells have loss of nuclei, a unique membrane structure and shape provide the red blood cells with an intrinsic ability to deform and pass through channels less than half their diameter. Blood viscosity is affected, as well, by the hematocrit; a decrease in hematocrit causes a decrease in viscosity. This compensatory mechanism is especially effective in the presence of narrowed vessels and a low shear stress.

The successful function of any closed circulation depends, in part, on diffusional constraints, which tend to minimize capillary and red blood cell diameters and increase red blood cell deformability. Elaborate hemostatic mechanisms must be established to avoid blood loss related to injury, and sufficiently high pressures must be generated to maintain flow through vessels.

The presence of a closed circulation in vertebrates has led to the evolution of microcirculation. This term refers to the smallest components of the cardiovascular system—arterioles, venules, and capillaries. In a closed circulatory system, tissue exchange is maximized by the small diameter of these vessels. Compensatory changes include the loss of nuclei during maturation of the mammalian red blood cells and possession of the remarkable ability to deform in order to pass through vessels half their size in diameter. The study of this aspect of circulation—how the blood and blood vessels interact and function as integral parts of the living organism—is referred to as *hemorrheology*.

It is becoming increasingly evident that the status of the cardiovasculature as a whole is critically dependent on the function of blood vessels, some of which are smaller than 0.1 mm in diameter. Capillaries are the smallest channels of the cardiovascular system; on an average, they have an inner diameter of 5 mm. They are lined with a single layer of flat endothelial cells joined by tight junctions. The network of capillaries—the capillary bed—forms the functional unit of tissue exchange. The simple, thin lining of capillaries facilitates exchange of respiratory gases, fluids, and metabolites between the circulating blood and surrounding tissues. Each organ has its own characteristic microcirculation varying in length, density, and architecture. Of the three types of capillaries—continuous, discontinuous, and fenestrated—the latter two have large pores in their endothelial cytoplasm, which facilitate transendothelial transport of large molecules.[10]

Arterioles are small arteries with an average width of less than 5 mm and with an inner lining of flat endothelial cells surrounded by one or two layers of smooth muscle cells.[11] Nonmyelinated nerves adhere closely to the arteriolar wall, and neurotransmitters control the flow of blood into the capillary bed. In hypertension, a generalized narrowing and rigidity of the arteriolar system occur, causing an increase in peripheral resistance.

The capillary bed is drained by venules that contain endothelial lining continuous with the capillaries. The venules further away from the capillaries are lined with smooth muscle cells.[12] The junctional regions of these endothelial cells can be made to open up under the influence of histamine and serotonin and facilitate emigration of leukocytes. Nonmyelinated nerves accompany all venules, but the contraction of venules is slow and limited in degree compared with that of the arterioles.

In addition to the channels described above, the microcirculation contains lymphatic capillaries, an integral part of the system, and numerous arteriovenous anastomoses and preferential channels, which lead from one capillary bed to another.[10]

The primary function of circulation is to deliver blood to various organs to facilitate oxygenation and nutrient exchange. The flow of blood through these small vessels depends on sufficient force (pressure) being generated proximally. This rate of blood flow through the microcirculation is determined by the pressure gradient between the arteries and veins and is inversely related to flow resistance.[2] The latter is governed by viscosity of the fluid and geometry of the blood vessels. Blood viscosity, in turn, relies on red blood cell concentration, red blood cell aggregation, red blood cell deformability, and plasma viscosity.[2] Integrity and successful functioning of the microcirculation rely on the complex interaction among these various factors. Failure or disease in one leads the compensatory mechanisms to facilitate normal functioning of the system.

Fluidity, an essential property of blood as a transport organ, depends on the uninterrupted presence of sufficient hemodynamic forces (*i.e.*, a normal cardiovascular system). Reduction in the driving forces (*e.g.*, generalized hypotension or a local obstruction) is compensated for by arteriolar vasodilatation, leading to increased vascular conductance, increased local driving pressure, and increased shear stresses. The vasomotor dilatory reserve of microcirculation is limited, and when this aspect of the system has been maximized, flow depends on the viscosity of blood.[6]

A critical reduction in flow forces, however, cannot be overcome by the fluidity of blood and leads to increased rouleaux formation, inability of red blood cells to deform, and a decrease in the plasma volume fraction. The end result is that the blood degenerates from a highly fluid emulsion to a viscous reticulated suspension with functional properties of a solid. In a vascular network, the longer, narrower channels with the lower conductance are affected preferentially.

On the other hand, an adequate shear stress can overcome

differences in rheologic properties of blood. These deficiencies would then manifest preferentially in areas where local shear forces are insufficient.

RED BLOOD CELL CONCENTRATION AND AGGREGATION

Under conditions of normal flow, the formation of red blood cell aggregation is a fully reversible physiologic event. It is highly dependent on the hematocrit level and shear stress. If, however, because of severe hemodynamic impairment the shear stress falls below a critical level, intensified aggregation occurs and the blood loses its Newtonian properties. A lowered red blood cell count reduces the collision probability of red blood cell-forming aggregates. At a hematocrit of less than 35%, no strong network of rouleaux exists. Bailey and colleagues showed that hemoglobin was significantly lower in diabetics who healed their amputations primarily.[1] The implication is that the flow in the microcirculation is critical for limb salvage. A decrease in viscosity of flow or a decrease in particulate matter is necessary for effective nutrient exchange and off-loading of oxygen to the tissue. Other investigators showed that lowering the hematocrit by means of hemodilution aided the healing of ulcers in patients with peripheral vascular disease.[8] The reduction in viscosity in low shear stresses beyond a vascular obliteration aids tissue perfusion.[14] The gain in fluidity exceeds the loss in oxygen transport capacity. It is felt that shear stress present at a higher hematocrit almost disappears totally at a hematocrit level of 35% or below. Besides the hemorrheologic effects, the low hematocrit leads to an increased stroke volume, increased cardiac output, and decreased total peripheral resistance. Overall, it leads to increased oxygenation of vital organs; however, it must be realized that the compensatory mechanisms are limited.[8] It is apparent that if the flow is decreased beyond a critical point, no therapeutic benefit can be achieved by reducing blood viscosity. In patients with an increased hematocrit, red blood cell aggregation and increased viscosity become manifest at significantly higher shear stresses than normal human subjects. Blood fluidity is jeopardized by high hematocrit values.[5] The plasma viscosity and fibrinogen content tend to be lower than normal, seeming to normalize fluidity. The patients have a high risk of cardiovascular decompensation and thromboembolic events.[3] If sufficient hemodynamic forces and shear stresses are present, passive flow adaptation and fluidity of the blood are maintained.

The relationship between red blood cell concentration and blood viscosity is an exponential one. A greater effect of hematocrit on blood viscosity occurs at low shear in flow rate. Several investigators have shown that an increased red blood cell concentration may be a primary risk factor, leading to an increased risk of hypertension, myocardial infarction, and cerebrovascular accident.[3,7,9] In the Framingham study, males with a hemoglobin concentration greater than 15 g/dl and females with a hemoglobin concentration greater than 14 g/dl had twice the risk of being hypertensive or suffering from a cerebrovascular accident.[7]

The increased red blood cell concentration increases aggregation and viscosity and causes a decreased blood flow at the same shear stresses. Under increased shear stress predisposing to thrombosis, increased platelet–endothelial contact, increased platelet adhesion, and release of adenosine diphosphate occur.

RED BLOOD CELL DEFORMABILITY

The rapid, unimpeded flow of concentrated cell suspension is a unique phenomenon based on the ability of the denucleated red blood cell to deform. The cell is endowed with a favorable ratio of surface area to volume and, thus, can be deformed without straining the membrane. The cells pass through the splenic circulation where red blood cells devoid of this property are sequestered and phagocytized. Consequently, all red blood cells found circulating in the peripheral blood are highly selected and capable of promoting flow in microvessels through their potential of change in shape and flexibility.

Forces exerted on the erythrocyte deform it into various shapes induced by motion of the membrane relative to its content. Dreissen and co-workers, in experiments injecting rigidified red blood cells into rats, showed that complete loss of red blood cell fluidity was incompatible with circulation and cell survival, whereas with reduced deformability, circulation is maintained so long as flow forces are sufficient to induce red blood cell deformation.[4] Fluidity of the red blood cells is responsible for rapid axial migration; produces marginal layer lubricating, low-viscosity plasma; and leads to a reduction in dynamic hematocrit. By microscopic observation, it was seen that blood flow at extremely low shear stresses is induced by shearing in a plasma layer surrounding a solid plug of red blood cell aggregate network, and fluidity is determined by the width and fluidity of the plasma layer. An added dividend of red blood cell fluidity is rapid and highly effective intracellular mixing, which induces complex intracellular laminar flow of hemoglobin, oxyhemoglobin, and dissolved oxygen. As a consequence, diffusive transport of oxygen in and out of red blood cells is augmented.[15] The advantage of this characteristic of human red blood cells is that mammalian capillaries are much smaller, the volume occupied by these capillaries is smaller, and the exchange area is much higher. The goal of therapeutic intervention would be to change the shape of the red blood cell to allow for passage flexibility without losing the ability to off-load oxygen.

PLASMA VISCOSITY

Elevations of plasma viscosity are generally associated with an enhanced tendency of red blood cell aggregation. It is uncertain whether the increased or abnormal plasma proteins adhere to red blood cell membranes and curtail their fluidity. Abnormal concentrations of high-molecular-weight proteins, such as fibrinogen, promote rouleaux formation. Several examples of this process are found in many chronic disease states associated with elevated sedimentation rates in which hepatic overproduction of this macromolecule compromises the fluidity of blood and promotes coagulation and thrombotic deposits. Increased fibrinogen levels have been found in patients with myocardial infarction, cerebrovascular accidents, diabetes, peripheral arterial disease, and hyperlipoproteinemias. Red blood cell aggregates become manifest at higher shear stresses, and blood flow declines in the presence of flow forces that would normally keep blood in a fluid state.[13] In the presence of polycythemia and other hyperviscosity syndromes in which blood fluidity is compromised, fibrinogen level and plasma viscosity decrease, thereby tending to normalize blood fluidity.

Functioning of the entire system depends on the presence of an elaborate hemostatic mechanism to avoid blood loss secondary to injury. Clotting depends on platelets and coagulation factors. The initial vascular phase decreases blood flow to the site of injury. The second phase involves platelets adhering to the subendothelial collagen fibrils and release of vasoactive factors, resulting in further vasoconstriction and platelet aggregation. The plasma factor phase is initiated and consists of a series of zymogen activation and regulated proteolysis, with multiple components acting in a contributory fashion. The end result is formulation of fibrin and a stable clot. The blood also contains factors that promote dissolution of clots with restoration of flow to normality.

SUMMARY

The successful functioning of a closed circulation depends on sufficiently high pressures being generated to maintain flow through these narrow channels. Diffusional constraints tend to minimize capillary and red blood cell diameters and increase red blood cell deformability. Elaborate hemostatic mechanisms have been established to prevent blood loss caused by injury. The entire system is not foolproof and is compromised frequently by both congenital and acquired deficiencies. Compensatory mechanisms within the system cover for these deficiencies. A combination of hemorrheologic abnormalities and a critical decrease in hemodynamic forces results in production of disease symptoms. A mechanism to facilitate red blood cell deformability may be the adjunct to fluidity and flow.

REFERENCES

1. Bailey MJ, Yates CJP, Johnston CLW et al: Preoperative hemoglobin as predictor of outcome of diabetic amputations. Lancet 2:168–170, 1979
2. Chin S: Progress in clinical hemorrheology. Fahraeus Lectures, 1981
3. Dormandy J: Progress in clinical hemorrheology. Fahraeus Lectures, 1983
4. Dreissen GK, Haest CWM, Heidtmann H et al: Effect of reduced red cell deformability on flow velocity in capillaries of rat mesentery. Pfleugers Arch 388:75–78, 1980
5. Dreissen GK, Heidtmann H, Schmid-Schonbein H: Effect of hematocrit on red cell velocity in capillaries of rat mesentery during hemodilution and hemoconcentration. Pfleugers Arch 380:1–6, 1979
6. Holger SS: Factors promoting and preventing the fluidity of blood. In Effros RM et al (eds): Microcirculation, pp 249–266. New York, Academic Press, 1981
7. Kannel WB, Jordon T, Wolf P et al: Hemoglobin and the risk of cerebral infarction. The Framingham Study. Stroke 3:409–420, 1972
8. Kessler M, Messmer K: Tissue oxygenation during hemodilution. Bibl Haemotol 41:16, 1975
9. Reiger H, Kholer M, Schoop W et al: Hemodilution as a therapy in occlusive vascular disease of the limb. In Effros RM et al

(eds): Microcirculation, pp 281–292. New York, Academic Press, 1981
10. Rhodin JAG: Anatomy of the microcirculation. In Effros RM et al (eds): Microcirculation, pp 11–17. New York, Academic Press, 1981
11. Rhodin JAG: Ultrastructure of mammalian arterioles and precapillary sphincters. J Ultrastruct Res 18:181–223, 1967
12. Rhodin JAG: Ultrastructure of mammalian venous capillaries, venules and small collecting veins. J Ultrastruct Res 25:452–500, 1968
13. Schmid-Schonbein H: Blood fluidity as a consequence of red cell fluidity: Flow properties of blood and flow behavior of blood in vascular diseases. Angiology 31:301–319, 1980
14. Yates CJP, Vivienne A, Berent A et al: Increase in leg blood flow by normovolemic hemodilution in intermittent claudication. Lancet 2:166–168, 1979
15. Zander R, Schmid-Schonbein H: Intracellular mechanisms of oxygen transport in flowing blood. Respir Physiol 19:279–289, 1973

CHAPTER TWO
Microvascular Changes in Diabetes
Julian L. Ambrus

The role that blood cells play in microvascular perfusion has been reviewed at length.[1-5,7-9,11-19,21-26,28,29,31] Figure 2-1 is an intraoperative picture of the microcirculation; the large capillary containing red blood cells branches into small capillaries with an average diameter of 3 μm. An average human red blood cell has a diameter of about 8 μm. An 8-μm ball can get through a 3-μm tube only if it squeezes, takes a cigar shape, and folds up on itself. A red blood cell flexing and slipping through in a modified shape in the microcirculation is shown in the lower right corner of Figure 2-1.

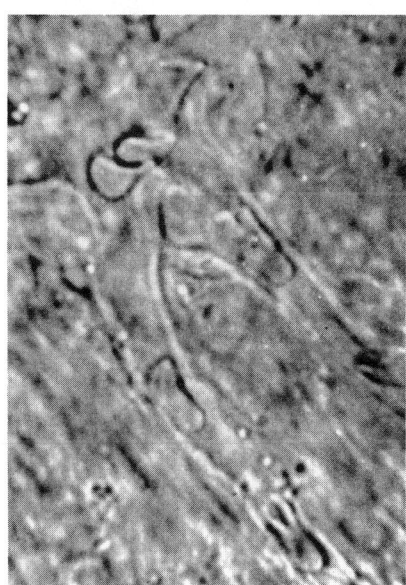

Figure 2-1. Mesenteric microcirculation by intraoperative microscopy shows shape change by red blood cells in the small capillaries.

When it gets into the large capillaries, it reverts back to its normal shape.

It is clear, therefore, that flexibility, or deformability, of the red blood cell membrane is an important attribute of the normal red blood cell. In several disease conditions, relatively nonflexible red blood cells are found. This condition is known as the "stiff red cell syndrome." Following is a list of diseases in which red blood cells are relatively stiff:

Hemoglobinopathies: Sickle cell disease, hereditary spherocytosis, thalassemia

Vessel wall and related disorders: Chronic obstructive arteriosclerotic disease (including Buerger's disease), Raynaud's syndrome, advanced diabetes mellitus (with ketoacidosis macro- and microangiopathy, retinopathy, nephropathy, neuropathy), toxemia of pregnancy

Red blood cell parasitism: Malaria, Nantucket fever (*Babesia microti*)

Miscellaneous disorders: Mountain sickness, brisket disease, emphysema suffered by heavy smokers, Behçet's disease, ankylosing spondylitis, advanced metastatic malignant melanoma

A prominent member of the stiff red cell syndrome family is diabetes. Figure 2-2 illustrates that when an 8-μm nonflexible red blood cell cannot get through a 3-μm capillary, it does one of two things: (1) it lodges in the narrowed area and obstructs the microcirculation, then also represents a surface on which platelets aggregate, stimulating clotting and producing a stable clot; or (2) it may bypass the microcirculation, which is too narrow for it to get

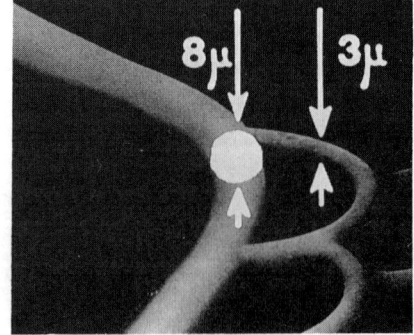

Figure 2-2. A red blood cell in the microcirculation.

into, and stay in the larger channels, leaving part of the tissue inadequately oxygenated.

RED BLOOD CELL DEFORMABILITY

Red blood cell deformability is the single most important factor in determining whole blood viscosity (Fig. 2-3). This is not commonly realized, because the average clinical laboratory is set up to measure plasma viscosity and recognize the hyperviscosity syndrome, but not to measure cellular deformability. Most modern laboratories will measure platelet aggregation using, perhaps, the Born-type aggregometer, but few laboratories are capable of measuring red blood cell deformability. The apparatus used is based on the simple principle that when one inserts membranes with various pore sizes into the apparatus and applies standard negative pressure, it measures speed of passage of cells through the membranes (Figs. 2-4 and 2-5). The results are proportional to the deformability of red blood cells, if red blood cell columns are measured. When working with whole blood, of course, other components are involved as well, including platelet aggregation, white blood cell deformability, and plasma viscosity.

Figure 2-6 is a scanning electron microscopic view of normal whole blood filtered through a 5-μm pore filter. Figure 2-7 depicts a normal red blood cell being filtered through a 3-μm pore filter.

Figure 2-8 shows red blood cell filtration from a patient in sickle cell crisis. Important to note is that not only are the patient's

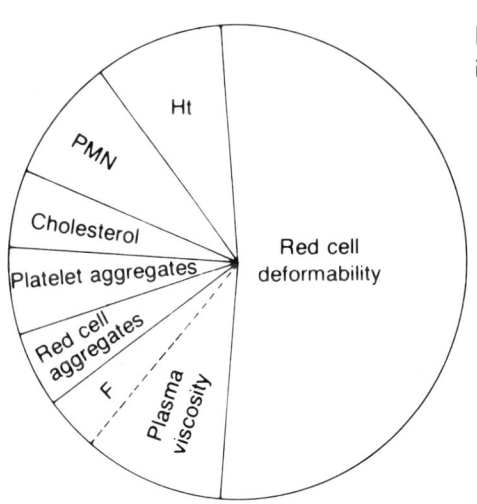

Figure 2-3. Factors that influence blood filterability.

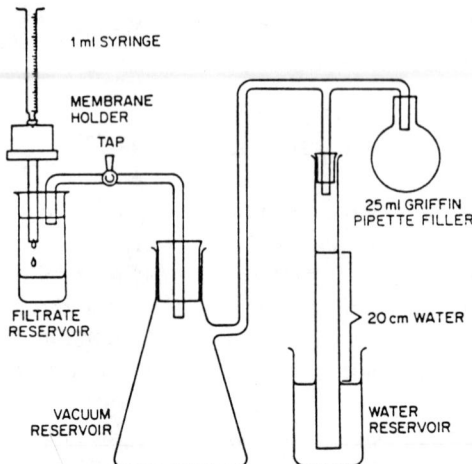

Figure 2-4. Apparatus to measure red blood cell deformability.

Figure 2-5. View of Pop-Top Holder, part of the apparatus in Figure 2-4.

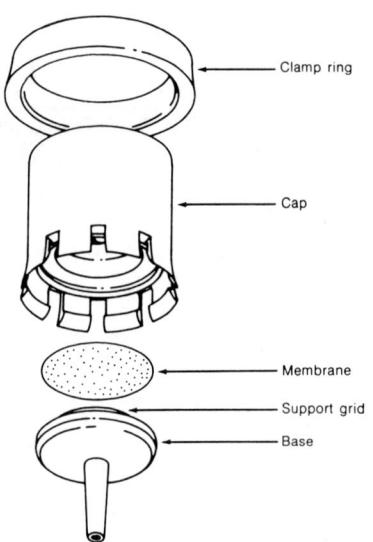

red blood cells abnormally shaped, but they are stiff and make no attempt at flexing and getting through the membranes. They actually block the way of normal red blood cells that might have been introduced into the patient with exchange transfusions.

The significance of the stiff red cell syndrome is shown by the examples in Figure 2-9. This child, a native of Uganda, had SS-genotype sickle cell disease and an overwhelming gram-negative

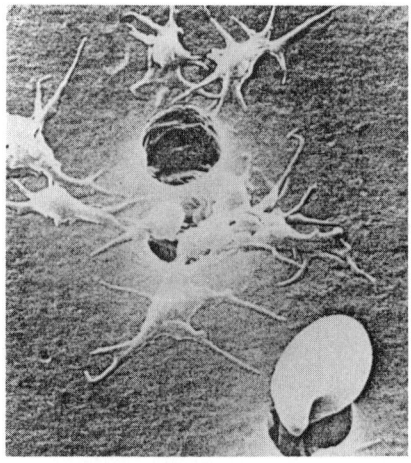

Figure 2-6. Scanning electron microscopic view of normal whole blood filtered through a 5-μm pore diameter filter.

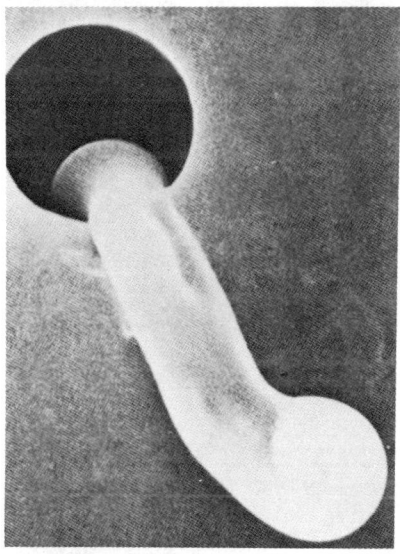

Figure 2-7. Scanning electron microscopic view of a normal human red blood cell filtered through a 3-μm pore diameter filter.

infection. During the evaluation, a macroaggregated human albumin scan of the liver and spleen was reported as normal. The patient was treated with antibiotics and released. Shortly thereafter, the child returned with another episode of gram-negative septicemia. On repeat scan the liver remained normal, but no spleen was seen. The child had obstructed splenic flow with stiff red cells, as well as platelets. The microcirculation of the spleen was overwhelmed until the spleen disappeared completely, which, of course, added to the susceptibility of the child to gram-negative

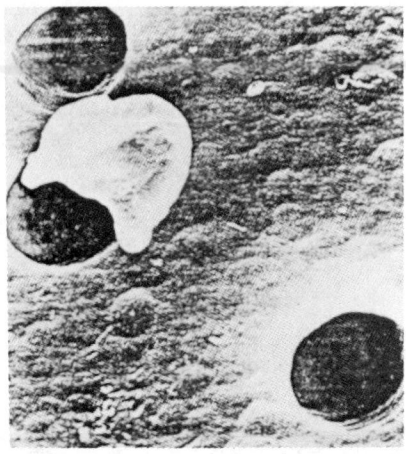

Figure 2-8. Scanning electron microscopic view of red blood cells from a patient in vaso-occlusive crisis of sickle cell disease.

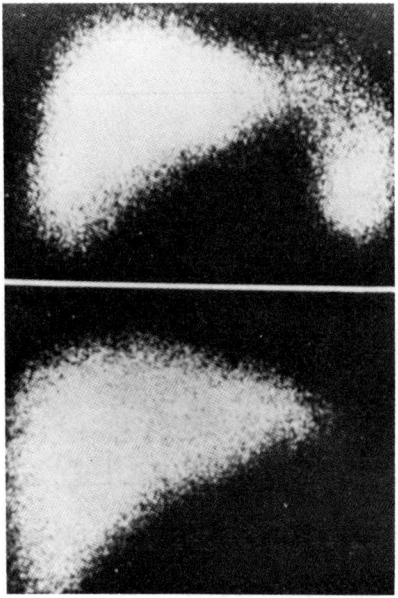

Figure 2-9. Liver-spleen scan of a SS-genotype infant before and after autosplenectomy.

infections. The child died and upon autopsy the bone marrow was found to be virtually empty. The capillaries of the bone marrow were clogged with aggregating red blood cells and platelets (Fig. 2-10).

The importance of the splenic circulation of this type of phenomenon is shown in Figure 2-11, which is an intraoperative picture of a patient who suffered splenic rupture as the result of a car accident. Shown are small pores, which present the same pic-

MICROVASCULAR CHANGES IN DIABETES

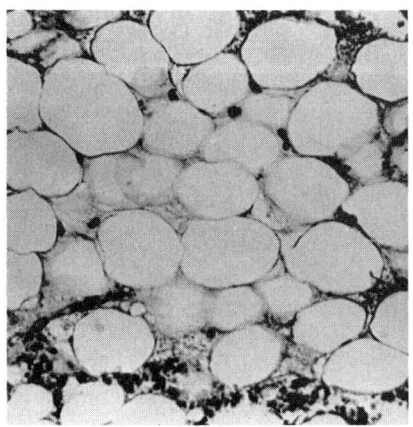

Figure 2-10. Bone marrow of an infant—the subject of Figure 2-9.

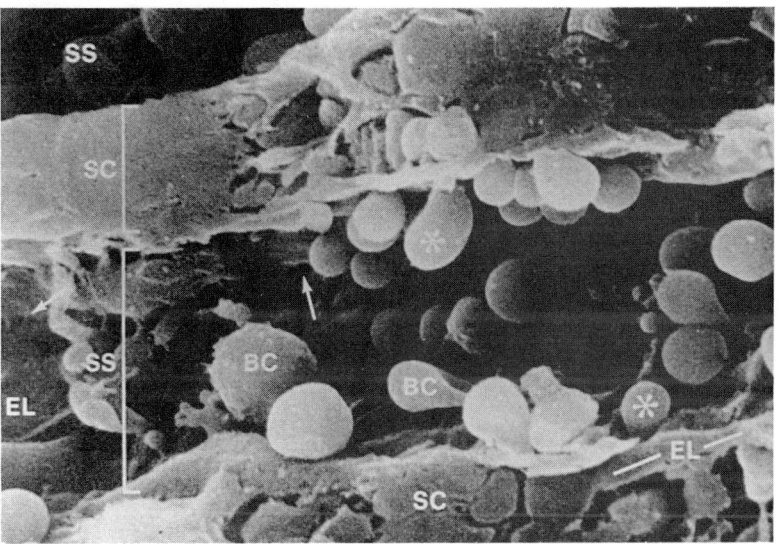

Figure 2-11. Scanning electron microscopic view of a normal spleen. (SS = splenic sinus; EL = endothelial cells; SC = splenic cortex—red pulp; BC = buffy coat elements—white blood cells; * = deforming red blood cells.)

ture as the filters in the apparatus shown above. Red blood cells deform and elongate in preparation to slip through the microcirculatory aspects of the spleen. Obviously, if the red blood cells are stiff and unable to deform, they block the microcirculation and produce splenic infarction.

Another important principle is illustrated in Figure 2-12. In this experiment, SS-genotype blood was put into a chamber, deoxygenated gradually, and observed with a scanning electron microscope. The red blood cell in the middle appears normal. It will eventually assume a sickle shape; however, some membrane changes occurred earlier. The membrane began to stiffen. As the abnormal membranes were touched by platelets, they started to put out pseudopodia and aggregate. This figure illustrates, therefore, that the stiff red cell syndrome brings about platelet aggregation.

Figure 2-13 illustrates another important principle, observed

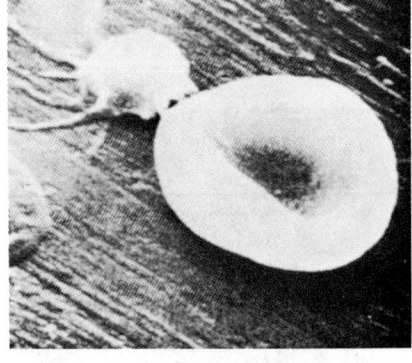

Figure 2-12. SS-genotype red blood cell being deoxygenated before significant morphologic changes develop (sickling). These membrane changes result in increased rigidity and platelet pseudopodium formation, with aggregation developing whenever the membranes are touched by platelets.

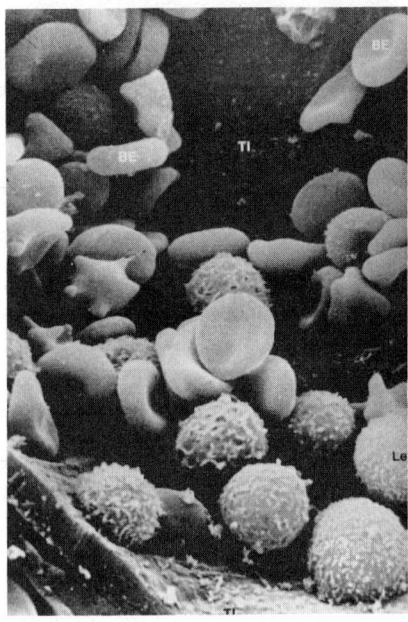

Figure 2-13. Scanning electron microscopic view of normal blood vessel.

with the scanning electron microscope. The figure shows a small blood vessel with normal hemic cells. This vessel wall is pricked with a needle. In the early phase of clot formation in the blood vessel, a loose fiber network is seen (Fig. 2-14). At that point, a contest ensues between the clotting factors and fibrinolysin system. The balance determines whether a clot will occlude the blood vessel or if these fibers will be dissolved as soon as the vessel wall regenerates and the patient will experience no problems. At this stage, the loose fibrin network acts as a filter, as in the research apparatus (Figs. 2-15 and 2-16). Red blood cells have to squeeze through pores in the fibrin network. If they are flexible, they will get through; if they are stiff, they will not. They will occlude the fibrin network, increasing the surface on which platelets aggregate and, thereby, will promote the thrombotic aspect of the equation as opposed to fibrinolytic factors. As the red blood cell's role alters fibrin-trapped stiff red cells and aggregating platelet masses, their membranes become injured, morphologically crenated, and functionally stiffer (see insert in Fig. 2-15). In some instances, this may represent a vicious circle. Stiff red cells and hyperaggregable platelets promote thromboembolic complications, as opposed to the resolution of incidentally forming thrombotic episodes.

An important question to ask is: What is the situation with red blood cell deformability in normal people? In a study with patients

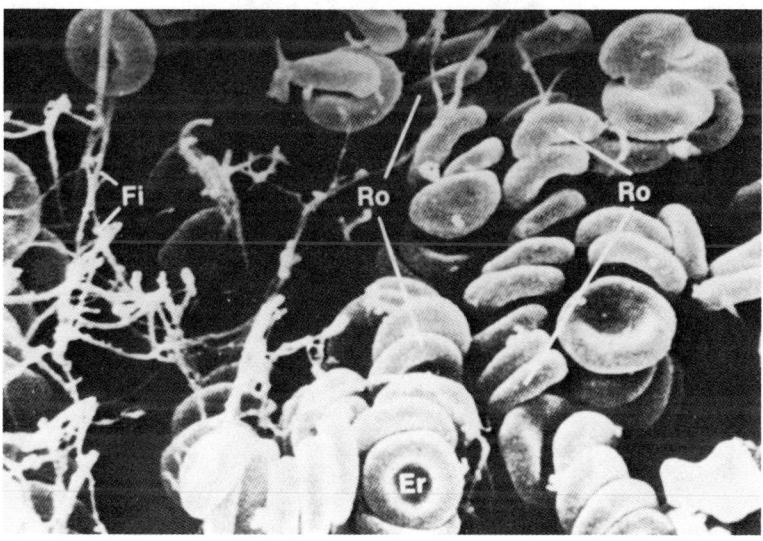

Figure 2-14. Blood vessel in Figure 2-13 immediately after being injured by needle prick.

DIABETES AND VASCULAR DISEASE

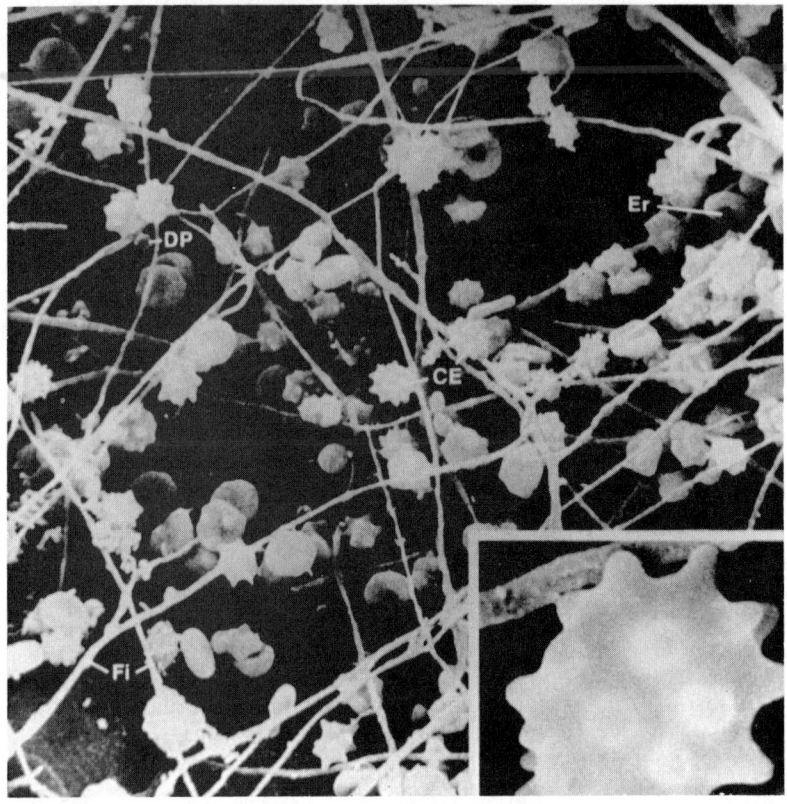

Figure 2-15. Blood vessel in Figure 2-13 one minute after being injured by needle prick. (Insert: crenated red blood cell.)

Figure 2-16. Blood vessel in Figures 2-13, 2-14, and 2-15 after 2 minutes.

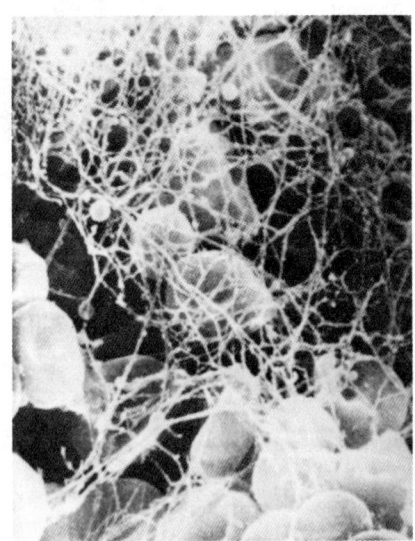

from 3 to 82 years of age, both males and females, no difference was found by sex, but a significant relationship to age was seen (Table 2-1).[26] The older the patients, the stiffer were their red blood cells. These findings may relate somehow to the increased incidence of skin ulcerations and other vascular problems seen in otherwise normal elderly people. In each person, older members of the red cell population were stiffer than younger members.

This same study also reviewed a number of disease processes.[26] Table 2-2 shows that when age- and sex-matched controls were compared, a significant increase was seen in red cell stiffness in the diabetics and patients with other types of chronic obstructive arterial disease, including its variations such as Buerger's disease.

In this group of patients, another interesting phenomenon was demonstrated (Table 2-3). If red blood cells are relatively stiff, they may cause platelet aggregation. This can be studied in the normal vascular system with a simple technique. A butterfly needle is inserted without a tourniquet into the antecubital vein of the patient and, after discarding the initial sample, blood is collected into two tubes. One tube contains ethylenediaminetetraacetate (EDTA) as an anticoagulant, and the second tube contains EDTA plus formaldehyde. If platelets occur in the form of platelet clumps rather than as individual platelets in the circulation, the clumps will fall apart in EDTA solution, but formaldehyde will fix the clumps.

Table 2–1

Relationship Between Age and Red Blood Cell Filterability by Normals and Patients with Peripheral Vascular Disease

Variables	Normal Persons	Peripheral Vascular Disease Patients
Age range	3–82	5–80
No.	20	20
FR mean*	7.14	3.82
SD	2.17	1.97
SE	0.48	0.44
Age–FR correlation	$r = 0.693$	$r = 0.427$

*Filtrate rate (FR), ml/min, of 20% red blood cell suspension in buffered saline through 5-μm nucleopore filters at 20 cm H_2O negative pressure and 22°C. (Ambrus JL, Ambrus CM, Taheri SA et al: Red cell flexibility and platelet aggregation in patients with chronic obstructive atherosclerotic disease (COAD) and study of therapeutic approaches. Angiology 35(7):418–426, 1984

Table 2-2
Red Blood Cell Filterability in Various Diseases Compared to Controls

Group	No.	Range	Mean	SD	SE	Statistical Significance	
						In Comparison With Control Group	In Comparison With Equal Number of Matched Controls
Control	20	2.9–11.0	7.14	2.18	0.050		
COAD	10	0.75–6.7	3.16	2.42	0.284	$p < 0.001$	$p < 0.01$
Buerger's disease	1		3.90				
Raynaud's syndrome	2	3.2–4.1	3.65	0.64	0.350	$p < 0.05$	$p < 0.05$
Diabetes	5	3.1–6.0	4.52	1.40	0.157	$p < 0.05$	$p < 0.05$
Thromboembolism	2	5.1–6.0	5.50	0.64	0.100	n.s.	$p < 0.05$
All disease groups	20	0.75–6.7	3.82	1.98	0.154	$p < 0.001$	$p < 0.05$

Filtration rates (ml/min) of 20% red blood cell suspension in buffered saline through 5-μm nucleopore filters at 200 cm H_2O negative pressure at 22°C.

COAD = chronic obstructive atherosclerotic disease.

Ambrus JL, Ambrus CM, Taheri SA et al: Red cell flexibility and platelet aggregation in patients with chronic obstructive atherosclerotic disease (COAD) and study of therapeutic approaches. Angiology 35(7):418–426, 1984

Table 2–3

Platelet Aggregate Ratios in Chronic Obstructive Atherosclerotic Disease (COAD) Patients and Controls

	Controls	COAD
	0.81	0.82
	0.72	0.71
	0.79	0.65
	0.85	0.61
	0.92	0.53
	0.88	0.81
	0.83	0.73
	0.78	0.81
	0.91	0.57
	0.83	0.65
Mean	0.832	0.689
SD	0.060	0.104

$t = 3.7446$
$p < 0.005$

Ambrus JL, Ambrus CM, Taheri SA et al: Red cell flexibility and platelet aggregation in patients with chronic obstructive atherosclerotic disease (COAD) and study of therapeutic approaches. Angiology 35(7):418–426, 1984

When the two tubes are centrifuged at a slow speed, the formaldehyde-fixed clumps will appear at the bottom. Consequently, the platelet count will be higher in the EDTA tube than in the EDTA-plus-formaldehyde tube. The ratio between the two expresses the incidence of platelet clumps in the patient's circulation. The ratio is approximately 0.8 in normal people, but in patients suffering from chronic obstructive arteriosclerotic vascular disease, the ratio is between 0.6 and 0.7. This suggests these patients not only have stiff red cells, but probably as a consequence some of their platelets have already aggregated and circulate in clumps.

STIFF CELL SYNDROME

A list of diseases where one may find the stiff red cell syndrome appears in the opening paragraphs to this chapter. It includes diabetes mellitus (types I and II), with ketoacidosis, macro- and microangiopathy, retinopathy, nephropathy, and neuropathy; the hemaglobinopathies; vessel wall diseases, including chronic obstructive arteriosclerotic disease, Buerger's disease, Raynaud's syndrome; several hypoxic conditions (*e.g.*, heavy smokers with advanced emphysema); and others. Dr. Clara Ambrus's group at the Children's Hospital in Buffalo, New York, which also has an obstetric unit, finds this an important pathophysiologic factor in toxemia of pregnancy. Patients with a large parasite in the red blood cell, whether it be a malaria parasite or *Babesia microti* in patients with Nantucket fever, all have relatively stiff red cells. The recent World Health Organization statistics show that the single major cause of death in the world today is drug-resistant falciparum malaria producing cerebral malaria, resulting in obstruction of the cerebral microcirculation because of stiff and disintegrating red blood cells related to malaria parasites.[37]

In a series of preliminary experiments, blood samples were taken from patients with stiff red cell syndrome (*i.e.*, arteriosclerotic vascular problems), and red blood cell deformability was compared with samples from age- and sex-matched controls using the apparatus shown previously in Figures 2-4 and 2-5.[27] Various agents were added *in vitro* to the blood samples to determine whether agents could be found that would reverse this phenomenon. Many of the active agents were xanthine derivatives; xanthines, which are used routinely in asthma, such as theophylline and aminophylline, had little effect. The most effective xanthine derivative was pentoxifylline (Trental) (Fig. 2-17).[6]

Figure 2-18 shows the results of an experiment in which red blood cells from normal blood samples and from samples of patients with chronic obstructive arteriosclerotic disease were tested for flexibility alone and together with increasing concentrations of pentoxifylline. Red blood cells from patients with disease were stiffer than control cells. Increasing doses of pentoxifylline increased red blood cell flexibility, more in the patient samples than in the normals. At optimal concentrations, the difference between the two groups disappeared. Higher doses were less effective,

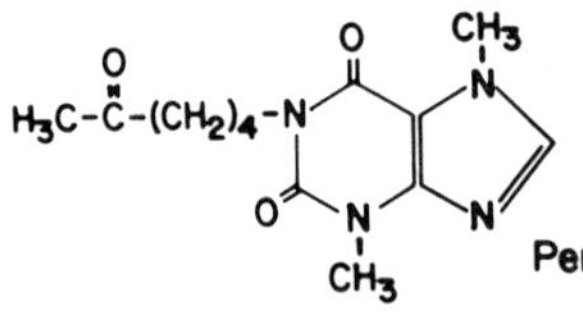

Figure 2-17. Blood vessel in Figures 2-13, 2-14, 2-15, and 2-16 after 3 minutes.

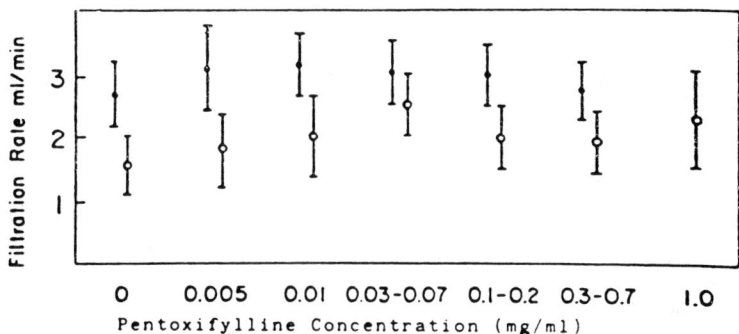

Figure 2-18. Filtration rates (ml/min) of 40% red cell suspensions in buffered saline through 5-μm nucleopore filters at 20 cm H_2O negative pressure and at 22°C.

resulting in a bell-shaped curve. A bell-shaped curve was also obtained when SS-genotype blood from a patient in vaso-occlusive crisis of sickle cell disease was studied under the same conditions (Fig. 2-19). This is probably not an important phenomenon clinically, because these high levels are never reached in the normal circulation. They may, however, be an interesting feature from the theoretic point of view.

After the chimp, which is too expensive for large-scale studies (about $5,000 each), the stump-tailed monkey (*Macaca arctoides*) is the species most similar to man in terms of platelet aggregation and red blood cell deformability (Fig. 2-20).[10,20] The apparatus shown in Figure 2-21 was inserted into an arteriovenous anastomosis. Included in the apparatus is a 20-μm pore size filter (see point *h* in Fig. 2-21), and we measured pressure before and after the filter with strain gauges. A small amount (1 μg) of adenosine diphosphate (ADP) or 1 μg serotonin per 10-kg monkey was injected intravenously. Platelet aggregates formed and tended to occlude the filter; therefore, pre-screen pressure increased and post-screen pressure decreased (Fig. 2-22). On the basis of these changes, an aggregation index can be calculated (the formula is shown in Fig. 2-22). The filter can also be removed and studied by scanning electron microscopy. Aggregating platelets tend to obstruct the microcirculation (Fig. 2-23). After a short time, these platelets undergo viscous metamorphosis, melt into each other, and form a viscous glue (Fig. 2-24). These animals were treated with various

Text continues on p. 27

DIABETES AND VASCULAR DISEASE

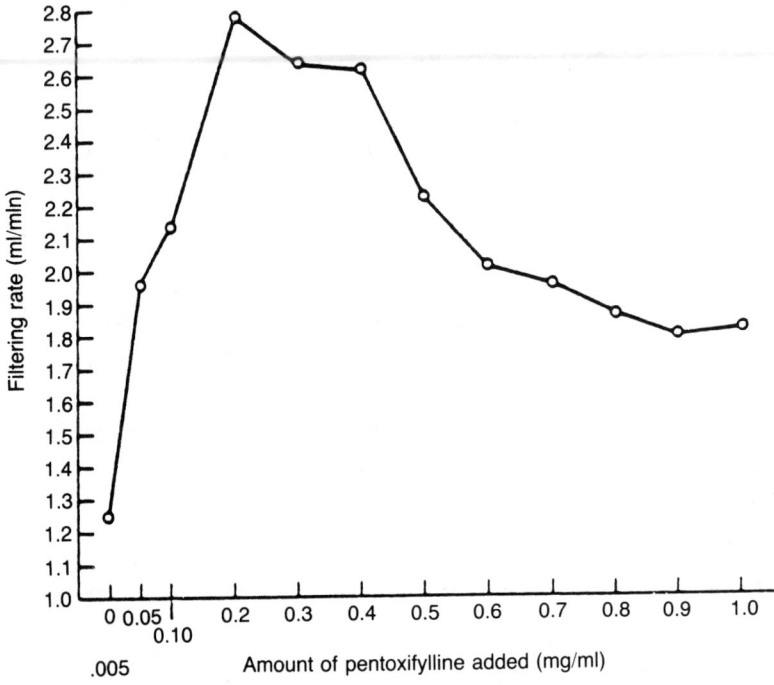

Figure 2-19. Effect of various doses of pentoxifylline on the filtration rate of blood obtained from a patient with sickle cell disease (10-μm pore size filter).

Figure 2-20. Stump-tailed monkey *(Macaca arctoides).*

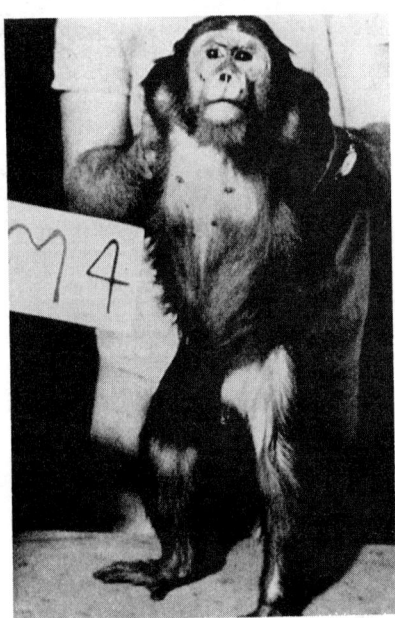

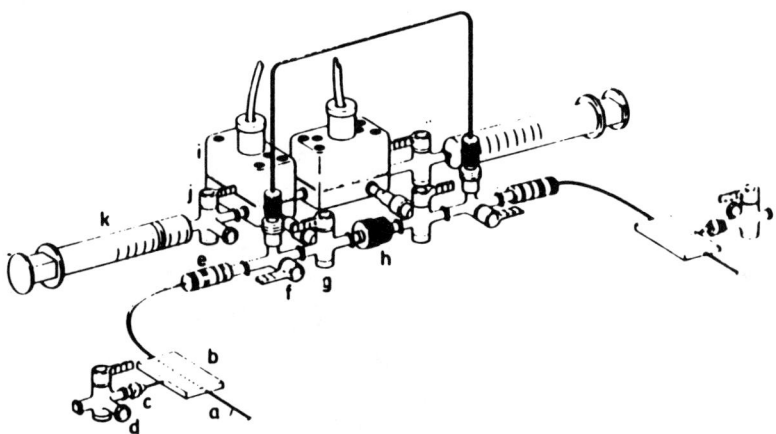

Figure 2-21. Measuring apparatus to determine *in vivo* platelet aggregation and red cell stiffness.

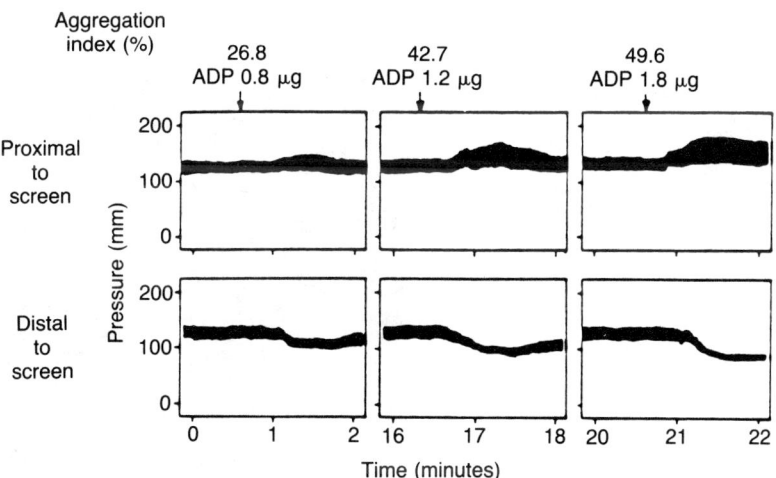

Figure 2-22. Effect of different doses of adenosine diphosphate.

Aggregation index $= 100 \times (1 - \left[\dfrac{EP_2}{RP_2} \times \dfrac{RP_1}{EP_1}\right]$

Where EP_2 = distal-to-screen pressure following challenge; RP_2 = proximal-to-screen pressure following challenge; EP_1 = distal-to-screen pressure before challenge; RP_1 = proximal-to-screen pressure before challenge.

DIABETES AND VASCULAR DISEASE

Figure 2-23. Scanning electron microscopic view of aggregating platelets in the apparatus in Figure 2-21.

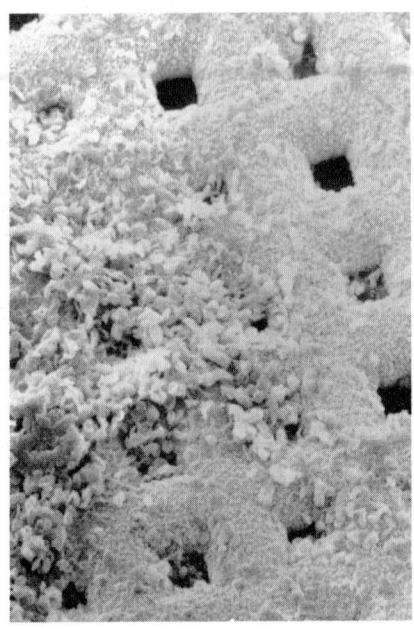

Figure 2-24. Scanning electron microscopic view of platelets undergoing viscous metamorphosis in the apparatus in Figure 2-21.

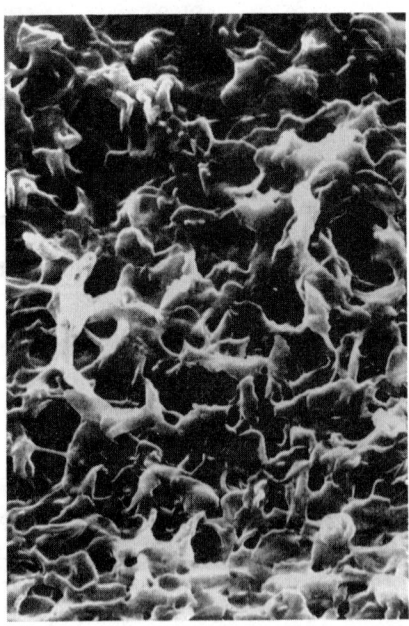

doses of pentoxifylline, and the optimal inhibiting dose was found to be 24 mg/kg intravenously. This dose resulted in significant inhibition of both ADP and serotonin-induced microvascular occlusion, a phenomenon that lasted for approximately 3 hours in this particular experiment (Fig. 2-25).

Red cell stiffness was also studied in this experiment. When sickle cell disease patients are in severe vaso-occlusive crisis, one usually does an exchange transfusion and the removed "bad blood" is discarded. Instead, the bad blood was cross-transfused into monkeys and low-oxygen tension was established for breathing. The red cells changed shape, became stiff, and occluded the microcirculation with partly deformed sickle-shaped, partly echinoid-shaped red blood cells, producing the same kind of pressure changes as in the previous experiments (Fig. 2-26). When these animals were pretreated with 24 mg/kg of pentoxifylline intravenously, a significant decrease of these changes was found as opposed to the control, untreated animals (Fig. 2-27).

BIOCHEMICAL MECHANISM OF PENTOXIFYLLINE ACTION

The following is a brief discussion of biochemical studies on the mechanism of action of pentoxifylline (Fig. 2-28).[3] In the red blood cell membrane, the spectrin–actin complex is a major structure responsible for membrane stiffness. Pentoxifylline acts

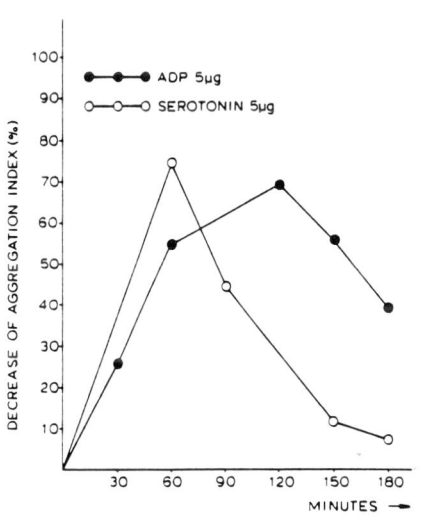

Figure 2-25. Effect of pentoxifylline on *in vivo* platelet aggregation.

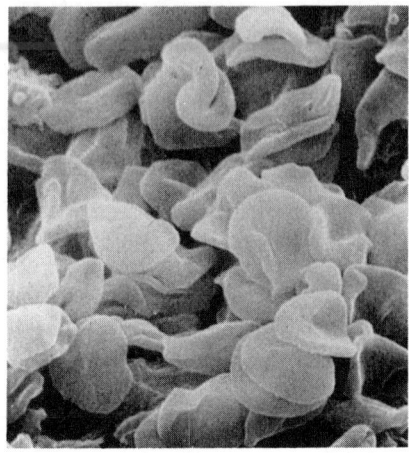

Figure 2-26. Stiff red cells occlude the pores (shown in the apparatus in Figure 2-21).

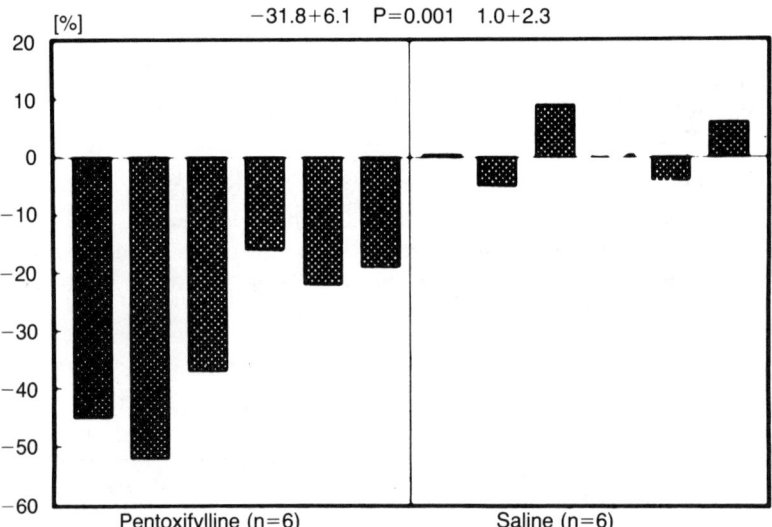

Figure 2-27. Pentoxifylline in an animal model of vaso-occlusive crisis of sickle cell disease. Reduction of aggregation index after pentoxifylline (24 mg/kg intravenously) or saline.

primarily on the endothelial wall, releasing both prostaglandin I_2 (PGI_2) and tissue plasminogen activator. PGI_2, in turn, binds to a receptor in the wall of the platelet, activates adenyl cyclase, and increases generation of cyclic adenosine monophosphate (c-AMP) from adenosine triphosphate (ATP). Cyclic AMP in the protoplasm

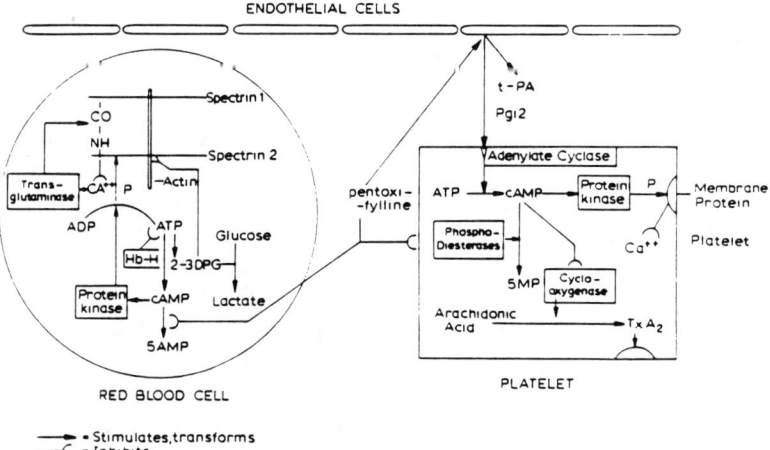

Figure 2-28. Present status of experiments on mechanism of action is summarized.

of these cells has two effects: it activates proteinkinases that phosphorylate the membrane proteins and binds ionized calcium; without it the platelets cannot aggregate. Cyclic AMP also inhibits intracellular cyclo-oxygenases, which are responsible for the generation of thromboxane A_2 (TxA_2) from arachidonic acid. TxA_2 is a major aggregation signal in the platelets. In addition, pentoxifylline acts directly on the cyclic AMP phosphodyesterases inhibiting them and, thus, interfering with the decomposition of cyclic AMP. Cyclic AMP generation is increased, and cyclic AMP decomposition is decreased; consequently, cyclic AMP levels become high and result in phosphorylation of membrane proteins binding free calcium and inhibition of the generation of TxA_2. In the red blood cells, the mechanism is somewhat similar. Phosphorylated membrane proteins will bind calcium, which is a co-factor for transglutaminases that cross-link spectrin-1, spectrin-2, and actin. If this is inadequate, the membrane proteins remain looser, membrane fluidity becomes greater, and the red blood cell is more deformable. In addition, by saving ATP an increase occurs in intracellular ATP levels, which, in turn, increases the 2–3 diphosphoglyceric acid level. This, in turn, interferes with the interaction between actin and spectrin, further increasing membrane fluidity, decreasing membrane stiffness, and increasing deformability of the red blood cell (Fig. 2-28).

ROLE OF CYCLO-OXYGENASE INHIBITORS AS AGENTS TO IMPROVE BLOOD FLOW

One of the questions often asked is: In the presence of microvascular disease, why not use cyclo-oxygenase inhibitors such as aspirin or indomethacin? Part of the explanation is shown in the metabolic chart of Figure 2-29. These agents inhibit cyclo-oxygenases and thereby inhibit the generation of TxA_2; they also inhibit generation of the prostaglandins, PGI_2 and PGD_2, which have the opposite effect—they inhibit platelet aggregation. With large doses of aspirin, therefore, what we gain on one metabolic pathway, we lose on the other. If a small dose of aspirin is given, the situation is different. The "good pathways" then regenerate more rapidly than the "bad pathways" and a therapeutic index is achieved, so far as the platelets are concerned. Aspirin and indomethacin have no effect on red blood cell flexibility. What is a small dose of aspirin? We consider it to be approximately 40 to 80 mg or one-half to one chewable baby aspirin. Another issue is that if cyclo-oxygenases are inhibited with aspirin, arachidonic acid metabolism is pushed over into the lipo-oxygenase pathway and more leukotriene C_4, D_4, and E_4 is synthesized. These together are the "slow reacting substance of anaphylaxis" and are responsible for aspirin-induced asthma.

The other problem with large doses of aspirin is that irreversible acetylation of the platelet membrane is produced and the only way to reestablish normal platelet function is by generating new platelets. On the other hand, pentoxifylline-induced platelet aggre-

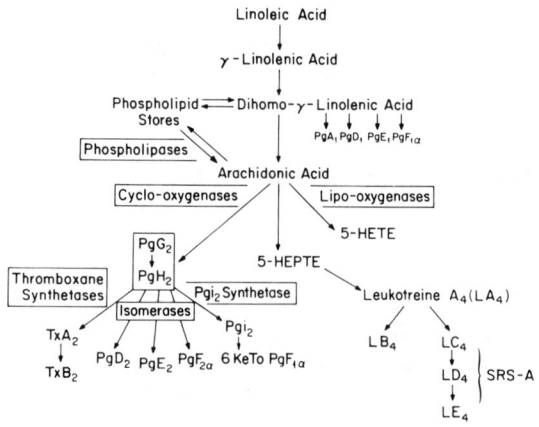

Figure 2-29. Arachidonic acid metabolism.

gation is readily reversible. Aspirin is also an important gastric irritant and ulcerogen.

Another interesting phenomenon is that pentoxifylline releases not only PGI_2, but also tissue plasminogen activator from the vessel wall. This, together with the platelet aggregation inhibitory effect of pentoxifylline, results in potentiation of thrombolytic therapy with streptokinase.[3,23]

Clinical studies were undertaken using Doppler ultrasonography, phonocardiography, platinum electrode measurement of tissue oxygen tension, and measurement of the disappearance of labeled ^{133}Xenon from the tissues (Fig. 2-30). The major criterion, however, was arteriography. Figure 2-31 shows a typical arteriogram, where one of the common iliac arteries has disappeared completely. In the upper left corner of the figure, narrowing is seen in the other iliac artery, and corresponding to that a significant change is seen in the phonocardiogram at the F-4 level.

PENTOXIFYLLINE TO FACILITATE PERFUSION

Pentoxifylline is metabolized partly by red blood cells and partly by the liver into seven metabolites (Fig. 2-32). Of these

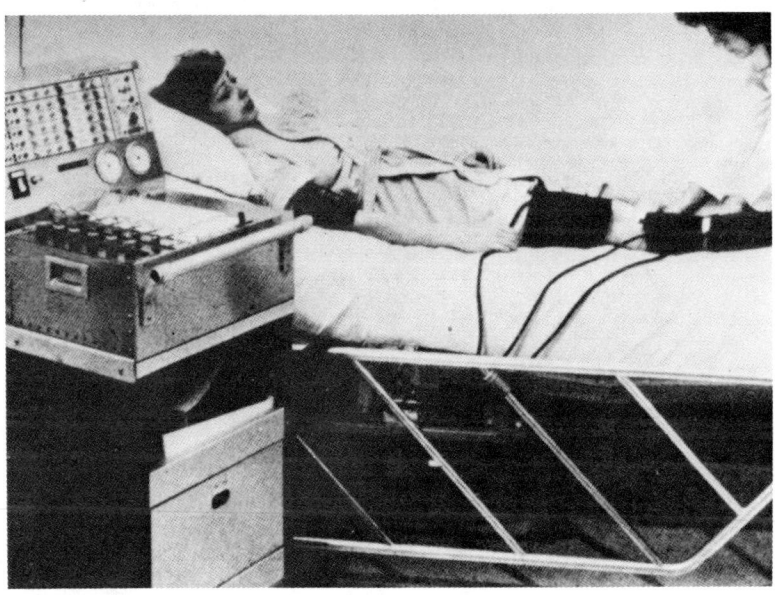

Figure 2-30. Patient under study.

DIABETES AND VASCULAR DISEASE

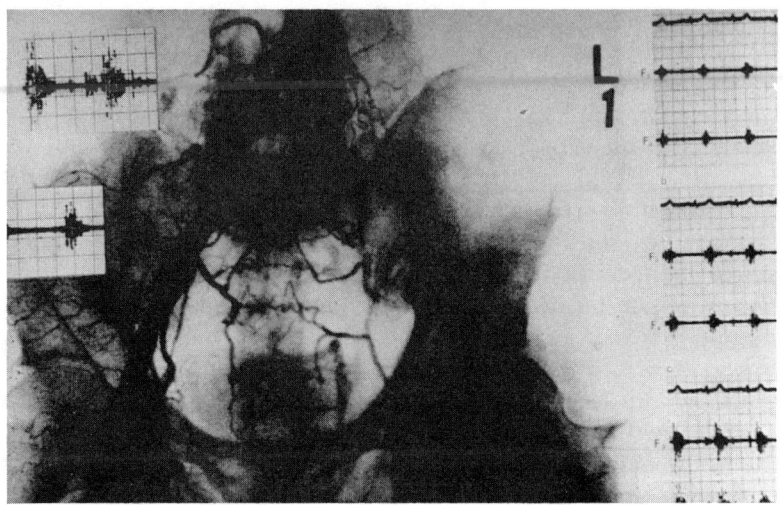

Figure 2-31. Arteriogram.

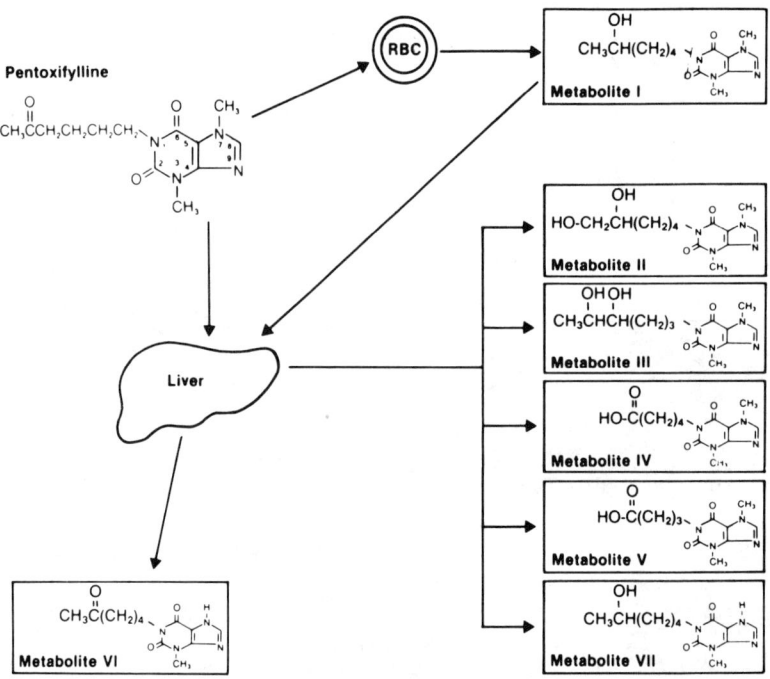

Figure 2-32. Metabolism of pentoxifylline.

metabolites, metabolite 1 and metabolite 5 are the most active hemorrheologic agents. They are more active than the parent pentoxifylline; metabolites 1 and 5 have the most important action in inhibiting platelet aggregation and increasing red blood cell deformability. When patients are treated with standard doses of pentoxifylline, one has to wait until an equilibrium is established between the parent compound and the most active metabolites. Tissue reserves are established and the hemorrheologically most active metabolites reach a steady state, establishing an adequate therapeutic level. The officially recommended dose is 400 mg t.i.d. When one measures red blood cell flexibility and platelet aggregation by the methods described previously, a few patients require higher doses. Doses can be adjusted on the basis of the laboratory studies described.

Pentoxifylline is a powerful red blood cell flexibility-increasing agent, but a somewhat weaker platelet aggregation inhibitor. For this reason, in patients with threatened amputation for serious vascular impairment, we combined oral pentoxifylline with intravenous infusion of prostaglandin E_1 (PGE_1). The latter is a powerful platelet aggregation inhibitor and vasodilator, which may synergize with pentoxifylline. PGE_1 somewhat increases red cell stiffness, but this is overridden by the simultaneous use of pentoxifylline.

A diabetic patient was seen with a significant vascular problem in the right foot and leg with some nonhealing ulcers, one on the heel and one on the ankle (Fig. 2-33). Consequently, the vascular surgeon decided to do a bypass and remove the contralateral saphenous vein and graft it into the diseased leg. Unfortunately, the postoperative situation did not improve adequately. The original ulcers did not heal, and both of the operative wounds showed poor healing. The patient was in danger of having to undergo a double amputation. The patient was administered a continuous three-day infusion of PGE_1 (10 ng/kg/min) and oral pentoxifylline (400 mg t.i.d.). After 3 days the patient got up and walked around for 2 days and then began another 3 days of continuous infusion. This cycle was repeated for a total of 6 weeks. At the end of 6 weeks the operative wounds as well as the original skin ulcers healed, and vascular perfusion and tissue oxygenation improved significantly; the patient was discharged in good condition (Fig. 2-34). It appears this type of desperately ill patient may be treated effectively with intravenous infusions of PGE_1, together with oral treatment of pentoxifylline.

A number of other investigators explored the various therapeutic possibilities that arise from the principles and preliminary

Figure 2-33.
Patient before treatment.

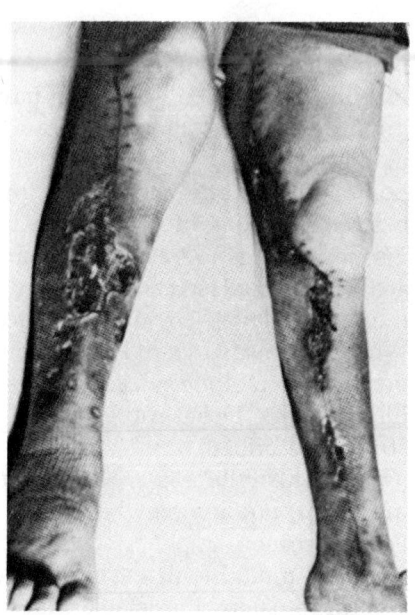

Figure 2-34.
Patient after treatment.

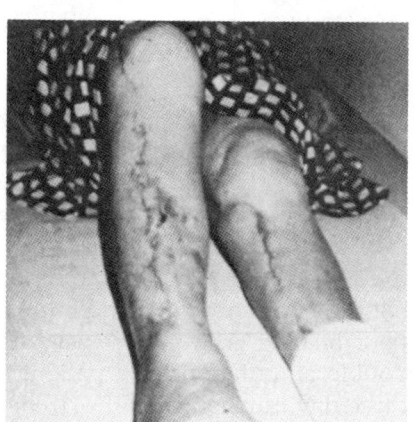

studies discussed above. A collaborative study was organized by Porter and associates for patients with intermittent claudication.[40–42] Both initial claudication and absolute claudication improved significantly in the group of patients treated with 400 mg of pentoxifylline orally t.i.d. compared with the placebo-treated patients.

A number of preliminary clinical studies found pentoxifylline effective in sickle cell disease.[32–38,39,45] In a recent report, we found pentoxifylline may prevent, but not abort, vaso-occlusive crisis of sickle cell disease.[28] Several investigators pointed out the value of pentoxifylline in diabetes with vascular complications.[30,37,43,44,46-48]

SUMMARY

The flexibility of normal red blood cell membrane is modified toward inflexibility in a number of disease states including diabetes. This stiffness is modified by the administration of pentoxifylline to increase passage of red blood cells through the narrowing compromised vessels.

REFERENCES

1. Ambrus CM, Ambrus JL: Platelet aggregation and erythrocyte deformability in sickle cell disease. Model experiments and pentoxifylline. In Manrique RV, Muller R (eds): Disorders of Blood Flow: New Therapeutic Aspects, pp. 129–135. Amsterdam-Oxford-Princeton, Excerpta Medica, 1981
2. Ambrus CM, Ambrus JL, Gastpar H et al: The role of fibrinolysis in the therapy of peripheral vascular disease. Angiology 35(7):436–442, 1984
3. Ambrus CM, Ambrus JL, Klein E et al: Study of factors in potentiating *in vivo* thrombolysis. Release of activators of the fibrinolysis system by phosphodiesterase inhibitors. Proceedings of International Conference on Fibrinolysis, Shizuoka, Japan, 1987
4. Ambrus JL: Chairman's concluding remarks to the session: Pharmacologic approaches in haemorheology. Proceedings of the Conference on Blood Rheology and Microcirculation, Capri, Italy. La Ricerca XI(Suppl 1):223–230, 1981
5. Ambrus JL: Chairman's introduction to the session: Pharmacologic approaches in haemorheology. Proceedings of the Conference on Blood Rheology and Microcirculation, Capri, Italy. La Ricerca XI(Suppl I):167–168, 1981
6. Ambrus JL: Editorial: Global health care. J Med 11(5,6):321–351, 1980
7. Ambrus JL: Chairman's introductory address to the workshop on Trental. Sing Med J 20(3 [Suppl 1]):I, 1979
8. Ambrus JL: Phosphodiesterase inhibitors in cerebrovascular disorders. Sing Med J 20(3 [Suppl 1]): I, 1979
9. Ambrus JL: Symposium on pentoxifylline (Trental). Chair-

man's introduction. Proceedings of the European Hematology Symposium on the Platelet Aggregation Inhibitor Pentoxifylline (Trental), Athens, Greece, 1978. J Med 10(5):305–306, 1979

10. Ambrus JL, Ambrus CM: Blood coagulation in neoplastic disease. In Gastpar H (ed): Onkohamostaselogie (Hematologic Problems in Cancer), pp 167–193. Stuttgart-New York, FK Schattauer Verlag, 1976
11. Ambrus JL, Ambrus CM, Bannerman R: Conduite a tenir devant une crise drepanocytaire. Medecine d'Afrique Noire 20:10, 1981
12. Ambrus JL, Ambrus CM, Bannerman R et al: Studies on the management and prevention of vasoocclusive crisis in sickle cell disease. J Med 15:385, 1984
13. Ambrus JL, Ambrus CM, Bannerman R et al: Effect of phosphodiesterase inhibitors and prostacyclin synthesis increasing agents on experimental sickle cell crisis and on the deformability of sickled red cells. Proceedings of the NIH-Airlie House Conference on Sickle Cell Disease, June 1981
14. Ambrus JL, Ambrus CM, Bannerman R et al: Studies on the management and prevention of crisis in sickle cell disease. Proceedings of the International Conference on Sickle Cell Disease, Abidjan, Ivory Coast, January 1981
15. Ambrus JL, Ambrus CM, Gastpar H: Effect of phosphodiesterase inhibitors on platelet aggregation and tumor metastasis. Proceedings of the Conference on Blood Rheology and Microcirculation, Capri, Italy. La Ricerca XI (Suppl 1):197–207, 1981
16. Ambrus JL, Ambrus CM, Gastpar H: The role of platelet aggregation in metastatic dissemination and thromboembolic complications in cancer patients. Prevention with pentoxifylline. In Manrique RV, Muller R (eds): Disorders of Blood Flow: New Therapeutic Aspects, pp 29–42. Amsterdam-Oxford-Princeton, Excerpta Medica, 1981
17. Ambrus JL, Ambrus CM, Gastpar H: New clinical indications for Trental. Sing Med J 20(3 [Suppl 1]):I, 1979
18. Ambrus JL, Ambrus CM, Gastpar H: Studies on platelet aggregation with pentoxifylline. Effect on neoplastic disorders and other new indications. Proceedings of the European Hematology Symposium on the Platelet Aggregation Inhibitor Pentoxifylline (Trental), Athens, Greece, 1978. J Med 10(5):339–345, 1979
19. Ambrus JL, Ambrus CM, Gastpar H et al: Studies on vasoocclusive crisis of sickle cell disease. I. Effect of pentoxifylline. J Med 10(6):445–456, 1979

20. Ambrus JL, Ambrus CM, Gastpar H et al: Study of platelet aggregation *in vivo*. I. Effect of bencyclan. J Med 7(6):439–447, 1976
21. Ambrus JL, Ambrus CM, Gurewich V et al: Pro-urokinase and prostaglandin I releasing phosphodiesterase inhibitors and the therapy of thrombolytic disease. Proceedings of the International Conference on Fibrinolysis, Shizuoka, Japan, 1987
22. Ambrus JL, Ambrus CM, Gurewich V et al: Pro-urokinase and prostaglandin I_2-releasing phosphodiesterase inhibitors in the therapy of thrombotic disease. Proceedings of the International Conference on Fibrinolysis, Hamamatsu, Japan, pp 171–195. Amsterdam, Elsevier, 1987; also: In Castelino FJ, Gaffney PJ, Samania MM et al (eds): Fundamental and clinical fibrinolysis. Exerpta Medica pp 185–195, 1987
23. Ambrus JL, Ambrus CM, Mahafzah M et al: Mechanism of the potentiation of thrombolysis by pentoxifylline (Trental). J Med 18:265–276, 1987
24. Ambrus JL, Ambrus CM, Odake K et al: Clinical and experimental studies on adenine, various nucleosides and their analogs in hematology. Ann NY Acad Sci 255:435–467, 1975
25. Ambrus JL, Ambrus CM, Sharma SD et al: Studies on platelet aggregation inhibitors *in vivo*. X. Relationship to thrombolysis. J Med 13(5,6):365–371, 1982
26. Ambrus JL, Ambrus CM, Taheri SA et al: Red cell flexibility and platelet aggregation in patients with chronic obstructive arteriosclerotic disease (COAD) and study of therapeutic approaches. Angiology 35(7):418–426, 1984
27. Ambrus JL, Meky N, Stadler S et al: Studies on the vasoocclusive crisis of sickle cell disease. IV. Mechanism of action of pentoxifylline (Trental). J Med 19:67–88, 1988
28. Gastpar H, Ambrus JL, Ambrus CM: Studies on platelet aggregation *in vivo*. II. Effect of pentoxifylline on circulating tumor cells. J Med 9(3):265–268, 1978
29. Gastpar H, Ambrus JL, Ambrus CM et al: Study of platelet aggregation *in vivo*. III. Effect of pentoxifylline. J Med 8(3,4):191–197, 1977
30. Goltseva SV: Comparative assessment of efficacy of various methods for treatment of diabetic retinopathies. Ophthalmologii Zhurnal 38:36–38, 1983
31. Gordon SW, Cohen HS, Williams J et al: Studies on platelet aggregation inhibitors *in vivo*. VIII. Effect of pentoxifylline on spontaneous tumor metastasis. J Med 10(6):435–443, 1979
32. Heilmann E, Laage HM, Zimmermann E et al: Therapeutic influence on flexibility of erythrocytes in sickle cell anemia. Innere Medizin 9:277–280, 1982

33. Keller F, Leonhardt H: Verbesserung der blutviskositat bei sichelzellanamie durch pentoxifyllin (Improvement of blood viscosity in sickle-cell anemia by pentoxifylline). Dtsch Med Wochenschr 105:898–900, 1980
34. Keller F, Leonhardt H: Amelioration of blood viscosity in sickle cell anemia by pentoxifylline: A case report. J Med 10:429–431, 1979
35. Khosla AA, Chintu C: A pilot study: An open clinical trial of pentoxiphylline in patients with painful sickle cell crises. East Afr Med J 61:829–836, 1984
36. Lee MV, Ambrus JL, DeSouza JML et al: Diminished red blood cell deformability in uncomplicated human malaria. A preliminary report. J Med 13(5,6):479–485, 1982
37. Masowezkij AH, Stoilov LD, Kukashina TV et al: The use of pentoxifylline in diabetes mellitus. Pharmatherapeutica 2(Suppl 1):105–108, 1978
38. M'Bensa A: Interet de la pentoxifylline dans le traitement de la drepanocytose. Medecine d'Afrique Noire 30:480–484, 1983
39. Ngandu-Kabeya D: Interet d'un medicament augmentant la deformabilite des globules rouges (pentoxifylline-Trental) dans le traitement de la drepanocytes. Medecine d'Afrique Noire 30:431–434, 1983
40. Porter JM: Pharmacologic approaches to intermittent claudication and vasospasm. In Spittell JA (ed): Pharmacologic Approach to the Treatment of Limb Ischemia, pp 179–195. Philadelphia, College of Physicians of Philadelphia, 1983
41. Porter JM, Cutler BC, Lee BY et al: Pentoxifylline efficacy in the treatment of intermittent claudication: Multicenter controlled double-blind trial with objective assessment of chronic occlusive arterial disease patients. Am Heart J 104:66–72, 1982
42. Reid HL, Barnes FS, Lock PJ et al: A simple method for measuring erythrocyte deformability. J Clin Pathol 10:855, 1976
43. Saldan IR: The usage of disaggregants for the treatment of diabetic retinopathy. Offtal'mologicheskii Zhurnal 7:395–398, 1984
44. Schubotz R: Double-blind trial of pentoxifylline in diabetics with peripheral vascular disorders. Pharmatherapeutica 1:172–179, 1976
45. Seiffge D, Berthold R, Berthold F: Effect of pentoxifylline on sickle cell thalassaemia: Haemorrheological and clinical results. Klin Wochenschr 61:1159–1160, 1983
46. Slijepcevic D, Devecerski M: The use of pentoxifylline in insulin dependent diabetics, with late complications. Curr Med Res Opin 6(Suppl 4):37–42, 1979

47. Solerte SB, Ferrari E: Diabetic retinal vascular complications and erythrocyte filterability: Results of a 2-year follow-up study with pentoxifylline. Pharmatherapeutica 4:341–350, 1985
48. Tartakovskaja AJ, Archangelskaja EN, Dudnikova LH: Disorders of erythrocyte and thrombocyte aggregation in the pathogenesis of diabetic retinopathy and the possibilities of disaggregating therapy. Vestnik Oftal'mologii (Moskova) 6:59–62, 1983

CHAPTER THREE
Natural History and Risk Factors in Peripheral Vascular Disease
D. Eugene Strandness, Jr.

HISTORICAL PERSPECTIVE

Before the availability of sensitive noninvasive diagnostic tests, the only reliable data with regard to arteriosclerosis obliterans were based on rates of limb loss. In fact, studies published in the 1950s and 1960s are still quoted widely in predicting the prognosis for patients with peripheral vascular disease.[4,6]

What is the risk of limb loss? The Boyd study showed that in a nondiabetic population, the limb loss rate was about 1.4% per year.[4] In diabetic patients, the figure increased approximately five times.

Most physicians recognize that patients with peripheral vascular disease have a shortened life span, but to what extent? Boyd found the life span to be 10 years shorter for patients with peripheral arterial disease than for a comparable age group from the general population.[4] A study of the 1950s by Silbert and Zazeela pointed out that the mortality rate for nondiabetics with peripheral arterial disease was about 1% per year; however, in diabetic patients, the mortality rate increased to about 3% to 4% per year.[6]

My own research and interest in this field began in the 1960s when I applied noninvasive ankle blood pressure measurements in a prospective fashion to the study of 60 patients with atherosclerosis obliterans seen at the Veteran's Administration Hospital in Seattle.[7] The follow-up period was 3 years. In patients with peripheral arterial occlusive disease, the rate of disease progression over an average 3-year follow-up was 43%, or about 14% per year—a striking figure. For the diabetic patients in this study, 83% of the limbs showed progression. Of importance was that 38% of the patients were unaware that progression had occurred. Amputations were required in 8 of 12 patients whose progression led to tissue necrosis, for a limb loss rate of about 3% per year.

PREVALENCE

More recent studies of the prevalence of peripheral arterial disease in a nonselected population of diabetics and nondiabetics have established a data base on arterial disease and its related risk factors.[1-3,5] The true prevalence of peripheral arterial disease in diabetics and nondiabetics is unknown, but the consensus is that it is much higher in diabetics. When the prevalence is established, it is important to determine the risk factors responsible for the disease. The methods used to document the prevalence of disease could also be used to examine the rates of progression and how this might be modified to reduce the incidence of limb loss. Currently, it is estimated that diabetics account for about 50% of all amputations done in this country when those done for trauma are excluded.

The carotid artery bifurcation was also studied in this cohort of patients. High-grade carotid stenosis (>50%) was found to be eight times more common in the type II diabetic than in the nondiabetic control subjects. The prevalence of atherosclerosis in the lower limbs was 20 times higher than in the nondiabetic population. For the lower limbs, one of the diagnostic end-points used was the ankle/arm systolic pressure index. The normal value for the ankle/arm index is 0.95 or greater. Because this index becomes positive only with high-grade lesions, the estimates of prevalence are undoubtedly lower than they should be. From these studies, patients with an ankle/arm index of 0.9 to 0.95 were classified as having mild occlusive disease and those <0.9 were placed in the moderate-to-severe occlusive disease category.

The control and diabetic patients who entered this prospective study were not selected from peripheral vascular clinics; rather they were recruited by informational mailings, posting of signs in drug stores, and so forth. The 101 community control subjects, who were age- and sex-matched to the diabetic population, had a mean age of 61 years. Surprisingly, the prevalence of peripheral arterial disease in the control subjects was only 1%; in the patients with diabetes, it varied depending on the treatment given.

The prevalence of arterial disease in the type II diabetic

patients ranged from a low of 12% in the insulin-treated group to a high of 28% in the diet-treated group. The prevalence rate in the type I diabetic patients was only about 6%, but the mean age of this population was considerably lower than that of the type II patient group.

Another interesting finding from the study was that patients classified as having elevated fasting plasma glucose, but not as diabetic (fasting blood sugar between 115 and 140 mg/liter on at least two occasions), had a prevalence of disease equal to that seen in the type II diabetic patients.

RISK FACTORS

Figure 3-1 is a bar graph of the prevalence of peripheral arterial disease (ankle/arm index <0.9 in cigarette-smoking diabetics). Cigarette smoking appeared to be one of the most important risk factors in the type II diabetic patients in this study. As noted in the figure, the prevalence rate appeared to be lowest in the insulin-treated patients. The prevalence rates of severe arterial disease ranged from 10% to 40% in the elevated fasting plasma glucose, diet-treated, sulfonylurea-treated, and insulin-treated groups.

A fact of great importance is the type of treatment of the diabetic state and its relationship, if any, to the prevalence of arterial disease. Is insulin important? To determine this, the patients would have to be followed from day one of diagnosis, randomized to insulin and no insulin, and then followed longitudinally. Clearly, this would be an impossible task. Nonetheless, the insulin-treated, diabetic smoker appeared to have a lower prevalence of arterial disease than did the cigarette-smoking patient treated with sulfonylurea, or by diet. In the cigarette-smoking diabetic patient treated by diet, the prevalence of arterial disease was two and one-half times that of the insulin-treated patient. In the sulfonylurea-treated patient, the prevalence of arterial disease was twice that of the insulin-dependent patient. These differences were statistically significant ($p<0.05$). Cigarette smoking is such a potent risk factor in the diabetic patient that it must be controlled, if at all possible.

The role of lipoproteins is important, particularly because data on this problem in atherosclerosis from the Lipid Research Clinic study showed that a 10% reduction in cholesterol can result in a 2% reduction in mortality from myocardial infarction. Data with regard to lipid in lower-limb arterial disease and lipid levels are sparse. In our studies, 12-hour fasting lipoprotein determinations yielded interesting facts.[1] For the diet-treated diabetics,

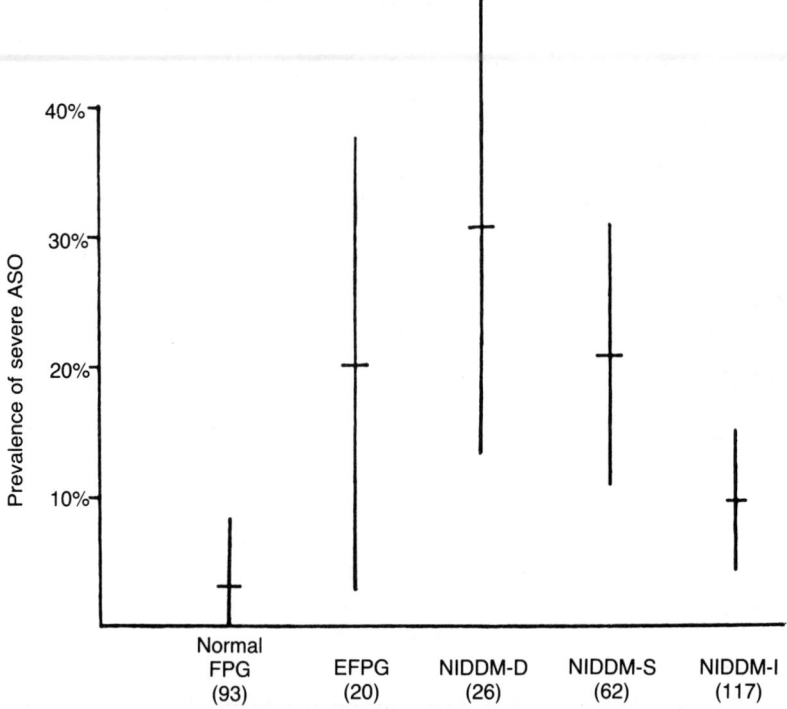

Figure 3-1. Prevalence of severe arteriosclerosis obliterans in subjects with a history of cigarette smoking. Error bars indicate 95% confidence limits. FPG = fasting plasma glucose; EFPG = elevated fasting plasma glucose; NIDDM-D = noninsulin-dependent diabetes mellitus—diet-treated; NIDDM-S = noninsulin-dependent diabetes mellitus—sulfonylurea-treated; NIDDM-I = noninsulin-dependent diabetes mellitus—insulin-treated. (Reproduced with permission of Beach KW, Brunzell JD, Strandness DE Jr: Prevalence of severe arteriosclerosis obliterans in patients with diabetes mellitus: Relation to smoking and form of therapy. Arteriosclerosis 2:275–280, 1982)

high-density lipoprotein (HDL) cholesterol was the most predictive for development of peripheral arterial disease; the lower the HDL cholesterol, the more likely the patient is to have peripheral arterial disease.

In the sulfonylurea-treated patients, we found no subfragments of lipoproteins that appeared to be predictive, but in the insulin-treated type I and type II diabetic patients, very low-density lipoprotein (VLDL) triglyceride and low-density lipoprotein (LDL) cholesterol had the highest association with arterial disease.[1] Also, female diabetics appeared to have the same prevalence of arterial disease as did their male counterparts, which is not the case in the nondiabetic population. We compared the lipoprotein patterns in diabetic patients with those from the Northwest Bell population control group.[1] The female diabetics, both noninsulin-dependent diabetes mellitus type I and type II, had consistently elevated median totals of VLDL triglyceride and LDL cholesterol, and a lower HDL cholesterol.[8] This may explain why the prevalence of disease in male and female diabetics appears to be the same.

Finally, what is the role of hypertension as it relates to peripheral arterial disease? In our diabetic patient population, 65% of the diet-treated, 82% of the sulfonylurea-treated, 74% of the insulin-treated, and 53% of the type I diabetics had a positive history of hypertension. This suggests that hypertension may also be an important contributing factor in the prevalence of peripheral arterial disease.

Diabetic patients, therefore, should never smoke; their lipoproteins should be monitored regularly; and if they have hypertension, this should be treated. These are the same risk factors associated with nondiabetic peripheral arterial disease. Perhaps the control of these risk factors should be emphasized more strongly rather than focusing on the form of therapy in the type II diabetic patient.

NATURAL HISTORY—PROGRESSION OF DISEASE

In our studies of disease progression, we used the following criteria to document worsening of the disease. Patients had to have an ankle/arm index of <0.95 at the time to be labeled as having atherosclerosis obliterans and a decrease of at least 15% at any visit to indicate progression. A change of 15% is outside the range of variability in the measurements (Beach KW and Strandness DE Jr, unpublished data).

The long-term follow-up study consisted of 246 type II diabetic and 156 nondiabetic control patients who had been followed for at least 2 years. An interesting fact from this study was that prevalence of medial calcification in our diabetic population was only about 1%. The usual incidence of medial calcification reported is as high as 16%, but these patients are seen in vascular clinics where selection bias is likely. Only two patients in the entire diabetic cohort of 246 had medial calcification; five had undergone previous amputations. During the 2-year follow-up period, 9% of the type II diabetics without atherosclerosis obliterans developed the disease, while 52% of those with the problem at the time of entry showed a >15% decrease in their ankle/arm index.

Given this apparent remarkable rate of progression, we reviewed the data to assess the factors that might have contributed to this occurrence. There were some surprises. For example, in the type II patients who had disease at the time of entry and progressed, none of the usually important risk factors appeared to apply. No correlation was found between cigarette smoking, hypertension, or problems with lipoproteins. We could show no relationships with the above in the progression of disease in this subset of patients. On the other hand, in those patients with ankle/arm indices >0.95 at the time of entry into the study, 9% had a decrease >15%. In these patients, the important risk factors included those mentioned earlier (cigarette smoking, hypertension, and lipoprotein abnormalities).[7]

The question, therefore, is why does this occur in the diabetic patient with established arterial disease who appears to progress rapidly? Currently, it is our feeling that thrombosis may be the event that leads to "apparent disease progression," resulting in a decrease in the ankle/arm index. Thrombosis does not appear to be related to the same factors responsible for initiation of the disease, which raises important questions concerning secondary intervention trials. Perhaps antiplatelet therapy may have an important role in this problem, which will require more intensive study with large groups of patients.

REFERENCES

1. Beach KW, Brunzell JD, Conquest LL et al: The correlation of arteriosclerosis obliterans with lipoproteins in insulin-dependent and noninsulin-dependent diabetes. Diabetes 28:836–840, 1979
2. Beach KW, Brunzell JD, Strandness DE Jr: Prevalence of severe arteriosclerosis obliterans in patients with diabetes mellitus: Relation to smoking and form of therapy. Arteriosclerosis 2:275–280, 1982
3. Beach KW, Strandness DE Jr: Arteriosclerosis obliterans and associated risk factors in insulin-dependent and noninsulin-dependent diabetes. Diabetes 29:882–888, 1980
4. Boyd AM: The natural course of arteriosclerosis of the lower extremities. Ann Roy Coll Surg Engl 28:36–52, 1962

5. Chan A, Beach KW, Martin DC et al: Carotid artery disease in NIDDM diabetes. Diabetes Care 6:562–569, 1983
6. Silbert S, Zazeela H: Prognosis in arteriosclerotic peripheral vascular disease. JAMA 166:1816–1821, 1958
7. Strandness DE Jr, Stahler C: Arteriosclerosis obliterans. Manner and rate of progression. JAMA 196:1–4, 1966
8. Walden CE, Knopp RH, Wahl DW et al: Sex differences in the effect of diabetes mellitus on lipoprotein triglyceride and cholesterol concentrations. N Engl J Med 311:953–959, 1984

CHAPTER FOUR

Role of Hyperglycemia in Development of Diabetes Complications

Philip Raskin

The relationship between microvascular complications of diabetes and diabetes control has been unclear for many years. There is considerable evidence that, at least in experimental diabetes of animals, some relationship exists between antecedent diabetic control and the subsequent development of a characteristic diabetic lesion in the eyes and kidneys. In human beings, this relationship is far from clear. Evidence exists on both sides of this issue. But it is difficult to arrive at a firm conclusion regarding the matter, because until recently it was almost impossible to provide treatment strategies that would result in normal or near-normal blood glucose levels for sustained periods of time in most patients with insulin-dependent diabetes. Thus, it was impossible to compare diabetic complications in large groups of patients with normal or near-normal blood glucose levels with those in whom blood glucose levels were elevated. The recent development of more effective treatment methods and the rapidly expanding use of self-monitoring of blood glucose levels have made it possible to achieve near-normal glycemia for prolonged periods of time.

This chapter will review the issue in detail. The more pertinent older data and most recently acquired information in this area will be discussed, much of which has been accumulated in a prospective fashion.

NATURAL HISTORY OF DIABETES

The results of two long-term studies of the occurrence of vascular complications in patients who have had diabetes for more than 40 years are shown in Table 4-1. The incidence of complications in this group of patients is low. These patients, who have survived diabetes for more than 40 years, may represent a special subset of patients who are different from those we usually see.

Other data suggest that the incidence of the various complication rates is higher than in these two long-term studies. Figure 4-1 shows the data of Palmberg and co-workers.[16] These data are, perhaps, the best available for two reasons: first, and most importantly, they show the increased ascertainment of diabetic retinopathy when fundus photography or angiography is used rather than just the ophthalmoscope; and second, they also show that 80% to 90% of patients after 20 years of diabetes have some form of retinopathy.

With respect to nephropathy, the data of Kussman and co-workers are of interest (Table 4-2).[8] They are the result of a retro-

Table 4–1

Vascular Complications in Diabetes After 40 Years

	Boston*	London†
Patients	72 (31 males, 41 females)	92 (32 males, 60 females)
Therapy	Insulin	Insulin
Complications (%):		
Retinopathy	75.3	60.8
Nonproliferative type	45.0	43.4
Proliferative type	17.8	10.8
Proliferative type (blind)	12.3	6.5
Nephropathy	41.0	8.6
Proteinuria only	28.7	6.5
Proteinuria and renal failure	8.2	2.1
Neuropathy:	48.0	16.3
Ischemic heart disease	20.5	45.6
Peripheral vascular disease	40.0	44.5

*Aronoff SL, Bennett PH, Williamson JR et al: Muscle capillary basement membrane measurements in prediabetic, diabetic, and normal Pima Indians and normal Caucasions (abstr). Clin Res 24:455, 1976
†Abouna GM, Dremer GD, Dadah SK et al: Reversal of diabetic nephropathy in human cadaveric kidneys after transplantation into nondiabetic kidneys. Lancet 2:1274–1276, 1983

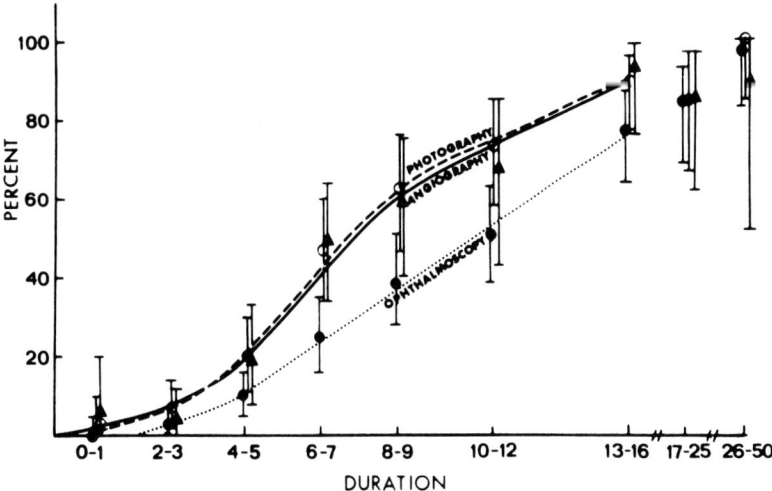

Figure 4-1. Prevalence of retinopathy. The prevalence of retinopathy is given for the modalities of (closed circle) ophthalmoscopy, (open circle) photography, (closed triangle) fluorescein angiography, at each duration of disease.

spective analysis of 112 type I diabetic patients listed in the death registry of the Joslin Clinic between 1962 and 1972, as well as patients diagnosed as having diabetic nephropathy from 1966 to 1967. It is evident that nephropathy was far more common and severe in this group of patients than in those in the 40-year studies.

What is important to note, and an issue that will be addressed later, is the group of patients with typical insulin-dependent diabetes mellitus, who despite many years of diabetes, never get the severe complications of the disease. This fortunate subset makes up approximately 20% to 25% of patients. Also of interest is the fact that an even smaller group of patients, perhaps 5%, get severe complications of diabetes in the presence of only mild elevation of blood glucose and a short duration of diabetes. These are the unfortunate people whose first indication that they have diabetes is when they seek medical attention because of one of the small blood vessel complications of diabetes.

Because of the widespread differences in the appearance of diabetic complications in patients, two major hypotheses have been advanced regarding their pathogenesis. The first, the genetic hypothesis, suggests that small blood vessel complications of diabetes are not related to the metabolic abnormalities of the disease,

Table 4–2
Development of Nephropathy in Type I Diabetes Mellitus

Number of Patients	Duration of Diabetes Onset of Proteinuria (Years)	Time Onset of Proteinuria to Renal Failure (Years)	Overall (%)	Renal Failure (%)	Mortality Cardiovascular Disease (%)
112	17.3 ± 6	4.0	53	59	36

Kussman MJ, Goldstein HH, Gleason RE: The clinical course of diabetic nephropathy. JAMA 236:1861–1863, 1976

but are somehow genetically predetermined as part of the diabetic syndrome. Thus, people with diabetes get diabetic complications because they are, in some way, genetically predisposed to do so. The second, the metabolic hypothesis, suggests that development of diabetic complications is a direct consequence of the hyperglycemia of diabetes. If one could prevent the hyperglycemia of diabetes, diabetic complications would not develop. Arguments between the proponents of these two seemingly opposite hypothesis are legion.

DIABETIC COMPLICATIONS: GENETIC INFLUENCES

The strongest evidence against the hypothesis that diabetic microangiopathy is the consequence of the metabolic abnormalities of the disease, and in support of the genetic hypothesis, has come from our department. Siperstein and co-workers, using a simple morphometric method for measuring the basement membrane thickness of quadriceps muscle capillaries, showed clearly that >90% of adults (19 years of age and over) with diabetes had an abnormal capillary basement membrane thickness compared to a group of normoglycemic controls with a negative family history of diabetes (Table 4-3).[20]

In addition, Siperstein and co-workers showed that of 30 genetic prediabetic (offspring of two overt diabetics) adults, whose

Table 4–3

Quadricep Capillary Basement Membrane Width in Normal, Diabetic, and Prediabetic Subjects

Subjects	Average Basement Membrane Width ($A°$)	Prevalence of Basement Membrane Thickening (%)
Normal (50)	1080 + 27	8
Diabetic (51)	2403 + 119	98
Prediabetic (30)	1373 + 44	53

Siperstein MD, Unger RH, Madison LL: Studies of muscle capillary basement membranes in normal subjects, diabetic, and prediabetic patients. J Clin Invest 47:1973–1999, 1968

glucose tolerance was normal, 53% had thickened capillary basement membranes compared to the control group. In these studies, no correlation was found between the severity or duration of the diabetes and thickness of the basement membrane. Mean capillary basement membrane thickness in 29 "mild" diabetics treated with diet or tolbutamide, or both, was 2410 + 167 A°, whereas in 22 "severe" diabetics requiring insulin therapy it was 2395 + 173 A°. Also, no differences were seen in basement membrane thickness when the patients were divided into those whose disease began before or after age 21. Additionally, no correlation was found between width of the basement membrane and duration of the disease. Lastly, they showed in eight patients with "secondary" diabetes caused by chronic pancreatitis, some of whom had long-standing fasting hyperglycemia, that only one (20%) patient had a thickened basement membrane.

These data have been criticized over the years for many reasons. Suffice it to say, although there has been considerable disagreement over the precise prevalence of the lesion of a thickened skeletal muscle capillary basement membrane in human diabetes as well as its relationship to the age of the subject or duration of the diabetes, a thickened basement membrane in skeletal muscle capillaries from diabetic patients is a finding confirmed on many occasions.

Finally, more evidence with respect to a genetic factor being operative in the development of a diabetic microvascular disease was provided by Marks and co-workers (Table 4-4).[11] They measured skeletal muscle capillary basement membrane thickness in 38 unaffected parents (*i.e.*, with normal oral glucose tolerance tests) of children with insulin-dependent diabetes mellitus and found a striking relationship between presence of the antigen HLA-DR4 and thickness of the skeletal muscle capillary basement membrane.

Dornan and co-workers compared the incidence of retinopathy in a group of 127 insulin-dependent patients in relationship to the HLA haplotype.[3] Interestingly, they found that HLA-DR4 was present in 70% of patients with background or proliferative retinopathy and in only 54% with no retinopathy. Also, the retinopathy tended to be more common in patients with "poor diabetic control" (Fig. 4-2).[3] The combination of poor diabetic control and HLA-DR4 increased the odds of having retinopathy to 33.3%. They concluded that genetically determined factors appear to influence susceptibility to retinopathy. This relationship between HLA-DR4 and a seemingly increased susceptibility to retinopathy has not been confirmed by other investigators.

Table 4-4
Correlation Between Basement Membrane Thickness and HLA-DR4

		Number	
HLA Phenotype of Parents	Mean Basement Membrane Thickness (A°)	Basement Membrane Thickness >2000	Basement Membrane Thickness <2000
HLA-DR4 positive	2026 ± 350*	12	8[†]
HLA-DR4 negative	1642 ± 373	2	6
Normal subjects	1628 ± 218	8	10

*p 0.001, t-test (DR4 positive versus negative)
[†]p 0.005, Fisher test (DR4 positive versus negative)
Marks JF, Raskin P, Stastny P: Increase in capillary basement membrane width in parents of children with type I diabetes mellitus; association with HLA-DR4. Diabetes 30:475–480, 1981

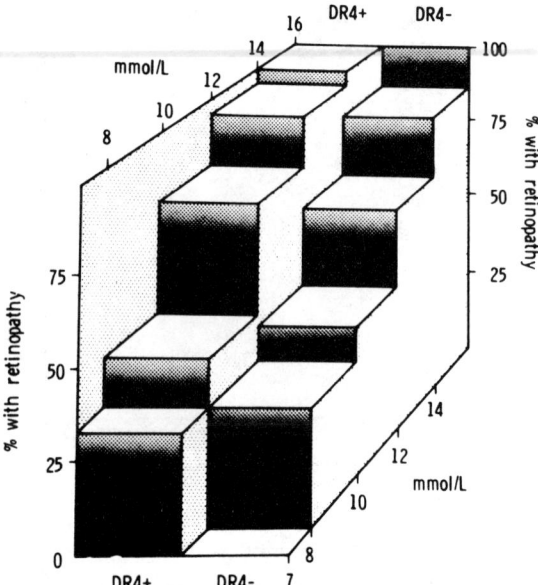

Figure 4-2. Patients with and without HLA-DR4 have been divided into five groups by mean blood glucose (8.0, 8.0 to 9.9, 10.0 to 11.9, 12.0 to 13.9, and 14.0 mmol/liter). Within each group, the proportion of patients with backgrounds of proliferative retinopathy is shown as a percentage.

DIABETIC COMPLICATIONS: METABOLIC INFLUENCES

When one discusses the metabolic influences on the development of diabetic microvascular disease, the following important questions should be considered. If we control hyperglycemia in diabetes, can we:

1. Prevent the development of diabetic complications?
2. Reverse established diabetic complications?
3. Slow the progression of established diabetic complications?

Studies using immunohistochemical techniques have added considerable information with regard to renal lesions in diabetes. Miller and Michael carried out a comprehensive immunofluorescent analysis on renal tissue from three groups of patients.[15] Group I consisted of 24 living normal renal allograft donors and two infants less than 1 week of age. Group II included 24 patients with severe nephropathy, who had diabetes mellitus for 16 to 30 years. Their ages ranged from 20 to 47 years. The last group (group III) consisted of 33 patients with chronic renal failure of diverse etiology other than diabetes. Their ages ranged from 5 to 63 years. Renal sections from patients with diabetes were easily distinguished from those of the other patients and normals by the intense linear staining of extracellular membranes. The most specific reaction was the presence of IgG and albumin lining the tubular basement membrane. The relative specificity of the immunofluorescence in the renal sections from patients with diabetes is shown in Figure 4-3.[15] Except for some minimal staining of the

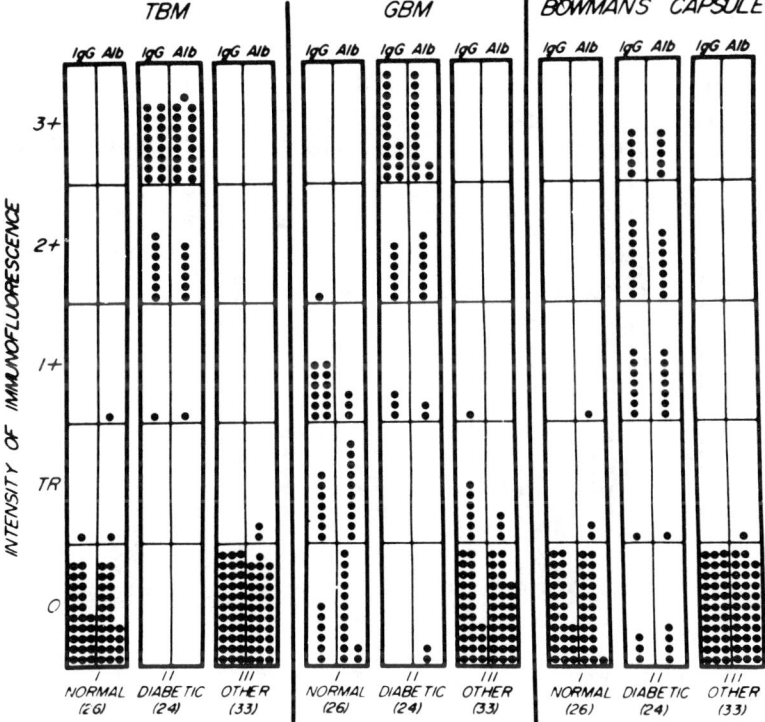

Figure 4-3. Immunofluorescence for IgG and albumin in tubular basement membranes, glomerular basement membranes, and Bowman's capsule in kidneys from normal subjects, and patients with chronic renal failure causing diabetic nephropathy and other renal disease.

DIABETES AND VASCULAR DISEASE

glomerular basement membrane from the normal kidneys, practically no overlap was found among these three groups.

In experimental diabetes in rats, exciting data are available regarding the role of hyperglycemia and diabetes. First, similar changes with respect to the immunofluorescent staining for rat IgG and complement C3 occur after 4 to 6 months of hyperglycemia. If kidneys from diabetic rats are transplanted into normal rats, the characteristic immunofluorescent lesion disappears in 2 months (Fig. 4-4).[10] If kidneys from nondiabetic rats are transplanted into diabetic rats, the lesion appears after 2 months (Fig. 4-5).[10]

Finally, if diabetic rats are made normoglycemic by islet cell transplantation, regression of the immunofluorescent changes occur (Fig. 4-6),[14] as well as a reduction in the glomerular volume (Fig. 4-7), and a reduction in the percentage of the mesangial volume occupied by the matrix component (Fig. 4-8).[21]

In human beings, experiments of a comparable nature have yielded results similar to those obtained in the experimental diabetes of animals. Mauer and co-workers examined kidney tissue obtained from 12 diabetic and 17 nondiabetic patients from 2 to 12 years after renal transplantation.[12,13] The frequency and intensity of IgG and albumin staining of the tubular and glomerular base-

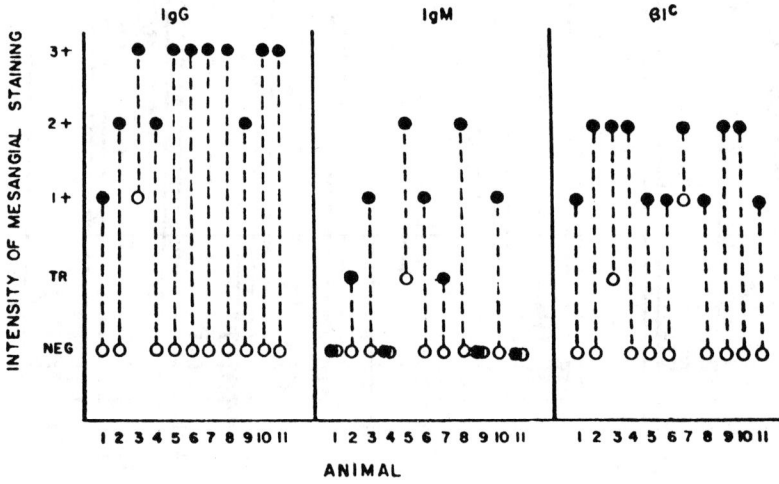

Figure 4-4. Results of immunofluorescent microscopy studies of kidneys transplanted from diabetic rats into normal recipients; biopsies before transplantation (closed circle), biopsies 2 months after transplantation (open circle).

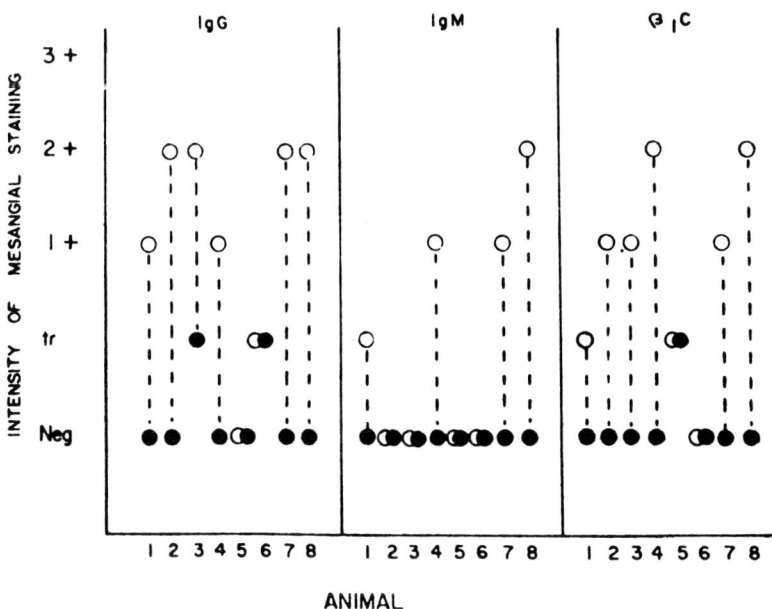

Figure 4-5. Results of immunofluorescent microscopy studies of kidneys transplanted from nondiabetic rats into diabetic recipients; biopsies before transplantation (closed circle), biopsies 2 months after transplantation (open circle).

ment membrane and Bowman's capsule were significantly greater in diabetic than in nondiabetic patients. Except for some staining of the glomerular basement membranes in the nondiabetic kidneys, practically no overlap was found between the two groups (Fig. 4-9).[14]

Although 9 of 12 diabetic patients received their kidney from a living-related donor, no immunofluorescence was observed in seven kidneys studied at the time of their transplantation into diabetic recipients.

Mauer and colleagues studied renal-transplant tissue from 12 diabetic and 28 nondiabetic patients who had a renal graft for at least 2 years (Table 4-5).[13] Ten of the 12 kidneys studied from diabetic patients showed arteriolar hyalinosis and in 6 of the 10, the hyaline change involved both the afferent and efferent limb of the glomerular arterioles. One diabetic patient developed typical nodular glomerulosclerosis 35 months after transplantation. Three of

Text continues on p. 63

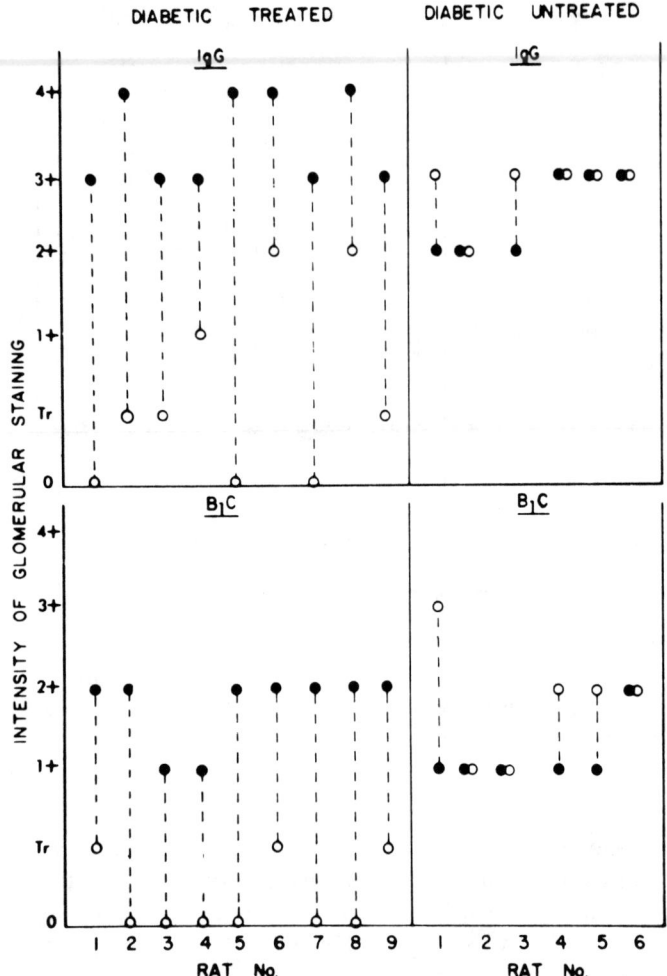

Figure 4-6. Results of immunofluorescent microscopy studies with staining for rat IgG and B_1C; biopsies before transplantation (closed circle), biopsies 3 months after transplantation (open circle).

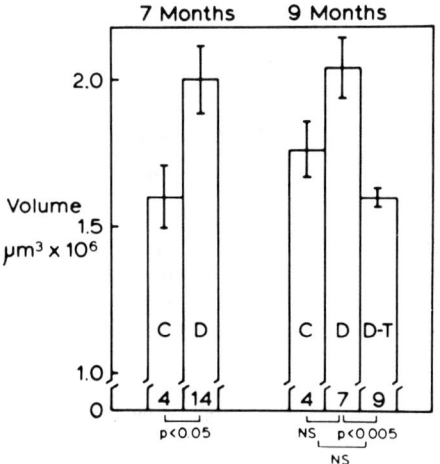

Figure 4-7. Glomerular volumes at the time of, and 2 months after, islet transplantation (intraportal distribution of neonatal pancreatic tissue after 7 months of diabetes; C = control, D = diabetic, D-T = diabetic transplanted).

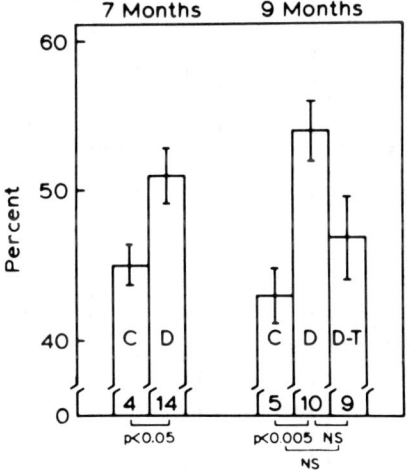

Figure 4-8. Percentage of the total mesangial volume occupied by the matrix component at the time of, and 2 months after, islet transplants.

Table 4-5
Incidence of Lesions of Arteriolar Hyaline

Group	Patients with Hyaline Deposits	
	2 to 10 Years After Transplantation	2 to 5 Years After Transplantation
Diabetic	10 of 12	10 of 12
Nondiabetic	3 of 38	0 of 23
P value*	0.001	0.0005

*By chi-square test.
Mauer SM, Miller K, Goetz FC et al: Immunopathology of renal extracellular membranes in kidneys transplanted into patients with diabetes mellitus. Diabetes 25:709–712, 1976

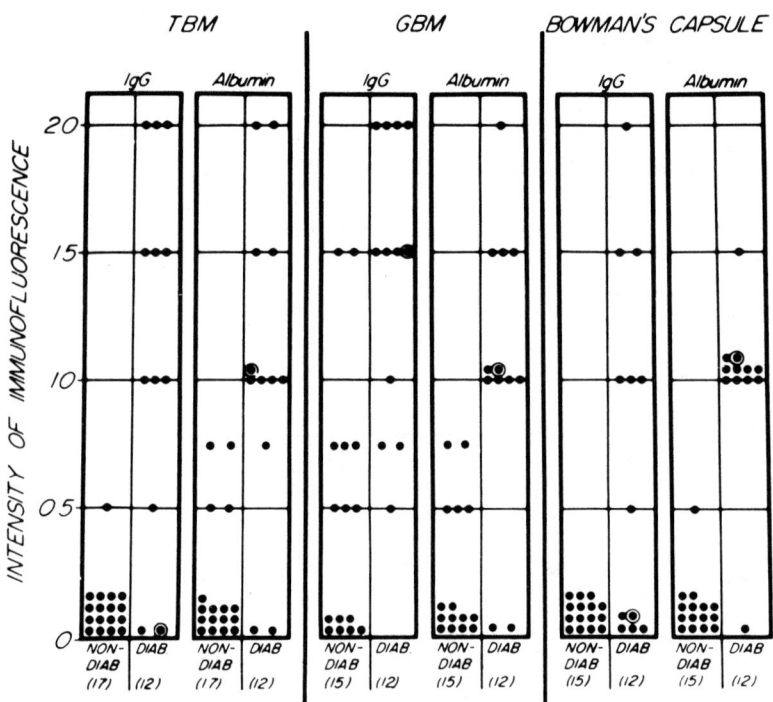

Figure 4-9. Immunofluorescence for IgG and albumin in tubular basement membrane, glomerular basement membrane, and Bowman's capsule of kidneys transplanted into diabetic and nondiabetic patients.

the 28 kidneys studied from the nondiabetic transplant recipients had hyaline vascular changes. These occurred only in rare vessels and did not appear until 5 years post-transplantation and never involved both afferent and efferent arterioles. None of the blood vessel changes was present in the kidneys transplanted into the diabetic recipients at the time of transplantation, although 10 of the 12 received living-related donor grafts.

There is another interesting human counterpart to some of the animal studies described above. Kidneys from a 37-year-old man with a 17-year history of insulin-dependent diabetes were offered for transplantation following his becoming comatose and brain dead. His urine was positive for both glucose and protein. All other laboratory tests were unremarkable. At donor nephrectomy, both kidneys were grossly normal. After some difficulty placing the organs, they were finally accepted by a transplant center in Kuwait. Both kidneys were transplanted successfully into two male recipients whose chronic renal failure was caused by polycystic kidney disease. After transplantation, both kidneys functioned well with standard immunosuppression. At the time of transplantation, both kidneys showed features of established glomerulosclerosis, an increase in the mesangial matrix, and a thickening of the glomerular capillary basement membranes. Renal biopsy specimens taken 7 months after transplantation showed complete resolution of the light microscopic abnormalities, and both patients had no proteinuria after an additional 7 months of follow-up (Fig. 4-10).[1]

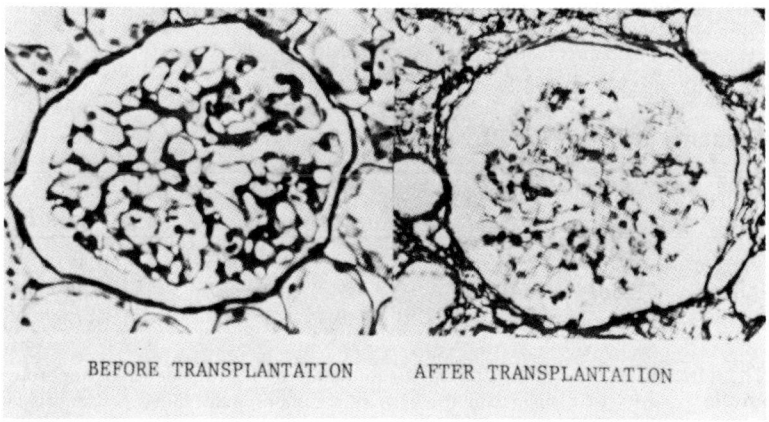

Figure 4-10. Biopsy specimen 7 months after transplantation showing (left) widely open glomerular capillaries with almost normal basement membrane and mesangium (PAS × 400) and (right) almost normal glomerular architecture (methenamine silver × 400).

CLINICAL TRIALS

If the metabolic abnormalities of diabetes are somehow responsible for the development of microangiopathy, in a cause and effect fashion, it should be possible to demonstrate that correction of these metabolic abnormalities prevents or delays the development of these vascular complications. Following is a description of clinical trials, whose data bear upon these issues. The first two of these studies are retrospective and, thus, suffer from all of the problems associated with retrospective analysis. Also, there is the problem of the appropriate assessment of overall diabetes control; most often, no objective data are available to judge diabetes control.

MALMO STUDY

Johnsson reviewed all diabetic patients in Malmo, Sweden, whose diabetes was diagnosed between 1922 and 1945 and who were less than 40 years of age at the onset of their disease.[6] The patients were divided into two groups or series. Series I consisted of 56 patients diagnosed from 1933 to 1945, who were treated with long-acting insulin and a less-regimented diet. The patients in series II had a much higher incidence of vascular complications than did those of series I.

Table 4-6 shows that, whereas the mean duration of the diabetes for the patients in series I was 10 years longer than series II, only 32% had nephropathy, compared with 56% in series II.[6] The

Table 4–6
Incidence of Nephropathy—Malmo Study*

	Series I	Series II
Number of patients	56	104
Duration of diabetes	24.5 years	15.9 years
Patients with nephropathy	18 (32%)	56 (54%)

*The difference is even more striking when one reviews the incidence of nephropathy in patients who have had the disease for more than 15 years (see Table 4–7).

Johnsson SL: Retinopathy and nephropathy in diabetes mellitus: Comparison of the effect of two forms of treatment. Diabetes 9:1, 1960

difference is even more striking when one reviews the incidence of nephropathy in patients who have had the disease for more than 15 years (Table 4-7).[6] Only 9% of patients in series I had nephropathy, compared with 61% of patients in series II. Similar striking differences were seen between the groups when the incidence of retinopathy was compared. Hypoglycemia was far more common in series I patients, reflecting attempts to achieve normoglycemia in the use of multiple daily insulin injections.

BELGIAN STUDY

The Belgian study is, perhaps, the largest of its kind.[17] Dr. Pirart has followed 4398 patients with diabetes from 1947, of which 2795 were followed since the initial diagnosis of their disease. Despite the obvious limitation of this study—the inability to accurately assess long-term diabetes control—Dr. Pirart's data suggest a strong relationship between the level of diabetic control and development of diabetic complications. Figure 4-11 demonstrates the prevalence of retinopathy as related to the level of diabetic control over the years of follow-up.[17] Clearly, the higher the level of blood glucose, the greater the prevalence of diabetic retinopathy. Of note, however, is that almost 30% of Dr. Pirart's patients, despite many years of poor diabetes control, had no diabetic retinopathy.

JOB STUDY

The study by Job and co-workers was designed in a prospective fashion (Table 4-8).[5] Diabetic patients were assigned randomly

Table 4–7

Incidence of Nephropathy in Malmo Study After 15 Years of Duration of Diabetes

	Series I	*Series II*
Number of patients	56	57
Patients with nephropathy	5 (9%)	35 (61%)

Johnsson SL: Retinopathy and nephropathy in diabetes mellitus: Comparison of the effect of two forms of treatment. Diabetes 9:1, 1960

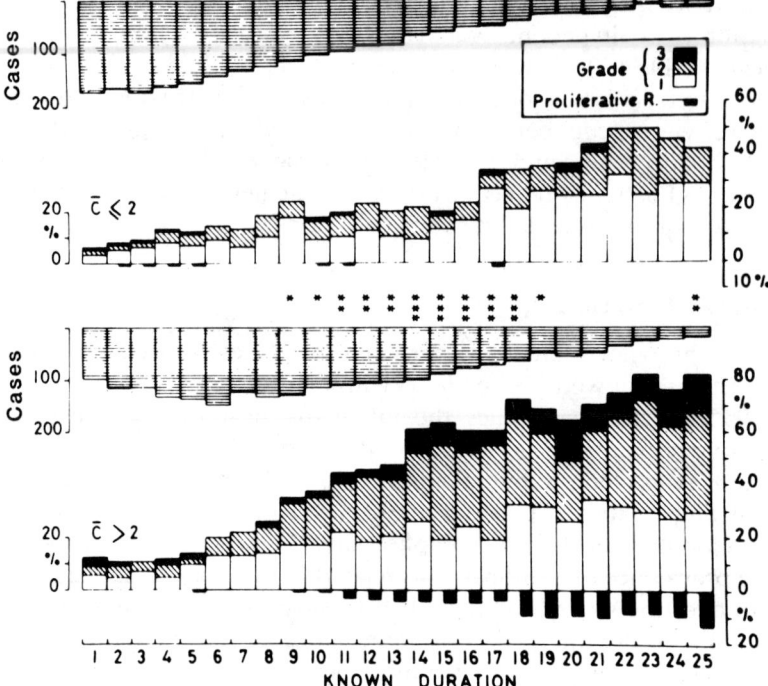

Figure 4-11. Ascending curves for different grades of retinopathy as a function of duration in severe diabetes with good (top) or poor (bottom) cumulative glycemia control.

to either a single-insulin-injection group or a multiple-insulin-injection (three times daily) group. Both groups were followed for a mean duration of 3 years. The progression of retinopathy was evaluated by fluorescein angiography and funduscopic examination. They reported a significantly greater increase in the number of microaneurysms in the single-injection group compared to the multiple-injection group. Unfortunately, this study suffers from an important defect, which makes the results difficult to evaluate. Of the 21 patients whose data were analyzed from the single-injection group, only 16 received one daily insulin injection for the entire period of study; the other five were changed either to two or three injections per day after the study began. In the multiple-injection group, only 5 of the 21 patients analyzed had three insulin injections daily for the entire period of the study. The others either accepted only two injections (4 patients) or some only one (4 patients) initially. Nine of the 13 patients who originally accepted three injections daily were reduced to two injections after 1 year.

Table 4-8
Comparison of Increase in Number of Microaneurysms Between the Two Groups (Means ± SEM)*†

	Single-Injection Group	Multiple-Injection Group	P Values
Number of microaneurysms			
At baseline	12.7 ± 3.5	9.0 ± 3.3	N.S.
At the last examination	33.3 ± 7.9	15.2 ± 3.3	0.05
Difference	20.3 ± 4.9	6.2 ± 2.5	0.02
Mean yearly increase in the number of microaneurysms	7.2 ± 1.9	1.8 ± 0.7	0.01
Mean yearly increase in the square root of the number of microaneurysms	0.85 ± 0.16	0.24 ± 0.13	0.01

*SEM = standard error of the mean.
†Nonparametric test. Because the variances of the mean yearly increases in the number of microaneurysms differed between the two groups, they were also compared by a nonparametric test (Mann and Whitney) and the square-root transformation, which equalized the variances.
Job D, Eschwege E, Guyat-Argenton C et al: Effect of multiple daily insulin injection on the cause of diabetic retinopathy. Diabetes 25:463–469, 1976

The small number of patients studied initially, coupled with the many crossovers in the protocol, probably make this study invalid.

CONTROLLED PROSPECTIVE TRIALS

As alluded to earlier, the past several years have brought great advances in the treatment of insulin-dependent diabetes mellitus. Included in these advances are the use of innovative treatment strategies such as multiple-insulin dose programs, portable-insulin-infusion devices, and the increased use of self-monitoring of blood glucose. As a result of these advances, it has been possible to design appropriate prospective studies to evaluate more fully the relationship between diabetic control and complications in human beings. Following are the results of some of these studies.

STENO STUDY

In the Steno study by Lauritzen and colleagues, 30 insulin-dependent diabetic patients with background retinopathy were given random assignment of either conventional treatment (two daily injections of insulin) or treatment with continuous subcutaneous insulin infusion and were followed prospectively for more than 2 years (Fig. 4-12).[9] Retinal examinations were done at 6-month intervals. Mean blood glucose levels and stable hemoglobin A_1C values were significantly lower in the continuous subcutaneous insulin infusion treatment group than the conventional treatment group. Retinal morphology deteriorated during the first year in both groups, but no significant differences were noted between the two. The frequency of deterioration, however, was highest in the continuous subcutaneous insulin infusion group, especially among patients with the best glycemic control. Retinal function (oscillatory potential, macular recovery time, and posterior vitreous fluorophotometry) improved significantly with continuous subcutaneous insulin infusion treatment and deteriorated significantly with conventional treatment. Changes in retinal function were most pronounced in patients with the best and poorest diabetic control. Table 4-9 shows the results of Steno study fundus photographs indicating that despite the apparent, although not statistically significant, deterioration of retinopathy after the

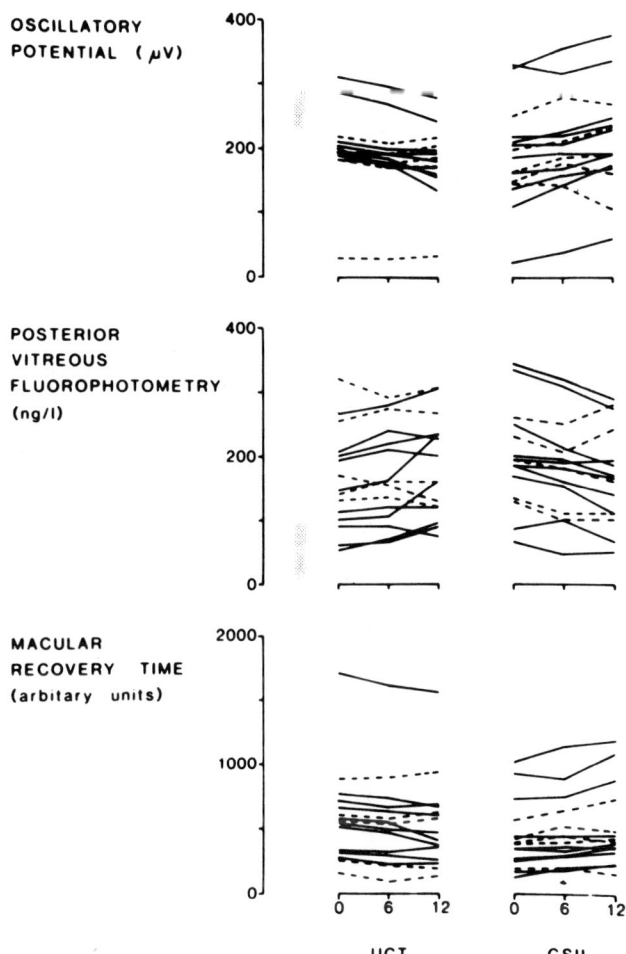

Figure 4-12. Oscillatory potential posterior vitreous fluorophotometry, and macular recovery time for conventional treatment and continuous subcutaneous insulin infusion patients. In the conventional treatment panel, solid lines indicate the ten poorest regulated patients; in the continuous subcutaneous insulin infusion panel, solid lines indicate the best regulated patients. In both panels, broken lines represent intermediately regulated patients. Each line represents the measurement for one patient at zero, 6, and 12 months. Shaded area indicates normal range (mean ± 2 SD).

Table 4-9
Steno Study—Fundus Photographs

	One Year		Two Years	
	Conventional Treatment	Continuous Subcutaneous Insulin Infusion	Conventional Treatment	Continuous Subcutaneous Insulin Infusion
Improved	3	3	2	7
No change	7	2	2	2
Worse	5	10	10	6

Lauritzen T, Frost–Larren L, Deckert T et al: Effect of one year of near-normal blood glucose levels on retinopathy in insulin-dependent diabetics. Lancet 1:200–203, 1983

first year of the study, there appears to have been a leveling off after 2 years of follow-up.[9] Several studies have reported a tendency toward an acceleration of diabetic retinopathy in patients treated intensively. The mechanism by which this reversible deterioration occurs is unknown.

In the Steno study, the effect of diabetic control on glomerular filtration rate and urinary albumin excretion rate was also evaluated. Lauritzen and co-workers showed that glomerular filtration rate can be reduced and frequently normalized with prolonged metabolic control, but this does not occur in patients on conventional treatment whose diabetes control is stable though unimproved. No effects were found on urinary albumin excretion with either treatment (Table 4-10).[9]

Several other studies report similar results (*i.e.*, little or no improvement in renal function despite several years of improved diabetes control). It appears that when significant diabetic renal disease develops, improved diabetic control does not cause reversal or even a slowing of the rate of progression. Aggressive management of patients' hypertension has been shown to be beneficial in terms of slowing the progression of diabetic renal disease.

BRITISH STUDY

In the British study conducted in diabetic clinics at Oxford and Aylesbury, 174 insulin-dependent diabetic patients with background retinopathy were randomized to continue with usual diabetic care (group U), or to a more intensive program (group A) using Ultralente insulin as a basal cover and soluble insulin before meals.[4] In addition, group A attended the clinic more frequently, received closer dietary supervision, and were taught self blood glucose monitoring. Group A had a significantly lower mean glycosylated hemoglobin level during the study, although the mean levels also fell in group U toward the end of year two (Fig. 4-13).[4] Renal and sensory nerve functions were significantly better preserved in group A than in group U (Fig. 4-14).[4] The rate of progression of retinopathy was similar in both groups. It was concluded that a modest improvement in diabetic control obtainable in most clinics is associated with a reduction in the progression of diabetic tissue damage.

NEW HAVEN STUDY

In the New Haven study, 30 eyes of 15 type I diabetic patients

Table 4–10
Steno Study—Renal Function Studies

	Glomerular Filtration Rate (ml/min × 1.73m²)			Urinary Albumin Excretion Rate (µg/min)		
	Zero	One Year	Two Years	Zero	One Year	Two Years
Continuous subcutaneous insulin infusion	131 ± 5*	117 ± 5	111 ± 4†	36 ± 9	43 ± 14	79 ± 43
Conventional treatment	114 ± 4	112 ± 4	112 ± 5	62 ± 18	195 ± 8	267 ± 98*

*p 0.05 continuous subcutaneous insulin infusion versus conventional treatment.
†p 0.05 2 years versus baseline.
Deckert T, Lauritzen T, Parving H et al: Effect of two years of strict metabolic control on kidney function in long-term insulin-dependent diabetics. Diabetic Nephropathy 2:6–10, 1983

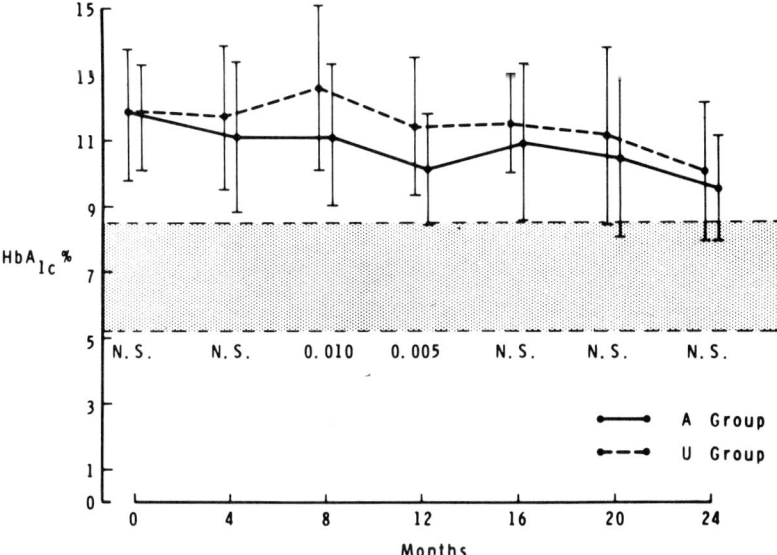

Figure 4-13. Mean HbA₁C levels (± SD) in each group. Shaded area = normal range. NS = not significant.

were evaluated prospectively before and after 11 to 23 months (mean: 18.1 months) of pump treatment. In each patient, plasma glucose and total glycosylated hemoglobin fell to normal or near-normal levels.[18] The ten eyes without diabetic retinopathy at entry remained without. Four of 20 eyes with diabetic retinopathy at entry advanced by modified Early Treatment Diabetic Retinopathy Study classification, including one eye that progressed from background to proliferative diabetic retinopathy. No eyes with diabetic retinopathy improved their modified Early Treatment Diabetic Retinopathy Study classification. One eye progressed to blindness; no other eye lost vision. Six eyes had laser treatment before insulin pump treatment; four of these and two others required laser treatment during pump treatment. Two eyes had vitreous hemorrhages before pump treatment; one of these and four others hemorrhaged during pump treatment. No eyes with diabetic retinopathy showed regression of microvascular changes (Table 4-11).[18] The data suggested to the authors that prolonged restoration of near-normal glucose metabolism with the insulin pump does not reverse established diabetic retinopathy (Fig. 4-15).[18]

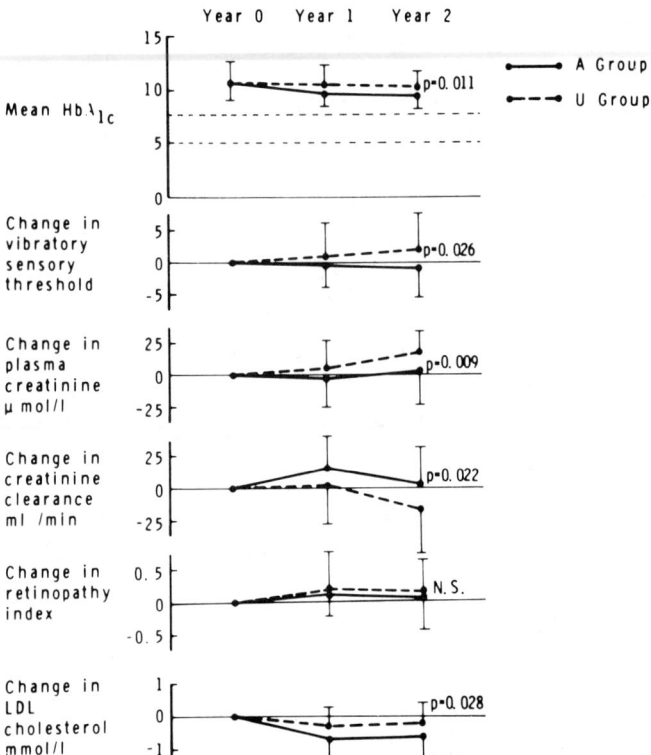

Figure 4-14. Changes from entry (year 0) to year 1 and to year 2, with the exception of HbA$_1$C for which values are given at entry and the mean of all values (excluding entry) over year 1 and year 2.

KROC STUDY

In the KROC prospective multicenter trial,[7] patients with nonproliferative diabetic retinopathy and absence C-peptide were randomly assigned to pump ($n = 35$) or conventional therapy ($n = 35$). Subsequently, glycemic control and retinopathy (fundus photography and fluorescein angiography) were assessed periodically over 8 months. At the start of the study, the age duration of diabetes, insulin dose, glycemic control, and degree of retinopathy were similar in the two groups. After randomization, mean blood glucose (175 ± 9 mg/dl) and glycosylated hemoglobin levels (10.0 ±

Table 4-11
**Summary: Diabetic Retinopathy Classification
(30 Eyes of 15 Patients)**

	Entry	*Current*
Number of diabetic retinopathy	10	10
Background retinopathy	9	8
Proliferative retinopathy	11	12
Total eyes	30	30

Puklin JE, Tamborlane WV, Felig P et al: Influence of long-term insulin infusion pump treatment of type I diabetes on diabetic retinopathy. Ophthalmology 89:735–737, 1982

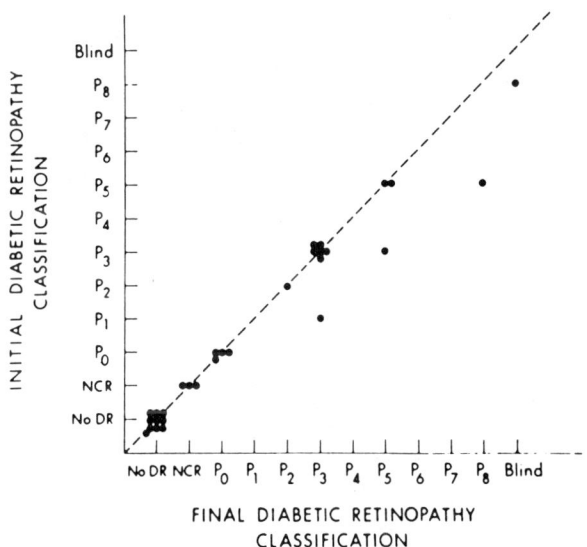

Figure 4-15. Plotting of the initial modified Early Treatment Diabetic Retinopathy Study classification of each eye on the ordinate with the final modified Early Treatment Diabetic Retinopathy Study classification on the abscissa. Dots falling on the 45° line represent no change; those below the line represent a progression of retinopathy.

0.3%) remained elevated in the conventional treatment group, but fell to near-normal values (117 ± 6 mg/dl and 8.1 ± 0.3%, respectively) during the entire period of pump treatment ($p < 0.001$ versus conventional treatment group) (Fig. 4-16).[7]

The frequency of biochemical hypoglycemia was similar in both groups, but ketoacidosis occurred only with pump therapy. The level of retinopathy assessed from photographs progressed in both groups. Continuous subcutaneous insulin infusion was associated with slightly more deterioration in diabetic retinopathy compared to the conventionally treated group, mainly because of the appearance of soft exudates and intraretinal microvascular abnormalities (Fig. 4-17).[7] In contrast, elevated albumin excretion rates fell during continuous insulin infusion, but not during conventional treatment (Fig. 4-18).[7] The conclusion from this study is that near-normal blood glucose level for 8 months does not retard progression of, and in fact may initially worsen, established retinopathy. The authors suggested the need for longer trials, particularly directed toward primary prevention.

DALLAS STUDY

Over the past several years, Raskin and his co-workers have been engaged in a prospective, nonrandomized trial of the effect of an experimental treatment program on diabetic complications in

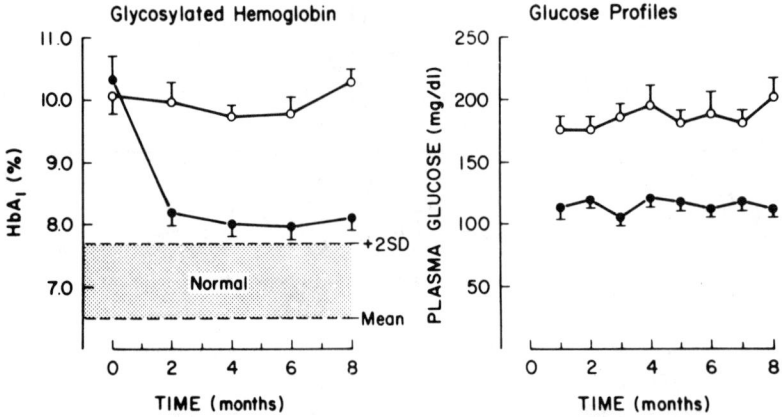

Figure 4-16. Home assessments of glycemic control in patients randomly assigned to continuous subcutaneous insulin infusion (closed circle) or unchanged conventional injection treatment (open circle).

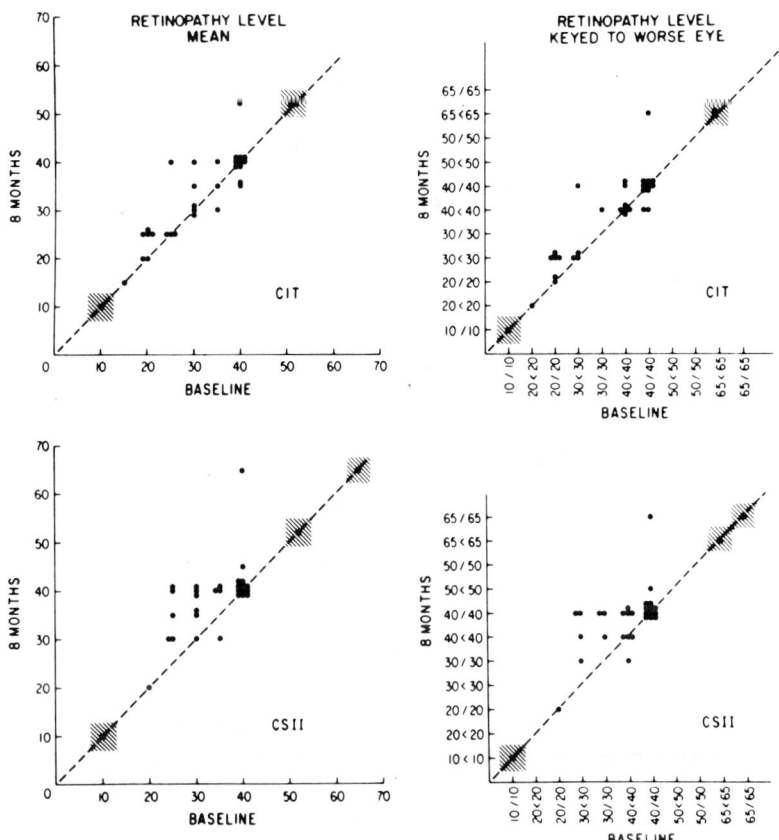

Figure 4-17. Retinopathy levels at baseline and at 8 months in individual patients assigned to the continuous subcutaneous insulin infusion or conventional treatment groups.

insulin-dependent diabetic patients (C-peptide negative).[19] This treatment program includes aggressive dietary instructions, self blood glucose monitoring, and continuous subcutaneous insulin infusion delivered by a portable insulin infusion device. Data were acquired from a group of patients who preferred to continue with their more conventional diabetes treatment rather than enter into the experimental treatment program. Over the years the experimental group has shown considerable advantage from the conventional treatment program with respect to many metabolic values such as plasma glucagon profiles, lipid and lipoprotein levels, and motor nerve conduction velocities.

Skeletal muscle capillary basement membrane width was also

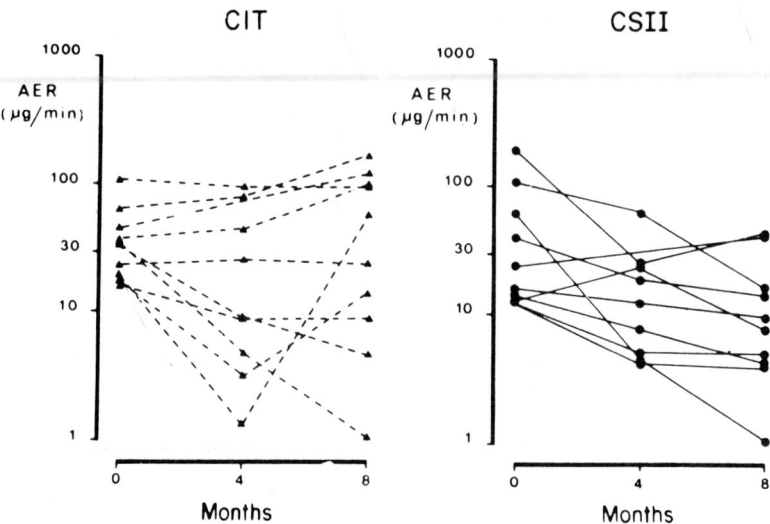

Figure 4-18. Changes in albumin excretion rate in the ten patients in each treatment group with supranormal baseline values (exceeding 12 μg/min).

measured in 51 of the patients in whom observations have been made from 1 to 3 years. Of these 51 patients, 26 entered the experimental treatment group and 25 were in the conventional treatment group. Data from diabetic patients were compared with those of a group of nondiabetic subjects, 43 of whom had glycosylated hemoglobin determinations and 21 who agreed to undergo a muscle biopsy for measurement of skeletal muscle capillary basement membrane width.

During the 3 years of improved diabetic control reflected by a decrease in glycosylated hemoglobin levels, using an experimental treatment program consisting of rigid dietary control, self blood glucose monitoring, and continuous subcutaneous insulin infusion, a significant reduction was found in skeletal muscle capillary basement membrane width (Fig. 4-19).[19] This reduction was not evident in the group of diabetic patients treated with a more conventional program who showed a stable, though unimproved, level of diabetic control (Fig. 4-20).[19] If capillaries in skeletal muscle are reflective of those in retinal or renal tissue, meticulous diabetic control for prolonged periods might be beneficial with respect to the microvascular complications of diabetes (Fig. 4-21).[19]

HYPERGLYCEMIA AND DIABETES COMPLICATIONS

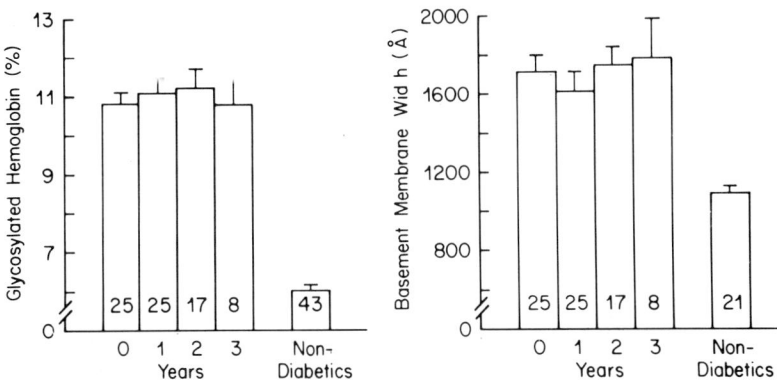

Figure 4-19. Quadriceps capillary basement membrane width and glycosylated hemoglobin levels in type I diabetic patients in the experimental treatment group. Values in nondiabetics are included for references.

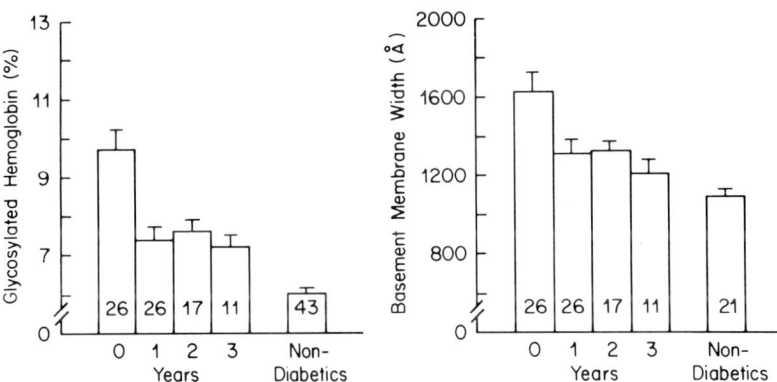

Figure 4-20. Quadriceps capillary basement membrane width and glycosylated hemoglobin levels in type I diabetic patients in the conventional treatment group. Values in nondiabetics are included for reference.

DIABETES CONTROL AND COMPLICATIONS TRIAL

The Diabetes Control and Complications Trial is the largest and most ambitious clinical trial to date. The multicenter study consists of 27 clinical groups, 25 of which are in the United States and 2

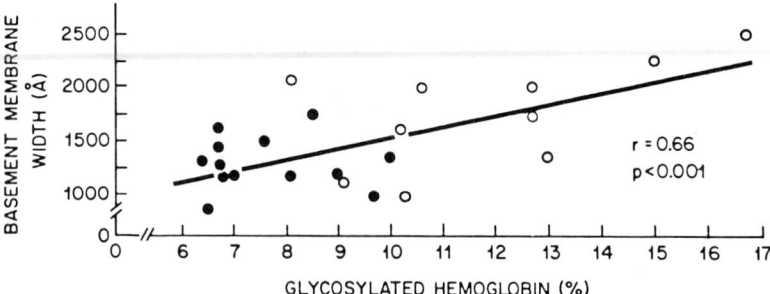

Figure 4-21. Relationship between capillary basement membrane width and glycosylated hemoglobin values in type I diabetic patients after 2 years of treatment.

in Canada. Two large groups of insulin-dependent diabetic patients will be followed for as long as 8 to 10 years. These patients will be assigned to treatment on a random basis. One group will receive conventional diabetes treatment; the other will receive an intensive experimental treatment designed to achieve euglycemia. The endpoint will be early diabetic retinopathy. This trial, if it continues as planned, should provide an unequivocal answer to this issue.

CONCLUSIONS

What are the overall conclusions to be drawn from the data presented? Which of the two hypotheses of the etiology of the microvascular complications of diabetes was the better supported? Given all the facts, it is difficult to arrive at a single answer. Alternatively, the small blood vessel complications of diabetes may be related to both genetic and metabolic influences. Figure 4-22 shows the interrelationship between genetic and metabolic factors in the development of diabetic complications.

INFLUENCE OF GENETIC PREDISPOSITION ON SEVERITY OF DIABETIC MICROANGIOPATHY

In 20% to 25% of diabetic patients, the genetic predisposition to develop diabetic complications is low. Thus, no matter how severe the metabolic abnormality (*i.e.*, how much hyperglycemia the patients have over the lifetime of their illness), they rarely develop significant complications. If we could identify this subset

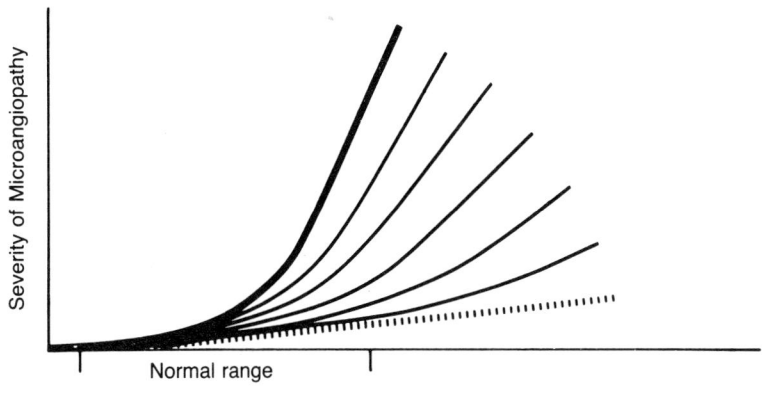

Figure 4-22. Influence of genetic predisposition on the severity of diabetic microangiopathy.

of patients at the beginning of their disease, our treatment recommendations would be simple, and we could keep them free of symptoms and avoid both hypoglycemia and severe hyperglycemia and ketoacidosis. These patients would not need expensive intensive diabetes management, which results in a higher impact on lifestyle. In another 5% of patients, the genetic predisposition to development of diabetic complications is so great that even a slight degree of hyperglycemia results in severe microvascular complications. Unfortunately, given our present treatment techniques, we may be unable to normalize the blood glucose level sufficiently to help this group of patients. Finally, the large remaining group of diabetic patients have varying degrees of genetic predisposition to develop the microvascular complications. In this group, improved diabetic control, which results in a lowering of the overall blood glucose level, might reduce the severity of microvascular complications.

SUMMARY

Although the data seem to support the suggested synthesis, it is not yet a proven fact. In those patients for whom we can do some good by intensive diabetes treatment with resulting long-term near-normal or normal glycemia, this should be considered as preventive in nature. It is possible that all we can do is prevent diabetic complications from occurring; however, when significant diabetic complications have occurred, no degree of normoglycemia will cause a reversal. Aggressive diabetes treatment should not be recommended for all patients with insulin-dependent diabetes mellitus in view of not having a definitive answer to this question, because complications can occur with this type of treatment. It is expensive both to the patient and health-care systems in general. There is the ever-present danger of insulin-induced hypoglycemia, which can have lethal consequence. Thus, we must continue to be careful whom we enter into an intensive diabetes treatment program.

REFERENCES

1. Abouna GM, Dremer GD, Dadah SK et al: Reversal of diabetic nephropathy in human cadaveric kidneys after transplantation into nondiabetic kidneys. Lancet 2:1274–1276, 1983
2. Aronoff SL, Bennett PH, Williamson JR et al: Muscle capillary basement membrane measurements in prediabetic, diabetic, and normal Pima Indians and normal Caucasians (abstr). Clin Res 24:455, 1976
3. Dornan TL, Ting A, McPherson CK et al: Genetic susceptibility to the development of retinopathy in insulin-dependent diabetics. Diabetes 31:222–231, 1982
4. Holman RR, Hayon-White V, Ored-Peckar C et al: Preventions of deterioration of renal and sensory-nerve function by more intensive management of insulin-dependent diabetic patients. Lancet 2:204–208, 1983
5. Job D, Eschwege E, Guyat-Argenton C et al: Effect of multiple daily insulin injection on the cause of diabetic retinopathy. Diabetes 25:463–469, 1976
6. Johnsson SL: Retinopathy and nephropathy in diabetes mellitus: Comparison of the effect of two forms of treatment. Diabetes 9:1, 1960
7. KROC Collaborative Study: Near normal glycemic control does not slow progression of mild diabetic retinopathy. Diabetes 32(Suppl 1):37A, 1983
8. Kussman MJ, Goldstein HH, Gleason RE: The clinical course of diabetic nephropathy. JAMA 236:1861–1863, 1976
9. Lauritzen T, Frost-Larsen L, Deckert T et al: Effect of one year of near-normal blood glucose levels on retinopathy in insulin-dependent diabetics. Lancet 1:200–203, 1983
10. Lee CS, Mauer M, Brown D et al: Renal transplantation in diabetes mellitus in rats. J Exp Med 139:793–800, 1974
11. Marks JF, Raskin P, Stastny P: Increase in capillary basement

membrane width in parents of children with type I diabetes mellitus; association with HLA-DR4. Diabetes 30:475–480, 1981

12. Mauer SM, Barbosa J, Vernier RL et al: Development of diabetic vascular lesions in normal kidneys transplanted into patients with diabetes mellitus. N Engl J Med 295:916–920, 1976
13. Mauer SM, Miller K, Goetz FC et al: Immunopathology of renal extracellular membranes in kidneys transplanted into patients with diabetes mellitus. Diabetes 25:709–712, 1976
14. Mauer SM, Sutherland DER, Steffes MW et al: Pancreatic islet transplantation. Diabetes 23:744–753, 1974
15. Miller K, Michael AF: Immunopathology of renal extracellular membranes in diabetes mellitus. Specificity of tubular basement membrane immunofluorescence. Diabetes 25:701, 1976
16. Palmberg PF, Smith M, Waltman S et al: The natural history of retinopathy in insulin-dependent juvenile-onset diabetes. Ophthalmology 88:613–618, 1981
17. Pirart J: Diabetes mellitus and its degenerative complications: A prospective study of 4,400 patients observed between 1947 and 1973. Diabetes Care 1:168–263, 1978
18. Puklin JE, Tamborlane WV, Felig P et al: Influence of long-term insulin infusion pump treatment of type I diabetes on diabetic retinopathy. Ophthalmology 89:735–737, 1982
19. Raskin P, Pietr A, Unger R et al: The effect of diabetic control on skeletal muscle capillary basement membrane width in patients with type I diabetes mellitus. N Engl J Med 300:1546–1560, 1983
20. Siperstein MD, Unger RH, Madison LL: Studies of muscle capillary basement membranes in normal subjects, diabetic, and prediabetic patients. J Clin Invest 47:1973–1999, 1968
21. Steffes MN, Brown DM, Basgen JM et al: Amelioration of mesangial volume and surface alterations following islet transplantation in diabetic rats. Diabetes 29:509–515, 1980

BIBLIOGRAPHY

Pickup JC, Viberti GC et al: Glycemic control in diabetic nephropathy. Br Med J 288:1187–1191, 1984

Bodansky HJ, Wolf A, Cudworth, AG et al: Genetic and immunologic factors in microvascular disease in type I insulin-dependent diabetes. Diabetes 31:70–74, 1982

Cataland S, O'Dorisio TM: Diabetic nephropathy. Clinical course in patients treated with the subcutaneous insulin pump. JAMA 249:2059–2061, 1983

Chazan BI, Balodimos MD, Ryan JR et al: Twenty-five to forty-five years of diabetes with and without vascular complications. Diabetologia 6:565–569, 1970

Christy M, Nerup J, Platz P et al: A review of HLA antigens in long-standing IDDM with and without severe retinopathy. Horm Metab Res 11:73–77, 1981

Dahl-Jorgensen K, Hanssen KR, Semland E et al: Long-term strict control in type I (insulin-dependent) diabetes mellitus: Effect on late diabetic complications. Diabetologia 25:149, 1983

Daneman D, Drash AL, Lobes LA et al: Progressive retinopathy with improved control in diabetic dwarfism (Mauriac's syndrome). Diabetes Care 4:360–365, 1981

Danowski TS, Fisher ER, Khurana C et al: Muscle capillary basement membrane in juvenile diabetes mellitus. Metabolism 21:1125–1132, 1972

Deckert T, Lauritzen T, Parving H et al: Effect of two years of strict metabolic control on kidney function in long-term insulin-dependent diabetics. Diabetic Nephropathy 2:6–10, 1983

Dunn FL, Pietri A, Raskin P: Plasma lipid and lipoprotein levels with continuous subcutaneous insulin infusion in type I diabetes. Ann Intern Med 95:426–431, 1981

Ellis D, Avner ED, Transue E et al: Diabetic nephropathy in adolescence: Appearance during improved glycemic control. Pediatrics 71:724–829, 1983

Eschwege E, Job D, Guyot-Argenton J et al: Delayed progression of diabetic retinopathy by divided insulin administration: A further follow-up. Diabetologia 16:13–15, 1979

Friberg TR, Rosenstock J, Sanborn M et al: The effect of long-term near-normal glycemic control in mild diabetic retinopathy. Ophthalmology 92:1051, 1986

Gray RS, Starkey IR, Rainbow S et al: HLA antigens and other risk factors in the development of retinopathy in type I diabetes. Br J Ophthalmol 66:280–285, 1982

Johnston PB, Kidd M, Middleton D et al: Analysis of HLA antigen association with proliferative diabetic retinopathy. Br J Ophthalmol 66:277–279, 1982

Johnston PB, Middleton D, Archer DB et al: HLA antigens in proliferative diabetic retinopathy. Int Ophthalmol 2:87–89, 1981

Kahn HA, Bradley RF: Prevalence of diabetic retinopathy. Age, sex, and duration of diabetes. J Ophthalmol 59:345–349, 1975

Kilo C, Vogler N, Williamson JR: Muscle capillary basement membrane changes related to aging and to diabetes mellitus. Diabetes 21:881–905, 1972

Klein BEK, Davis MD, Segal P et al: Diabetic retinopathy: Assessment of severity of progression. Ophthalmology 91:10–17, 1984.

Lawson PM, Champion MC, Canny C et al: Continuous subcutaneous insulin infusion (CSII) does not prevent progression of proliferative and preproliferative retinopathy. Br J Ophthalmol 66:762–766, 1982

Mathiesen ER, Oxenboll B, Johansen K et al: Incipient nephropathy in type I (insulin-dependent) diabetes. Diabetologia 26:406–410, 1984

Mauer SM, Barbosa J, Vernier RL et al: Development of diabetic vascular lesions in normal kidneys transplanted into patients with diabetes mellitus. N Engl J Med 295:916–920, 1976

Mauer SM, Michael AF, Fish AJ et al: Spontaneous immunoglobulin and complement deposition in glomeruli of diabetic rats. Lab Invest 27:488–494, 1972

Mauer SM, Steffes MW, Sutherland DER et al: Studies of the rate of regression of the glomerular lesions in diabetic rats treated with pancreatic islet transplantation. Diabetes 24:280–295, 1975

Oakley WG, Pyke DA, Tattersall RB et al: Long-term diabetes. Q J Med 18:145–156, 1974

Osterby R, Lundbaek K: The basement membrane morphology in diabetes mellitus. In Ellenberg M, Rifkin H (eds): Diabetes Mellitus: Theory and Practice. New York, McGraw-Hill, 1970

Palmberg PF: Diabetic retinopathy. Diabetes 26:703–711, 1977

Pardo V, Peres-Stable EL, Alzamor DB et al: Incidence and significance of muscle capillary basal lamina thickness in juvenile diabetes. Am J Pathol 68:67–77, 1972

Paz-Guevara ET, Hsu TH, White P et al: Juvenile diabetes mellitus after 40 years. Diabetes 24:559–565, 1975

Peterson CM, Jones RL, Esterly JA et al: Changes in basement membrane thickening and pulse volume concomitant with improved glucose control and exercise in patients with insulin-dependent diabetes mellitus. Diabetes Care 3:586–589, 1980

Raskin P: Treatment of insulin-dependent diabetes with portable insulin infusion devices. Med Clin North Am 66:1269–1283, 1982

Raskin P: Treatment of type I diabetes mellitus with portable insulin infusion devices. Diabetes Care 5:48–52, 1982

Raskin P: Diabetic regulation and its relationship to microangiopathy. Metabolism 27:235–251, 1978

Raskin P, Marks JF, Burns H et al: Capillary basement membrane width in diabetic children. Am J Med 58:365–372, 1975

Seiss EA, Nathke HE, Dexel T et al: Dependency of muscle capillary basement membrane thickness on the duration of diabetes. Diabetes Care 2:472–478, 1979

Siperstein MD: Capillary basement membranes and diabetic microangiopathy. In Stollerman GH (ed): Advances in Internal Medicine, pp 18:325–344. Chicago, Year Book Medical Publishers, 1972

Siperstein MD, Raskin P, Burns HL: Electron microscopic quantification of diabetic microangiopathy. Diabetes 22:514–527, 1973

Sosenko JM, Miettinen OS, Williamson JR et al: Muscle capillary basement-membrane thickness and long-term glycemia in type I diabetes mellitus. N Engl J Med 311:694–698, 1984

Tamborlane WV, Puklin JE, Bergman M et al: Long-term improvement of metabolic control with insulin pump does not reverse diabetic microangiopathy. Diabetes Care 5:58–60, 1982

Van Ballegooie E, Johanna MM, Timmerman A et al: Rapid deterioration of diabetic retinopathy during treatment with continuous subcutaneous insulin infusion. Diabetes Care 7:236–242, 1984

Viberti GC, Bilous RW, Macintosh D et al: Long-term correction of hyperglycemia and progression of renal failure in insulin-dependent diabetes. Br Med J 286:598–602, 1983

Vracko RL: Skeletal muscle capillaries in diabetics. A quantitative analysis. Circulation 41:271–283, 1970

Walton C, Dyer PA, Davidson JA et al: HLA antigens and risk factors for nephropathy in type I (insulin-dependent) diabetes mellitus. Diabetologia 27:3–7, 1984

West LM, Erdreich LJ, Stober JA: A detailed study of risk factors for retinopathy and nephropathy in diabetes. Diabetes 29:501–508, 1980

White MC, Kohner EM, Pickup JC et al: Reversal of diabetic retinopathy by continuous subcutaneous insulin infusion: A case report. 65:307–311, 1981

White N, Waltman SR, Krupin T et al: Reversal of abnormalities in ocular fluorophotometry in insulin-dependent diabetes after five to nine months of improved metabolic control. Diabetes 21:80–85, 1982

Williamson JR, Rowold E, Hoffman P et al: Influence of fixation and morphometric technics on capillary basement-membrane thickening prevalence data in diabetes. Diabetes 25:604–613, 1976

Wiseman M, Viberti G, Macintosh D et al: Glycemia arterial pressure and micro-albuminuria in type I (insulin-dependent) diabetes mellitus. Diabetologia 26:401–405, 1984

CHAPTER FIVE

Association Between Glycemic Control and Degenerative Complications of Diabetes Mellitus: A Brief Review of Current Concepts

Steven B. Leichter

Few clinical questions in diabetology are as important as whether metabolic control prevents or retards diabetic complications. In recent years, an increasing body of literature suggests good control is important. This has motivated a large number of clinical diabetologists to pursue metabolic control more aggressively in their patients. Other reviews, however, consider this question with more conservatism.[4,24,37] These uncertainties encourage a broad perspective about this issue because of its relevance to design of the clinical approach to diabetes.

The continued debate about the benefits of metabolic control may be ascribed to two common aspects of the previous literature: differences in results or interpretation of *in vitro* and *in vivo* studies, and the lack of a "smoking gun" study, which directly implicates hyperglycemia in the pathogenesis of clinical complications of diabetes mellitus. Of the two, the latter has been invoked as a more important caveat about the influence of metabolic control on complications.

CLASSIFICATION OF DIABETIC COMPLICATIONS

To consider this complex issue, it is important to understand the classification of diabetic complications, which have been grouped into two broad categories: microvascular and macrovascular (Table 5-1).[9] This classification has developed because there may be differences in the occurrences of these complications in different forms of diabetes. Patients with type I diabetes mellitus may be more likely to suffer microvascular complications, whereas patients with type II diabetes may be more likely to have macrovascular complications. These occurrences, however, are not invariable. Any complication may occur in any diabetic patient, regardless of the type of diabetes.[1,9,18] The classification also reflects the suggestion that metabolic factors, which influence the incidence or progression of complications, may differ for the microvascular versus macrovascular complications.[1,4,9,11,18,24,33,37] Although some or all of these specific postulated associations remain controversial, the relationships proposed by prior studies suggest that clinically important distinctions may exist in the mechanisms by which the metabolic abnormalities of diabetes may influence either group of complications. These differences may suggest differences in aims of treatment and approach in type I versus type II diabetes.

METABOLIC FACTORS AND MICROVASCULAR COMPLICATIONS

The differences in interpretation of similar data have been argued dramatically in considerations about control and microvascular complications. Over 25 years ago, Siperstein and co-workers demonstrated that the protein-based basement membrane of small

Table 5–1
Current Classification of Degenerative Complications of Diabetes Mellitus

Microvascular	*Macrovascular*
Neuropathy	Myocardial infarction
Nephropathy	Stroke
Retinopathy	

blood vessels (capillary basement membrane) thickened in patients with diabetes mellitus.[34] These investigators denied any direct, demonstrable links between the degree or duration of hyperglycemia and the degree to which the basement membrane thickened. Their studies implied that the vascular changes of diabetes were a concomitant problem with the disease itself and were not related to the degree of metabolic control. A contrasting view was published 4 years later by Kilo and co-workers.[21] They confirmed the capillary basement membrane thickened in persons with diabetes, but concluded that associations existed between the duration of disease and degree of thickening. The Kilo data, therefore, implied that the duration and degree of hyperglycemia influenced the rate or severity of capillary basement membrane thickening.

More recent investigations tend to support the hypotheses of Kilo and co-workers. Biochemical alterations of the protein matrix of the capillary basement membrane in diabetes have been identified, and may explain, in part, the altered basement membrane function.[2,5] These alterations may be associated with hyperglycemia. At least one other study by Camerini-Davalos and co-workers confirms this impression.[6] They reported a reversal of capillary basement membrane thickening in patients with impaired glucose tolerance who had long-term reduction in mean serum glucose levels with the sulfonylurea, glipizide. Some conclusions of that study are controversial, however, and its findings await further confirmation.

The evidence in favor of metabolic influences on diabetic microvasculopathy extends to other aspects of vascular physiology as well. A second focus of association between hyperglycemia and microvascular complications is abnormal platelet function in diabetes. Various adverse changes in platelet physiology have been described in diabetes.[20] These include an increased tendency for spontaneous platelet aggregation and increased platelet adhesiveness.[4] Some studies have linked this increased platelet adhesiveness to hyperglycemia.[8,26] Hyperglycemia may cause the enhanced platelet production of a prostaglandin-like factor, thromboxane A_2, which, in turn, may cause the changes in platelet physiology.[39]

A recent area of research, especially pharmaceutical research, is the aldose reductase pathway.[7] Hyperglycemia may cause large increases in intracellular glucose concentrations in certain tissues that transport glucose by simple osmosis, independent of the action of insulin. In these tissues, the high concentrations of intracellular glucose may overwhelm the normal catabolic pathways for glucose, such as the glycolysis pathway. The tissues activate a vestigial pathway, the sorbitol pathway, and by means of an enzyme, aldose reductase, convert glucose to sorbitol. Unlike glucose, the sorbitol is impermeable and, when formed, remains in the cell unless metabolized. The metabolic pathway for sorbitol catabolism acts at a much slower rate than the aldose reductase pathway. In the presence of poor control of hyperglycemia, therefore, the production of intracellular sorbitol in these tissues may be extremely high. The sorbitol may alter cell function and may be directly toxic to the cell.

Sorbitol formation has been postulated as a possible cause of certain diabetic complications, including neuropathy and cataracts.[16] It has also been suggested that it may affect cells in small blood vessels and possibly influence the progression of microvascular complications.[35] Because of this possibility, a number of drugs that inhibit aldose reductase and block the formation of sorbitol in susceptible cells are being tested to determine if they influence the progression of microvascular complications.

IN VIVO EVIDENCE ABOUT METABOLIC CONTROL AND DIABETIC MICROVASCULAR COMPLICATIONS

Some studies within the last decade have related hyperglycemia to the progression of microvascular complications. Thus far, the largest study is that of Pirart.[27] Pirart, a Belgian diabetologist, prospectively studied 4400 diabetic patients for 25 years to determine the incidence and prevalence of different complications among the patients, when grouped according to the degree of glycemic control. For all three microvascular complications (retinopathy, neuropathy, and nephropathy), Pirart demonstrated that their prevalence was up to 6.5 times greater in patients in poor glycemic control than in those in good glycemic control. He reported similar results for the incidence of these problems.

Pirart's findings have been questioned by more conservative views on two grounds. First, he did not demonstrate an elimination of microvascular complications in the subgroup maintained for 25 years in good control. Second, the study suggested, but did not prove, an association between poor glycemic control and complications. An alternative explanation is that the patient with a form of diabetes that permitted good control had a lower risk of complications, not because of the degree of glycemic control, but rather because of the less aggressive nature of his condition.

These questions may be softened, in part, by subsequent

data, which appear to support the results of the Pirart study at least with reference to retinopathy. Three separate studies published in the last 5 years have all shown a positive association between poor glycemic control and risk of diabetic retinopathy. This has been suggested for the occurrence of retinopathy.[22] It also has been suggested for the progression of established background retinopathy.[10,14] The data about established retinopathy have, at times, been confusing. Initially, the investigators reported a worsening of retinopathy in the first year of establishing glycemic control; however, this progression stabilized or reversed after 1 year of glycemic control.

Animal studies seem to demonstrate similar results. Bloodworth and Engerman noted that diabetic dogs developed fewer retinopathic lesions if their glycemic control was good versus those dogs kept in poor glycemic control.[3] Retardation of diabetic microvascular complications with glycemic control has been found in other animal models.

QUESTIONS ABOUT STRICT GLYCEMIC CONTROL AND MICROVASCULAR COMPLICATIONS

These persuasive arguments in favor of glycemic control have to answer important questions raised by more conservative observers. One question about strict glycemic control is whether the risks are acceptable. Unger reviewed these risks and noted that they are not always negligible.[41] Adverse experiences caused by hypoglycemia in patients using subcutaneous insulin infusion pumps have been reported by more than one group.[23,38]

Another set of questions relates to evidence suggesting that the degree of glycemic control does not, by itself, completely predict the risk of microvasculopathy. Raskin and Rosenstock argued that data also exist suggesting risks based on genetic factors such as HLA phenotypes.[28] One implication of these data is that both hyperglycemia and genetic factors influence the risk for each patient, and the degree of glycemic control is not invariably the predominant determinant.

A third group of questions, noted previously, is why *in vivo* studies on occurrences of complications versus glycemic control show positive associations. Positive associations may be demonstrated because of a direct causal relationship or the association of these two variables with another independent factor that determines them both. For example, genetic factors may determine which subjects achieve good glycemic control more easily, and the same factors may independently determine which subjects are more likely to avoid complications.

DIABETES CONTROL AND COMPLICATIONS TRIAL

These unresolved issues could only be solved conclusively by a controlled clinical trial.[13] The National Institutes of Health, therefore, recently launched a complex, multicenter trial known as the Diabetes Control and Complications Trial. It is hoped that this randomized, long-term study will demonstrate whether direct links exist between hyperglycemia and macrovascular complications.

This extraordinary undertaking is an honest and positive effort. Patients in the study with type I diabetes mellitus are randomized to a treatment group maintained in meticulous control of hyperglycemia, or to a "standard" group maintained in "adequate" glycemic control with traditional treatment methods. The study hopes to show that these moderate differences in levels of control, maintained over many years, reveal differences in rates of complications.

A question is whether serious assumptions about the effect of hyperglycemia on microvascular complications should be entertained before the results of this study become clear. Many respected investigators are placing faith in this undertaking. On the other hand, there are cogent reasons to view this important effort as a part of the larger, evolving perspective on control and complications. First, the differences in levels of glycemic control may not be sufficient to demonstrate convincing differences in rates of complications; therefore, a negative result may not necessarily exclude a positive association. Second, participation in the study, particularly in the experimental group, may be so demanding that a high "washout rate" of participants occurs. Whether the Diabetes Control and Complications Trial answers this question completely, its progress deserves close monitoring by all interested clinicians.

METABOLIC CONTROL AND MACROVASCULAR COMPLICATIONS

Whereas direct associations between hyperglycemia and microvascular complications have been postulated, similar relationships are not generally considered likely for macrovascular complications.[17,27] Instead, the possible metabolic influences on macrovascular complications are thought to be a more complicated matter.

Abnormalities in lipid metabolism have been proposed as important factors. These abnormalities are prevalent in diabetic patients and may be related pathogenically to metabolic changes induced by diabetes.[18,19,32] They are also associated with higher risks of macrovascular atherosclerosis.

Hyperinsulinism has been advocated as another possible risk factor.[29,36] Hyperinsulinism appears as a possible independent variable in certain epidemiologic studies on heart disease in diabetic patients.[12,31] There are also biochemical studies that seem to implicate insulin excess in accelerated atherogenesis.[29]

Currently, only some confusing evidence is reported in favor of an association between glycemic control and macrovascular complications. An exciting initial article proposing a positive association has not always been substantiated.[25] Instead, most studies have demonstrated only a partial relationship.[15] Some data published recently, however, suggest that glycemic control may influence certain risks of recurrent myocardial disease in different groups of patients with established atherosclerotic heart disease.[30,40]

SUMMARY

Each clinician must individually assess the clinical significance of this growing body of literature. Its complexity seems to preclude simple assessments of the subject, which may be based on a study or hypothesis of only one segment of the data. The increasing number of studies in the area make this aspect of diabetology an important focus for future clinical interest.

At present, it is my opinion that the data argue in favor of a tentative conclusion that metabolic control may yield positive clinical influences on the occurrence or progression of diabetic complications. This assessment is structured according to the distinction between microvascular and macrovascular complications, and in consideration of the proposed associations between each set of complications and their postulated metabolic risk factors. The important questions raised about the risks of strict glycemic control or the possible influences of other risk factors, unrelated to metabolic abnormalities, must be taken into account. This opinion implies, therefore, that the risks of strict glycemic control outweigh the potential risks of persistent, severe hyperglycemia. The opinion also assigns an important relative weighting to metabolic risk factors as one of the possible influences on diabetic complications.

My advocacy of a broad perspective, however, implies that it is important to listen sincerely to opposing arguments. Until this issue is clearly settled, rigid orthodoxy has no place in the necessary open consideration of the many possible aspects of this problem. Open discussion and consideration of all reasonable views seem to be the only appropriate course.

REFERENCES

1. Aiello LM, Rand LI, Briones JC et al: Diabetic retinopathy in Joslin Clinic patients with adult-onset diabetes mellitus. Ophthalmology 88:619–623, 1981
2. Birkeland AJ, Christensen TB: Resistance of glycoproteins to proteolysis ribonuclease, A and B compared. J Carbohydr Nucleosides Nucleotides 2:83–90, 1975
3. Bloodworth JMB Jr, Engerman RL: Diabetic microangiopathy in the experimentally diabetic dog and its prevention by careful control with insulin. Diabetes 22(Suppl 1):290, 1973
4. Brownlee M: Microvascular disease and related abnormalities: Their relation to control of diabetes. In Marble A, Krall LP (eds): Joslin's Diabetes Mellitus, pp 185–216. Philadelphia, Lea & Febiger, 1985
5. Brownlee M: 2-macroglobulin and reduced basement membrane degradation in diabetes. Lancet 1:779–780, 1976
6. Camerini-Davalos RA, Velasco C, Glasser M et al: Drug-induced reversal of early diabetic microangiopathy. N Engl J Med 309:1551–1556, 1983
7. Clements RS Jr: Diabetes neuropathy—new concepts of its etiology. Diabetes 28:604–611, 1979
8. Colwell JA, Halushka PV: Platelet function in diabetes mellitus. Br J Haem 44:521–526, 1980
9. Colwell JA, Halushka PV, Sarji KE et al: Vascular disease in diabetes: Pathophysiological mechanisms and therapy. Arch Intern Med 139:225–230, 1979
10. Dahl-Jorgensen K, Brinchmann-Hansen O, Hanssen KF et al: Effect of near normoglycaemia for two years on progression of early diabetic retinopathy, nephropathy, and neuropathy: The Oslo study. Br Med J 1195–1199, 1986
11. Deckert T, Poulsen JE, Larsen M: Prognosis of diabetics with diabetes onset before the age of thirty-one. I. Survival, causes of death, and complications. Diabetologia 14:363–370, 1978

12. Ducimetiere P, Eschwege E, Papoz L et al: Relationship of plasma insulin levels to the incidence of myocardial infarction and coronary heart disease mortality in a middle-aged population. Diabetologia 19:205–210, 1980
13. Editorial Announcement: Diabetes Control and Complications Trial. Clin Diabetes 1:10–11, 1983
14. Friberg TR, Rosenstock J, Sanborn G et al: The effect of long-term near normal glycemic control on mild diabetic retinopathy. Ophthalmology 92:1051–1058, 1985
15. Fuller JH, McCartney P, Jarrett RJ et al: Hyperglycemia and coronary heart disease: The Whitehall study. J Chronic Dis 32:721–728, 1979
16. Gabbay KH: Hyperglycemia, polyol metabolism, and the complications of diabetes mellitus. Annu Rev Med 26:521–536, 1975
17. Ganda OP: Pathogenesis of macrovascular disease including the influence of lipids. In Marble A, Krall LP (eds): Joslin's Diabetes Mellitus, pp 217–250. Philadelphia, Lea & Febiger, 1985
18. Ganda OP: Pathogenesis of macrovascular disease in the human diabetic. Diabetes 29:931–942, 1980
19. Gordon T, Castelli WP, Hjortland MC et al: Diabetes, blood lipids, and the role of obesity in coronary heart disease risk for women. Ann Intern Med 87:393–397, 1977
20. Jones RL, Paradise C, Peterson C: Platelet survival in patients with diabetes mellitus. Diabetes 30:486–489, 1981
21. Kilo C, Volger N, Williamson JR: Muscle capillary basement membrane changes related to aging and to diabetes mellitus. Diabetes 21:881–905, 1972
22. Klein BEK, Moss SE, Klein R: Longitudinal measure of glycemic control and diabetic retinopathy. Diabetes Care 10:273–277, 1987
23. Leichter SB, Schreiner ME, Reynolds LR et al: Long-term follow-up of diabetic patients using insulin infusion pumps. Arch Intern Med 145:1409–1412, 1985
24. Lippe BM: Insulin action and the insulin receptor. In Kaplan SA (moderator): Diabetes Mellitus. Ann Intern Med 96:635–649, 1982
25. Ostrander L, Francis T Jr, Hayner NS et al: The relationship of cardiovascular disease to hyperglycemia. Ann Intern Med 62:1188–1198, 1965
26. Peterson CM, Jones RL, Koening RJ et al: Reversible hematologic sequelae of diabetes mellitus. Ann Intern Med 86:425–429, 1977
27. Pirart J: Diabetes mellitus and its degenerative complications: A

prospective study of 4400 diabetic patients observed between 1947 and 1973. Diabetes Care 1:168–188, 1978
28. Raskin P, Rosenstock J: Blood glucose control and diabetic complications. Ann Intern Med 105:254–263, 1986
29. Reaven GM: Role of insulin resistance in human disease. Diabetes 37:1595–1617, 1985
30. Rytter L, Troelsen S, Nielsen HB: Prevalence and mortality of acute myocardial infarction in patients with diabetes mellitus. Diabetes Care 8:230–234, 1985
31. Santen EJ, Willis PW, Fajans SS: Atherosclerosis in diabetes mellitus. Arch Intern Med 130:833–843, 1972
32. Saudek C, Eder H: Lipid metabolism in diabetes mellitus. Am J Med 66:843–852, 1979
33. Scott RC: Diabetes and the heart. Am Heart J 90:283–289, 1975
34. Siperstein MD, Unger RH, Madison LL: Studies of muscle capillary basement membranes in normal subjects, diabetic, and prediabetic patients. J Clin Invest 47:1973–1999, 1968
35. Sochor M, Baquer NZ, McLean P: Glucose overutilization in diabetes: Evidence from studies on the changes in hexokinase, the pentose phosphate pathway and glucuronate-xylulose pathway in rat kidney cortex in diabetes. Biochem Biophys Res Commun 86:32–39, 1979
36. Stout RW: Diabetes and atherosclerosis—the role of insulin. Diabetologia 16:141–150, 1979
37. Tchobroutsky G: Relation of diabetic control to development of microvascular complications. Diabetologia 15:143–152, 1978
38. Teutsch SM, Herman WH, Dwyer DM et al: Mortality among diabetic patients using continuous subcutaneous insulin-infusion pumps. N Engl J Med 310:361–368, 1984
39. Thomas G, Skrinska V, Lucas FV et al: Platelet glutathione and thromboxane synthesis in diabetes. Diabetes 34:951–954, 1985
40. Ulvenstam G, Aberg A, Bergstrand R et al: Long-term prognosis after myocardial infarction in men with diabetes. Diabetes 34:787–792, 1985
41. Unger RH: Meticulous control of diabetes: Benefits, risks, and precautions. Diabetes 31:479–483, 1982

CHAPTER SIX

Hormones, Sugar Alcohols, and Diabetic Complications

Joseph R. Williamson
Charles Kilo

HISTORIC COMMENTARY

Diabetes has been known for over 3000 years, yet little progress was made in treating diabetics until the discovery and use of insulin in 1921. In the 1940s and 1950s, the oral hypoglycemic agents became available. The next significant advancement, in the 1960s, was self blood glucose monitoring. We are now entering an entirely new era of research that, in our opinion, may lead to the next major advancement in diabetes treatment.

Today, the most pressing problem in diabetes is how to prevent the late complications that are responsible for loss of vision and other nonfatal complications in large numbers of diabetics and that cause diabetics to die prematurely of cardiovascular disease. These complications of diabetes are so common that, for many years, research focused on whether the complications were hereditary (*e.g.*, the tendency to develop diabetes) or caused by metabolic and hormonal imbalances secondary to insulin deficiency. To make matters even more confusing, some investigators have suggested that vascular complications of diabetes may be promoted by high plasma insulin levels associated with insulin resistance in noninsulin-dependent diabetics, and occur transiently after each insulin injection in insulin-dependent diabetics.

The weight of evidence available today strongly favors the view that late complications of diabetes are largely the consequence of relative or absolute insulin deficiency. It is also clear, however, that other factors independent of insulin deficiency are important in the pathogenesis of late complications. It is well-known, for example, that increased blood pressure accelerates the progression of all forms of diabetic vascular disease. Many studies indicate that both retinopathy and nephropathy occur more frequently after puberty than in prepubertal diabetics, even with diabetes of the same duration and severity.[12] Unfortunately, however, progress in elucidating the pathogenesis of diabetic vascular disease has been painfully slow.

Thickening of capillary basement membranes is widely considered to be the ultrastructural hallmark of diabetic microvascular disease. It has been demonstrated in virtually every tissue examined including the retina, ciliary epithelium, and choriocapillaris in the eye, skeletal muscle, skin, and kidney. The basement membrane thickness of the capillary can be increased 10 to 20 times in a diabetic.

The thrust of this review is, first, to consider briefly some muscle capillary basement membrane studies in human diabetics that have yielded two important new clues to the pathogenesis of diabetic vascular disease. Some recent findings in an animal model will then be discussed, which indicate that diabetes-mediated vascular injury is linked to increased metabolism of glucose by the polyol pathway and also provide an explanation for the increased frequency of vascular complications in postpubertal diabetics.

BASIC STUDIES IN DIABETIC ANIMAL MODEL

Sosenko and co-workers have demonstrated a highly significant correlation between muscle capillary basement membrane width and the level of glycemia in postpubertal diabetics followed at the Children's Hospital in Boston.[10] The subjects were divided into three groups according to their growth increment during the 2 years preceding the muscle biopsy. The first group had grown over 7.5 cm during that time interval and were considered to be prepubertal; the second group grew between 1 and 7.5 cm and were considered to be pubertal; the third group had grown less than 1 cm during the 2-year period and for the purpose of this study were considered to be postpubertal.

Data on the postpubertal subjects indicated a striking increase in basement membrane width, with increasing levels of glycemia reflected in the glycosylated hemoglobin levels. In contrast, the prepubertal group presented an inverse relationship. These observations have been confirmed in an independent study on subjects in the Diabetes Registry at Washington University in St. Louis.[8]

These findings, coupled with evidence mentioned earlier regarding the frequency of retinopathy and nephropathy in postpubertal diabetics, suggest vascular metabolism of glucose, in general, may be different in pre- and postpubertal diabetics. In the postpubertal diabetic subjects studied in the St. Louis Registry, a highly significant correlation was also seen between muscle capillary basement membrane width and bone age.[8] Because bone age is related primarily to sex steroid levels in postpubertal diabetics with normal thyroid and pituitary function, this finding of changes in basement membrane width suggests that increased sex steroid production at the time of puberty may have an important role in initiation and progression of the vascular complications of diabetes. This relationship is only evident in postpubertal diabetics.

One of the reasons for the slow progress in elucidating the pathogenesis of diabetic vascular disease has been the lack of an animal model in which the characteristic features of human diabetic vascular disease can be readily produced and quantified in a reasonably short time period. Without such a model, it is virtually impossible to sort out which of the large numbers of biochemical, metabolic, and hormonal balances associated with diabetes are central to the pathogenesis of the functional abnormalities associated with late vascular complications, and which are of no functional consequence and should be regarded as epiphenomena.

Because functional changes undoubtedly precede capillary basement membrane thickening and other morphologic and clinical manifestations of vascular injury, we have sought to develop an animal model in which functional vascular changes identical to those in human diabetics can be produced and quantified readily. Perhaps the most characteristic functional abnormality demonstrable in human diabetics is increased vascular permeability. This phenomenon, like capillary basement membrane thickening, has been observed in every tissue examined, including the eyes, skin, muscle, and kidney.[5] It is seen most dramatically in the eyes of human diabetics with neovascularization of the retina or optic disk. If such a patient is given an intravenous injection of fluorescein, the dye will leak profusely from these new vessels, while relatively little dye leaks from neighboring vessels formed before the onset of diabetes. The explanation for the increased leakiness and fragility of these new vessels is not known, and, unfortunately, there is no diabetic animal model in which significant angiogenesis takes place in the eye.

EXPERIMENTAL MODEL

If increased leakiness of these new vessels is a consequence of the diabetic milieu, perhaps new vessels formed in any tissue of a diabetic may be more leaky than new vessels in corresponding tissues in the nondiabetic. To test this hypothesis, we performed a simple experiment. A piece of sterile polyester fabric was implanted under the skin of a rat. This fabric served to stimulate angiogenesis and proliferation of fibroblasts, which grow into the interstices of the fabric. An important advantage of performing studies on tissue recovered from such fabric is that the age and history of the tissue are known.

The collagen produced in this model in the diabetic rat reflects the same kinds of biochemical changes seen in human diabetics (increased cross-linking, increased nonenzymatic glycosylation, and so forth).[2] To assess the permeability characteristics of these vessels, the following protocol was used.[5] Three weeks after implanting the fabric and injecting streptozotocin to produce chemical diabetes, the animal was anesthetized, the trachea was cannulated for maintenance on a mechanical respirator, and an artery was cannulated to monitor blood pressure and withdraw blood samples. Three radiolabeled tracers (chromium-labeled red cells, iodinated albumin [bovine serum albumin], and cobaltic ethylenediaminetetraacetate [EDTA] as an extracellular space marker)

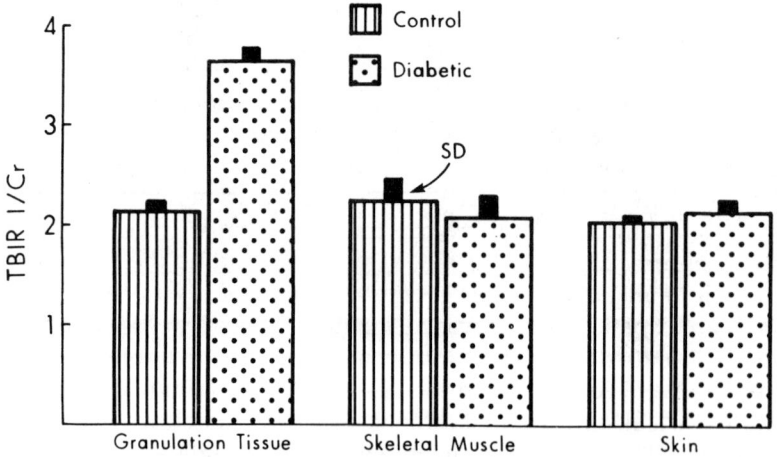

Figure 6-1. Effects of diabetes on ^{125}I-albumin permeation (TBIR-I/Cr) in new granulation tissue, skeletal muscle, and skin (mean ±SD for eight rats) 8 minutes after injection of tracers.

were injected. Six or 28 minutes later, a blood sample was drawn and at 8 or 30 minutes the heart was removed, stopping blood flow to all tissues. The new tissue with the fabric, as well as many other tissues, was sampled to quantify the tracer content in the blood and these tissues to derive an index of albumin permeation, which we refer to as the tissue-to-blood isotope ratio (TBIR).

The index was derived from the ratio of radiolabeled albumin to chromium-labeled red cells in the tissue, divided by the corresponding ratio in the sample of blood obtained just before removing the tissue. If no leakage of albumin occurs from the blood vessels, this equation would give a TBIR of one. To the extent that albumin leaks out of the vessels and into the tissue, the TBIR would be greater than one and would imply increased albumin permeation of the vessels. Figure 6-1 shows data from granulation tissue, skin, and muscle examined 8 minutes after injection of radiolabeled albumin. The index of albumin permeation is increased about 1.5 times normal in granulation tissue of diabetic rats, but not in skin or muscle or in aorta, eye, or kidney (other tissues known to manifest vascular complications in human diabetics)—the ratio one being the controls. The only other tissue in which an increase in albumin permeation is evident is the cecum, a tissue that undergoes marked hypertrophy in diabetic rats. This finding is consistent with the model and concept because, as a part of the hypertrophy of the cecum, one would expect new vessels to be formed as well. The absence of any increase in albumin permeation in the skin or skeletal muscle is of interest, because the vessels in new granulation tissue must be derived from vessels in either overlying skin or underlying muscle. This observation suggests that new vessels formed in the diabetic environment are more susceptible to injury produced by the diabetic environment. This situation is analogous to what one sees in the eyes of the human diabetic with neovascularization, where the new vessels leak to a much greater extent than pre-existing vessels.

The time allowed for the tracer to circulate in these animals was quite short—only 8 minutes. Thus, it could be that vessels formed before the onset of diabetes might manifest more subtle changes that would require a longer tracer circulation time to demonstrate. When the tracer is allowed to circulate for 30 minutes, in addition to increased albumin permeation in granulation tissue, significant increases occur in the eye, kidney, aorta, and sciatic nerve.[12] No increase is observed in the brain, testes, or skin (Fig. 6-2).

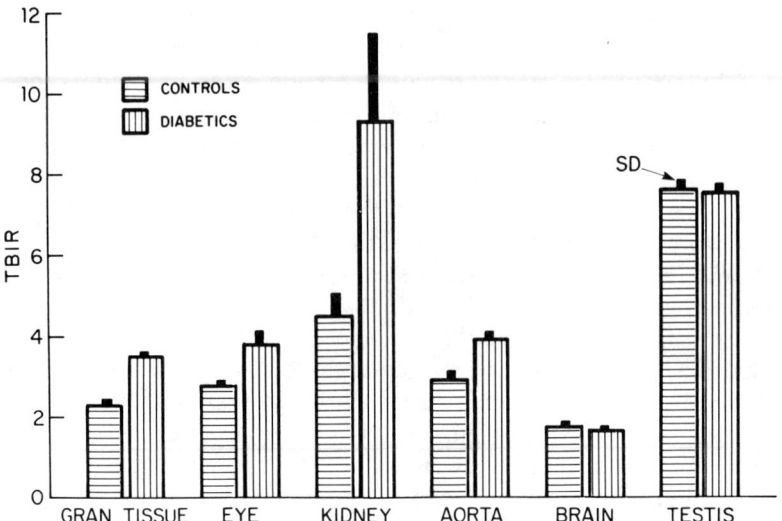

Figure 6-2. Effect of diabetes on ^{125}I-albumin permeation (TBIR) in various tissues (mean ±SD) 30 minutes after injection of tracers.

CLINICAL APPLICATIONS OF THE RESEARCH MODEL

In this model, vascular permeability is increased in the same tissues affected by complications in the poorly controlled human diabetic. For the first time in an animal model, this work demonstrates that diabetes causes increased vascular permeability in arteries. Thus, one explanation for the mechanism whereby diabetes might accelerate atherosclerotic vascular disease is an increase in permeability of arteries to atherogenic lipoproteins. More cholesterol could leak into the vessel walls and accelerate the progression of atherosclerosis.

These findings indicate that new vessels formed in the diabetic milieu are permeated by albumin more readily than vessels that antedate the onset of diabetes. Some of the implications of this finding are interesting. The magnitude of diabetes-induced increases in vascular permeability (*i.e.*, functional impairment) may be linked to the proportion of vascular constituents formed in the diabetic milieu. A corollary would be that vascular injury, of whatever cause, whether it be hypertension or cigarette smoking (if occurring in a diabetic and causing a proliferative repair response in the diabetic milieu), might be predicted to accelerate the rate of progression of diabetic vascular disease. That is exactly what one sees in the human diabetic.

ENZYMATIC ACTIVITY

Further studies indicated that diabetes-induced increases in vascular permeability in this model are linked to imbalances in polyol metabolism. Two enzymes are involved. Aldose reductase facilitates the conversion of glucose to sorbitol, a sugar alcohol. This reaction requires a co-factor, NADPH. The second step involves the conversion of sorbitol to fructose by the enzyme, sorbitol dehydrogenase. This reaction requires the co-factor, NAD. In the early studies of the role of polyol metabolism in diabetic cataract formation in animals, Kinoshita interpreted the data to indicate that the mechanism of injury was linked to osmotic effects related to the accumulation of sorbitol.[6] Studies in nerve and other tissues have led investigators to suggest that the mechanism of injury in these tissues may not be linked to osmotic effects, as much as to metabolic imbalances linked to alterations in the balance of the redox state of these pyridine nucleotides and, ultimately, to the capacity of cells to produce energy.[1]

Another hexose, galactose, is metabolized by the same enzyme to its corresponding sugar alcohol, galactitol or dulcitol. Animals fed diets enriched with galactose develop the same complications of cataracts and neuropathy seen in diabetic animals. They even develop them at a faster rate than in the diabetic animal. This may be related, at least in part, to the fact that aldose reductase has an even greater affinity for galactose than for glucose. Because of these findings, many investigators have postulated that one should be able to produce diabetes-like complications in an animal fed a diet enriched with galactose if such complications are the consequence of increased hexose metabolism by way of the polyol pathway.

At least three variables might influence the amount of polyol produced in a diabetic: glucose level, amount of aldose reductase enzyme present, and availability of the co-factors. Several chemicals that are inhibitors of aldose reductase prevent the accumulation of polyols and also completely prevent cataracts and nerve damage in experimental animals. Some recent studies in humans suggest these compounds may benefit neuropathy.[4]

When diabetic animals were fed a diet containing a chemical inhibitor of aldose reductase (*i.e.*, sorbinil), the increased albumin permeation seen typically in the new vessels in untreated diabetics was completely prevented; the tissue levels of sorbitol were also normalized by the drug.[11] Interestingly, the drug has no effect on blood glucose levels. Thus, if these drugs are efficacious in humans, it may be possible to prevent complications without having to normalize blood glucose levels. The inhibitors also prevented the increases in albumin permeation in tissues of rats fed galactose-enriched diets.[1] Thus, all of the vascular permeability increases present in diabetic and galactose-fed rats are prevented by the inhibitors of aldose reductase. The inhibitors of aldose reductase have also been shown to prevent capillary basement membrane thickening and other structural changes in vessels in both rats and dogs with experimentally induced diabetes.

Susceptibility of the vasculature to injury (manifested by increased permeability) linked to aldose reductase activity varies greatly in different tissues.[1,12] This may explain the predilection for the vessels in certain tissues and organs in human diabetics to develop complications, while others appear to be relatively spared.

INFLUENCE OF RISK FACTORS ON THE DIABETIC ANIMAL MODEL: HORMONAL INFLUENCES

Having developed a model in which one can produce permeability changes identical to those seen in humans, it is now possible to examine the influence of various risk factors associated with the development of clinically significant human diabetic vascular disease. Does the finding that diabetes-induced increased vascular permeability in diabetic rats is an aldose reductase-linked phenomenon provide any clues to an explanation for the clinical observation that complications are uncommon in prepubertal diabetics? It is a simple matter in the animal model to castrate the rat before implanting the fabric; castration has no effect on (granulation tissue) vascular permeability in the nondiabetic, but completely normalizes permeability in diabetic rats without decreasing blood glucose levels. Castration also normalizes granulation tissue polyol levels in diabetic rats.[13] Thus, these findings indicate that diabetes-induced increases in vascular permeability and tissue polyol levels are modulated by sex steroids. Because aldose reductase was first discovered in the reproductive tissues of male animals, perhaps it is not surprising that it should be a sex steroid-dependent enzyme.

A number of studies attest to the importance of the role of androgens in a variety of complications of diabetes. A much higher frequency of proliferative retinopathy occurs in men compared with women; the ratios range from 1.6 to over twofold higher in men than women.[14] In a recent study published by Sosenko and co-workers, it was noted that diabetic neuropathy is linked to diabetes control or blood glucose levels as reflected in hemoglobin A_1C levels only in postpubertal diabetics, not in prepubertal diabetics.[9] Greene and co-workers presented evidence that neuropathy is more frequent in postpubertal males than in females.[3] In our own animal studies we found castration of the male diabetic rat reduced the polyol levels in the sciatic nerve by 50%.[12]

If sex steroids were affecting complications, one might expect to see differences in tissue levels of polyols, perhaps even in red cells, which correlate with sexual maturation and diabetes. In prepubertal type I diabetics, no significant difference is seen in red cell polyol levels of males and females; however, levels are about three times higher after puberty in males than females.[7] Of course, a corresponding difference is noted in prepubertal diabetic males compared with postpubertal diabetic males. Blood glucose levels and hemoglobin A_1C levels were identical in all four groups. These kinds of observations suggest that the role of sex steroids in the pathogenesis of diabetic complications may be far more important than recognized previously.

One last question concerns the role of insulin itself. Does insulinopenia, independent of secondary hormonal imbalances in hyperglycemia, play a role in the pathogenesis of diabetic complications? A number of observations in the animal model suggest this may be the case; some studies on retinopathy in human diabetics also support this hypothesis. Several studies indicate that insulinopenia, independent of hyperglycemia, is a contributory factor to the development of retinopathy.

SUMMARY

The findings in the animal model support the hypothesis that imbalances in polyol metabolism mediated by the enzyme aldose reductase are responsible for most of the late complications of diabetes including neuropathy, cataracts, microangiopathy, and possibly macroangiopathy. These studies also suggest the hypothesis that diabetes-induced increases in collagen cross-linking and vascular permeability are mediated by enzymes (lysyl oxidase, which facilitates collagen cross-linking, and aldose reductase), whose activities are induced by sex hormones at the time of puberty. Insulin deficiency has a major role, which leads to an increase in blood glucose levels; this, in turn, increases the substrate available for the polyol pathway. In the adult with normal tissue levels of aldose reductase, increased flux of glucose to sorbitol results, which leads to a variety of other metabolic imbalances that produce delayed complications. In the prepubertal diabetic, before sex steroid levels reach critical levels, it would appear that insufficient flux of glucose exists through the polyol pathway to cause complications. This could explain the scarcity of complications in prepubertal diabetics.

REFERENCES

1. Chang K, Tomlinson M, Jeffrey JR et al: Galactose ingestion increases vascular permeability and collagen solubility in normal male rats. J Clin Invest 79:367–373, 1987
2. Chang K, Uitto J, Rowold EA et al: Increased collagen cross-linkages in experimental diabetes: Reversal by B-aminopropionitrile (BAPN) and D-penicillamine. Diabetes 29:778–781, 1980
3. Greene DA, Brown M, Gilbert P et al: Age and gender are factors in the development of diabetic neuropathy: Baseline neurologic assessment in the Diabetes Control and Complications Trial. Diabetes 35(Suppl 1):12A, 1986
4. Judewitsch RG, Jaspan JB, Polonsky KS et al: Aldose reductase inhibition improves nerve conduction velocity in diabetic patients. N Engl J Med 308:119–125, 1983
5. Kilzer P, Chang K, Marvel J: Albumin permeation of new vessels is increased in diabetic rats. Diabetes 34:333–336, 1985
6. Kinoshita JH: Concept of aldose reductase and diabetic cataracts. Ann Intern Med 101:82–91, 1984
7. Rogers D, Deren S, Sherman W et al: Sex and puberty-related differences in red blood cell polyol levels (RBC-P) in type I diabetics. Diabetes 35(Suppl 1):105A, 1985
8. Rogers DG, White NH, Santiago JV et al: Glycemic control and bone age are independently associated with muscle capillary basement membrane width in diabetic children after puberty. Diabetes Care 9:453–459, 1986
9. Sosenko J, Boulton A, Kubrusly D et al: The vibratory perception threshold in young diabetic patients: Associations with glycemia and puberty. Diabetes Care 8:605–607, 1985
10. Sosenko JM, Miettinen OS, Williamson JB et al: Muscle capillary basement membrane thickness and long-term glycemia in type I diabetes. N Engl J Med 311:694–698, 1984
11. Williamson JR, Chang K, Rowold E: Sorbinil prevents diabetes-induced increases in vascular permeability, but does not alter collagen cross-linking. Diabetes 34:703–705, 1985
12. Williamson JR, Chang K, Tilton RG et al: Increased vascular permeability in spontaneously diabetic BB/W rats and in rats with mild versus severe streptozotocin-induced diabetes: Prevention by aldose reductase inhibitors and castration. Diabetes 36:813–821, 1987
13. Williamson JR, Rowold E, Chang K et al: Sex steroid-dependency of diabetes-induced changes in polyol metabolism,

vascular permeability and collagen cross-linking. Diabetes 35:20–27, 1986
14. Yuen K, Kahn H. The association of female hormones with blindness from diabetic retinopathy. Am J Ophthalmol 81:820–822, 1976

CHAPTER SEVEN

Modern Treatment of Type II Diabetes

Leo P. Krall

Many believe that the type II diabetic is the most neglected and least well-treated patient in the world. There are at least 100 million people in the world with type II diabetes, previously called "adult onset diabetes." In the United States and other developed nations, patients worry about insulin pumps, home glucose monitoring, and other exotic phases of diabetic therapy. In about a third of the world, however, the supply of insulin is inadequate. In Nepal, for instance, insulin is only available in the hospital. Kenya, for many decades, was reported to have no juvenile onset diabetics; however, if a child became ill, had fever, and was dehydrated in several days and died, they assumed it was a jungle disease or a curse someone had put on them. Now type I diabetes is being found much more often. In Santa Domingo, a group of American doctors found inadequately treated diabetes similar to that seen before the days of insulin. China, with the largest population in the world, has between 20 and 40 million diabetics, and reports claim that only 5% of these need insulin. These diabetics do not use insulin because often the disease may not be identified until complications are apparent.

Table 7-1 lists trends in causes of death of approximately 35,000 patients.[3] Before insulin, half of the patients who died among the Joslin Clinic and New England Deaconess Hospital patients died of ketoacidosis and coma. When insulin was found in 1921, the situation began to improve. This figure has now dropped to about 1% and will probably never be lower because these are older patients with more complications. Death from infection has dropped, and tuberculosis and gangrene have nearly disappeared. Patients now die of cancer, cerebrovascular complications, and cardiac complications; hypertension is a leading killer of diabetics. In other words, the life span of diabetics has improved to the point

Table 7-1
Trends in Causes of Death (34,499 Patients of Joslin Clinic)

Causes	1898–1922 (1,162) (%)	1922–1949 (11,877) (%)	1950–1964 (12,450) (%)	July 1969–1979 (4,290) (%)
Diabetic coma	44.7	4.5	1.0	1.2 (Hyper-osm. = 0.2)
Vascular	22.6	63.6	77.0	75.6
Cardiac	9.9	36.1	53.3	54.5
Renal	3.8	5.1	9.0	7.0
Nephropathy			5.5	5.4
Cerebral	4.9	10.1	12.5	11.1
Gangrene	4.2	10.4	1.3	0.9
Infections	11.2	9.4	5.8	4.3
Tuberculosis	4.9	2.2	0.3	
Cancer	3.2	9.2	10.1	12.0

Percentage of distribution; principal causes of death: Diabetic patients in specific periods.
Adapted from Marble A, Krall LP (eds): Joslin's Diabetic Mellitus, 12th ed. Philadelphia, Lea & Febiger, 1985

MODERN TREATMENT OF TYPE II DIABETES

where they now die of many of the same causes as do the rest of us.

Management of the diabetic, therefore, includes treating kidney and heart disease, care of the feet and limbs, treating nervous system complications, and managing many other problems. The current leading causes of death in diabetics are almost the same as in nondiabetics except infection rates remain too high.

MANAGEMENT

Ideally, "control" of diabetes involves maintaining blood glucose at levels as normal as possible. This, however, is difficult to achieve with present day treatment tools. The objective is not to treat blood glucose levels, but to make certain enough active insulin is always available. The blood glucose level should be kept as close as possible to a realistic level of about 150 mg/dl; this goal can be achieved in many, but not all, patients. Occasionally, normal blood glucose levels will be achieved without severe hypoglycemic reactions. One attempts control that is as ideal as possible.

SHORT-TERM (ACUTE) EFFECTS OF "CONTROL"

Almost everyone understands the fact that acute complications (hypoglycemic reactions, ketoacidotic episodes, electrolyte imbalance, dehydration, undue infections, and so forth) can be avoided. What is not as well understood is that lack of control causes a decreased resistance to infection. In fact, every blood component is involved and the phagocytes do not function effectively, which is one reason for nonhealing in the presence of badly treated or uncontrolled diabetes. The following are reasons for the *short-term control of diabetes:*

Prevents ketoacidosis and hyperosmolar acidosis
Prevents cellular dehydration
Prevents electrolyte imbalance
Prevents decreased phagocytosis
Improves immunologic action
Improves wound healing
Prevents lipid abnormality
Improves lifestyle

There is no uncontroversial proof, but there is increasing belief that many of the long-term complications (*e.g.*, complications of eyes and kidneys) can be averted or ameliorated. Neuropathy is, however, still something of a question mark. The current feeling is that neuropathy may be related to long-term hyperglycemia, which results in the aldose reduction effect, causing the end-product, sorbitol, to accumulate in inappropriate tissues including the nerve sheaths. An attempt is now being made to use aldose reductase inhibitors to block this effect and ameliorate neuropathy. The most dramatic improvement has taken place in preventing perinatal morbidity and mortality. Obstetricians are now more zealous about normoglycemia in their diabetic patients than are many internists and general physicians. These stigmata have dropped from about 10% to often less than 2% in the last two decades. The following are reasons for the *long-term control of diabetes:*

- Ameliorates nephropathy
- Favorably influences retinopathy
- Favorably affects neuropathy
- Prevents early cataracts
- Improves perinatal mortality
- Prevents vascular complications and saves limbs
- Prevents or improves microvascular changes

CONTROL

Optimal control of diabetes is not easy. If control is too tight, severe reactions may result; if it is too loose, there may well be any of the complications listed above.

What, then, is good control? "Normal" blood glucose levels are difficult to achieve on a life-long basis. The fasting blood glucose should be kept under 120 mg/dl, and the 2-hour postprandial level should not be much above 150 mg/dl, where possible. It is often necessary to compromise these goals in active patients or children whose activities and metabolism are widely fluctuant. Besides this, normal weight and strength should be maintained with reasonable freedom from hypoglycemic reactions.

Glycosylated hemoglobin should be as nearly normal as possible, under 9%. Blood cholesterol and triglycerides should be normalized. In general, most of these "control" standards aim for as normal as possible when compared to the nondiabetic. The nondiabetic has a remarkable system, with about 100,000 islets of

Langerhans, and each with 100 beta cells. This remarkable system can measure the blood sugar in 10 to 20 seconds and respond accordingly. The blood glucose cannot be raised more than appropriate in the normal person, who secretes 40 to 50 units a day and stores about 200 units to be used as needed. The homeostatic mechanism put there by nature to take care of a person's diabetes is amazing.

TREATMENT

Any treatment used for diabetes depends on insulin. In the obese patient, the receptors are insufficient or defective—there is more patient than insulin to support the body mass. When the patient diets and loses weight, the body's own sufficient insulin is used, which is preferable to exogenous insulin. It is not only in correct increments, but also has fewer antibodies and costs less. If oral agents are successful, once again the patient uses his own insulin. Obviously, exogenous insulin is used as necessary. Exercise also helps use endogenous insulin. Not only does it use body glucose, but also sensitizes the cell receptors so available insulin is more effective. Insulin, therefore, is the basis of all and any treatment.

PANCREATIC FUNCTIONS

The problem of diabetes is not necessarily that the body does not produce enough insulin. While beta cells produce insulin, various other endocrine functions are anti-insulin in effect, whether pituitary, thyroid, or adrenal. Also, the alpha cell releases glucagon, which is likewise anti-insulin. Copious amounts of glucagon are present during surgery and release during stress. However, the delta cells found in the pancreas and other areas make somatostatin, which blocks the growth hormone, glucagon, as well as other hormones and maintains a balance between insulin and the other hormonal secretions. The problems of diabetes, therefore, are not simply related to insufficient insulin, but also to other anti-insulin or homeostatic mechanisms.

When a person begins to eat, the body releases a primary wave of insulin. Even before that, however, in preparation for eating, the gastrointestinal phase of insulin release begins. For example, as food passes into the gut during digestion, another hormone (GHIP) is released to trigger that first wave of insulin; then, as the blood glucose begins to rise, more insulin is released in response to this. With these homeostatic mechanisms in place, it is amazing that blood glucose is ever outside of normal limits.

RECEPTOR SYSTEM

The cell receptors are another phase in achieving euglycemia. These receptors are present on every cell, and each one is a lock that requires a particular hormonal key. Insulin does not go into the cells, but when it attaches to the proper receptors, it triggers the action within the cell by way of the "second messenger." Without sufficient receptors in numbers and sensitivity, insulin is not effective.

In treating diabetes, the stage of maximal therapeutic effectiveness must be determined. Insulin is synthesized, released, and distributed by the bloodstream. It seeks the receptors on the cells. Many early diabetics produce excessive insulin, but without adequate receptors, it is not effective. Sometimes obese persons have more insulin than they need, but with insufficient receptors this insulin is ineffective, and the blood glucose level will often remain about 330 mg/dl, regardless of whether the daily insulin is 40, 50, 60, or more units. Treatment in these persons must consist of finding ways to make the receptors more effective in numbers and sensitivity. Diet, exercise, tighter control, or oral hypoglycemic agents can all make the receptors more responsive.

TREATMENT CHOICES

Many therapies used commonly for diabetes are not effective. Among these are: (1) the common practice of giving one daily injection of insulin to many diabetics, (2) giving more insulin to obese persons who already have superfluous unused insulin, and (3) giving increasingly more oral agents to persons in whom they are not effective.

The target areas for treatment of diabetes are: (1) insufficient insulin release, (2) interference by other hormones, (3) insulin antibodies, (4) not enough, or insensitive receptors, and (5) finally, insulin resistance. Type I diabetes usually relates to inadequate insulin availability, while type II diabetes is most often caused by insulin resistance possibly aided by a defective receptor system.

CLASSIFICATION OF DIABETES

The two currently accepted types of diabetes are shown in

MODERN TREATMENT OF TYPE II DIABETES

Table 7-2. Typing is often difficult and some patients fit between types. Type I patients are usually young and dependent on insulin for life; type II patients (about 90% of the world diabetic population) are not ketosis-prone *under basal conditions*. If a severe infection develops in type II diabetics, however, they may become insulin-dependent. Some of the noninsulin-dependent diabetics, therefore, do need insulin and cannot be treated with oral agents alone. While they may not progress to a ketoacidotic state, the blood glucose levels can become grossly elevated, which may result in complications such as infections in the short term, and more severe long-term problems if not treated. While many type II patients can be treated with diet or oral hypoglycemic agents, some also require insulin.

Table 7–2
Classification of Diabetes Mellitus*

Type I—Insulin-Dependent Diabetes Mellitus (IDDM)	Type II—Non-Insulin-Dependent Diabetes Mellitus (NIDDM)
1. Insulinopenic and depends on exogenous insulin for life (most important)	1. Insulin levels increased, decreased, or normal (most important)
2. Ketosis-prone under *basal* conditions (most important)	2. Not ketosis-prone under basal conditions (most important)
3. Onset generally in youth, but possible at any age	3. Onset generally after age 40, but found at any age
4. Islet cell antibodies found frequently at diagnosis	4. May require insulin for symptoms or elevated fasting blood glucose
5. Associated with certain HLA[†] types	5. 60% to 90% obese, but not all
	6. Includes families with autosomal dominant inheritance of NIDDM

*The Expert Committee of the World Health Organization–International Diabetes Federation has now classified a third type, not ordinarily found in the United States, but widely found in a belt around the world, in the tropics, and among malnourished populations of underdeveloped countries, known as Malnutrition Diabetes.
[†]HLA = human lymphocyte antigen.

MALNUTRITION DIABETES (TYPE III)

Another type of diabetes may be appearing in certain parts of the world, so-called tropical or malnutrition diabetes. It is a strange phenomenon, found in developing countries with poor nutrition consisting of a high-carbohydrate diet with almost no protein. Many of these diabetics develop liver problems, pancreatic fibrosis, and occasionally calcification of the beta cells as seen on x-ray. The problem often begins in childhood. Although these patients are generally ketosis-resistant, they can develop complications and need treatment with insulin. This is thought to be caused by poor nutrition with lack of protein, dysfunction of the liver, and a diet that consists largely of certain root plants like Kasava (or tapioca root) that appear to contain cyanide and other trace metals. Consumed over many years, these may be additive. While malnutrition diabetes is not yet an official classification, it is under consideration by the World Health Organization.

TREATMENT OF TYPE II DIABETES

DIET

Dieting is not easy and is unpopular with most patients when you consider that it is a life-long problem. Many patients are noncompliant because their prescribed diets are too complex. Today, however, diets are much more liberal than they were in the past. The elements are simple: (1) eat approximately the same amount of food each day; (2) spread the meals during the waking hours to avoid hypoglycemic reactions; (3) make certain the overall diet has good nutritional balance; (4) avoid rapidly absorbed carbohydrates (*e.g.*, orange juice is absorbed most quickly, potatoes a bit more slowly, and rice—a complex carbohydrate—even more so); and (5) aim the caloric total at the desired body weight.

Timely patient education is important. The physician should not try to cram in a lot of information on the first patient visit. One does what is first needed for the patient and then gradually, as the patient accepts the diabetes and permits the treatment to become as involved as it must be. Certainly some patients on the verge of acidosis, for example, need insulin quickly, while the niceties of diet can be delayed. One of the problems with the obese diabetic patient is not necessarily hereditary, but often is the result of ethnic lifestyle or diet. In much of the world, obesity is still considered a sign of good health; this idea is difficult to overcome in certain cultures. If persons require a diet, at least the type of food they are accustomed to should be prescribed. The diet should consist of food they understand and enjoy.

INSULIN

Insulin, while almost always effective, can be difficult to prescribe and use. This is one of the few therapeutic instances in medicine where the physician must estimate the optimal dose 24 or more hours in advance for each patient. The patient's activities, emotions, diet, and potential infections must be considered. Most patients in the world are still treated with insulin from porcine or bovine sources. These cause antibodies in the recipients and make the insulin less effective. Human-like (genetically engineered) insulin has fewer antibodies, although some will still form. The newer insulins are pure and have made insulin allergies or insulin-caused dystrophies almost nonexistent. Most diabetic patients require insulin twice daily.

The older patient may be less active, but a major activity may be eating. If one has the choice, therefore, of prescribing an absolutely rigid, stringent diet to maintain adequate control or a more enjoyable diet with the use of oral agents, the choice is obvious. Duration of life is important, but so is lifestyle. If insulin is needed, its use is obvious, but if it can be prudently avoided, so much the better with these patients.

ORAL AGENTS

Oral agents are no longer controversial—many are available. None of these are miracle drugs that will eliminate diabetes; they are often useful, however. The first- and second-generation agents have certain similarities. They require viable beta cells to function. They all stimulate the release of insulin, some more than others. This effect continues beyond the life of the compound. In fact, the original compounds may disappear from the body, but their effect may continue for a long time, which is an important factor. Both the first- and second-generation oral agents have an effect on receptors and the postreceptoral state, which may be useful in type II diabetes patients.

The second-generation agents act directly on beta cells, increasing insulin secretion, although sometimes not as much as the first-generation agents. They are more effective, however, in increasing cell receptor sensitivity and decreasing insulin resistance. In research on second-generation oral agents in our clinic, almost no effect was found on insulin receptor numbers, but evidence of increased sensitivity existed.

With decreased insulin resistance, insulin levels can be more effective even with less insulin release. What is the ideal dose of insulin? The correct answer is "enough," no more and no less. The amount of insulin released is not as important as its effectiveness, which is one of the advantages of the second-generation agents.

In this group, essentially no antidiuretic effect is found, which is useful. Chlorpropamide, for example, retains sodium. While this is no great problem for most patients, there may be a tendency to increase edema.

Displacement at binding sites is important. The first-generation agents are displaced readily from binding sites by any number of medications. The second-generation agent, having a nonpolar group, is weakly charged, causing it to bind to a site not competitive with other medications. The second-generation agents, therefore, are effective without influencing or being influenced by other medications. In a study published recently, first- and second-generation oral agents were injected intravenously into laboratory animals.[5] Using tolbutamide, a short-acting agent, the compound was still widely present after 1 hour. It was everywhere: liver, adrenals, kidney, heart, blood, and pancreas. On the other hand, glyburide had completely dissipated, being found in the liver and gut during the process of elimination. For an agent to be effective, it has to be effective and disappear; therefore, glyburide could be considered a "hit and run compound."

Both second-generation agents, glipizide and glyburide (Table 7-3), are effective compounds in lowering blood glucose levels. By the manufacturer's own specifications, glyburide is effective

Table 7-3

Differences in Second-Generation Compounds*

Glyburide		*Glipizide*
Dosage:	Usually once daily 1.25 mg–20 mg/daily	One to two times daily 10 mg–40 mg/daily
Excretion:	50% gastrointestinal tract and 50% genitourinary tract	92% urinary tract alone

*Both glyburide (DiaBeta and Micronase) and glipizide (Glucatrol) are effective compounds that lower blood glucose by making insulin available and effective.

in a 5-mg to 20-mg daily dosage while, with glipizide, 10 mg to 40 mg daily is effective. Another difference between these is that glyburide is destroyed in the body, 50% by the gastrointestinal tract and 50% in the urinary tract. On the other hand, glipizide is excreted largely by the urinary tract, which might be important in patients with renal excretion deficiency. Another difference is that glyburide is usually a once-daily dosage, whereas glipizide is often needed twice daily. This might make a difference in patient compliance.

Camerini-Davalos and co-workers did a 3-year study of 41 patients with chemical diabetes (elevated blood glucose levels, but not diabetic).[1] Increased thickened capillary basement membranes were found in these patients. This is true of diabetics, but not in normals; these were treated with glipizide, and the condition was reversed and improved. Raskin and co-workers achieved this with type I insulin-requiring diabetics using continuous subcutaneous insulin injection as compared to controls.[6] Was it the oral agent per se, or was it control? In an editorial, Siperstein stated these two studies may provide evidence that meticulous diabetic control for prolonged periods may be beneficial with respect to the microvascular complications of diabetes.[7]

If first-generation agents are effective, there is no need for a change, but second-generation agents might be preferable, because they:

> Are more effective with much smaller doses because of increased potency per dose size.
>
> Are more effective in receptor and postreceptor areas; therefore, they decrease insulin resistance.
>
> Cause no sodium/water retention.
>
> Cause essentially no disulfiram effect.
>
> Are nonpolar, weakly charged, and do not bind at a site competitive with other medications.
>
> Are sometimes eliminated from the body by *both* gastrointestinal and urinary tract.
>
> Are quickly removed from the body; the "hit and run" effect.
>
> Form a possible combination with insulin in patients refractive to insulin.

Both require viable beta cells for the release of insulin and have an effect on sensitizing insulin receptors as well as decreasing insulin resistance.

COMBINED ORAL AGENTS AND INSULIN

For many years, especially with the first-generation agents, combination with insulin was considered to be a useless exercise. With the knowledge of second-generation influence on the receptors and postreceptoral areas, however, there has been increased interest in combined treatment.[2,4] For example, the patient who may be overweight, but continues with grossly elevated blood glucose levels regardless of the amount of insulin given, should probably *not* be given increasingly large amounts of insulin. Superfluous amounts of insulin are already present. This patient might be a candidate for second-generation oral agents plus insulin.

This treatment will not be effective in all patients, but can be in some. The method used would be to determine a fixed and adequate insulin dose daily, then gradually add the oral agents (*e.g.*, 5 mg daily) and increase as needed. It may take a month or two to demonstrate effectiveness, because the beneficial result does not occur immediately. The danger of insulin reactions is almost non-existent, and if not severe, would be welcome, indicating a successful effect of treatment by lowering the dose. What are the goals? Stability of therapy and better blood glucose control with less insulin.

SUMMARY

The choices of treatment of type II diabetics, therefore, are diet, oral agents, exercise, and sometimes insulin. Type I diabetes presents no choice problem. If insulin is needed with the older patient, there is a choice of diet, or diet and oral agents. Sometimes insulin is necessary, but the less complicated the treatment, the better. If the oral agents are effective, this is a treatment of choice.

One should not wait to start treatment of these patients, but should begin when the patient experiences frequent blood glucose elevation postprandially. Treatment does not necessarily require insulin. The first treatment method should be diet and then, if needed, the appropriate oral agents.

Knowledge and treatment of diabetes have improved tremendously. Dr. Priscilla White, when retiring after 50 years of practicing diabetes, was asked if she became discouraged with her long-term patients with diabetes. She said this might be true if you looked at the single, individual patient; however, as a group, diabetics are doing so much better than they did, not only 10 or 20, but even 5 years ago! Patients get depressed with the need for constant monitoring of their blood and urine and, of course, the dieting. The message to them should be, "Yes, diabetes is difficult, but if you must have diabetes, this is absolutely the best time in history to have it. So much has been accomplished and so much more is prospect!"

REFERENCES

1. Camerini-Davalos RF, Velasco C, Glaser M et al: Drug-induced reversal of early diabetic microangiopathy. N Engl J Med 309:1551–1556, 1983
2. Draznin B, Kao M, Sussman KE: Insulin and glyburide increase cytosolic free-Ca^{2+} concentration in isolated rat adipocytes. Diabetes 36:174–178, 1987
3. Entmacher PS, Krall LP, Kranczer SN: Diabetes mortality from vital statistics. In Marble A, Krall LP (eds): Joslin's Diabetes Mellitus, 12th ed, p 296. Philadelphia, Lea & Febiger, 1985
4. Lebovitz HE: Update of all hypoglycemic agents. In Krall LP, Alberti KGMM (eds): World Book of Diabetes in Practice, vol 2, pp 72–79. Amsterdam, Elsevier, 1986
5. Marble A, Krall LP (eds): Oral hypoglycemic agents. In Joslin's Diabetes Mellitus, 12th ed, pp 412–452. Philadelphia, Lea & Febiger, 1985
6. Raskin P, Pietri AO, Unger R et al: The effect of diabetic control on the width of skeletal-muscle capillary basement membrane in patients with type I diabetes mellitus. N Engl J Med 309:1546–1550, 1983
7. Siperstein MD: Diabetic microangiopathy and the control of blood glucose. N Engl J Med 309:1577–1579, 1983

CHAPTER EIGHT
Newer Modes of Treating Type II Diabetes

Alan M. Reich

There is reason to believe type II diabetes and type I diabetes mellitus are two separate diseases. Obviously, they have common characteristics (*e.g.*, hyperglycemia occurs in both). The long-term complications are similar in both, although a preponderance of macrovascular complications is seen with type II diabetes (*i.e.*, peripheral vascular, cerebrovascular, and coronary artery disease being predominant) and in type I, or insulin-dependent diabetes, the microvascular complications predominate (*i.e.*, diseases of the retina and kidney). A distinction does exist between these two diseases, however, because the genetics are known to be different. It has been shown on chromosome 6 (the HLA locus) that certain disease-related antigens are common in type I, or insulin-dependent diabetes, which are not seen in noninsulin-dependent (type II) diabetes. Similarly, it has been shown in gene blotting that near the promoter region of the insulin gene, pertubations in coding exist commonly in type II diabetes. The inheritance of these two entities is known to be different.

Furthermore, the population susceptible to these diseases is different, although recognizable overlapping occurs. The type I diabetic is usually younger, and the type II diabetic is usually older.

Probably the most important characteristic that separates these two diseases is the pathology. In type I diabetes, clearly an insulinitis occurs; a marked infiltration of lymphocytes occurs; and to some degree eosinophils. Obviously, studies proving this are difficult to come by, but if a young, newly diagnosed diabetic patient has an automobile accident, for example, and one is able to get tissue quickly enough, upon evaluation of the pancreatic islets one can see the insulinitis occurring. This is in contrast to what one sees in type II diabetes, where the pancreas can have any number of different characteristics. There is really nothing pathognomonic in looking at the islets of Langerhans in a patient with type II diabetes.

Because type I and type II diabetes are separate diseases, one might expect the treatment to be different. The treatment of type I diabetes has been, and continues to be, insulin. Diet is structured so that the portions and timing coincide with activity of the exogenous insulin administered. Type II diabetes, however, is more complex, requiring different methods of treatment. Insulin is one form of treatment, as well as diet and weight control. Exercise and the oral sulfonylurea agents, used singly or in combination, are others.

PATHOPHYSIOLOGY

Before discussing the different methods of treatment, a review of the pathophysiology of type II noninsulin-dependent diabetes follows, because herein lies the rationale for the various treatments.

Figure 8-1 is a schematic diagram plotting insulin secretion as a factor of glucose intolerance in people without diabetes, patients with noninsulin-dependent diabetes, and patients with insulin-dependent (or type I) diabetes mellitus.[4] A heterogeneity is seen in the normal group in that insulin secretion can be fairly low to fairly high. Similarly, with insulin-dependent diabetes a drop-off in insulin secretion is seen, but of importance is the group with noninsulin-dependent diabetes mellitus. Here, too, some degree of heterogeneity occurs, in that the insulin secretion mirrors that in normal nondiabetic people. The insulin secretion can, in fact, be supernormal, confirming that type II diabetic patients can have supernormal insulin levels. This indicates that if a patient has an abundance of insulin, yet is hyperglycemic, obviously some decrease occurs in the effectiveness of insulin (*i.e.,* an antagonism of insulin action exists known as insulin resistance).

Over the years, it has been shown that insulin resistance is one of the characteristic features of type II diabetes; however, defects are noted in insulin secretion as well. Perhaps one of the striking problems in insulin secretion abnormalities and type II diabetes is the loss of first-phase insulin release. When a glucose stimulus for insulin secretion occurs, insulin is secreted in a biphasic or bimodal fashion, and a rapid rise occurs in insulin secretion in the first 20 to 30 minutes, which is thought to reflect preformed insulin; a later sustained rise in insulin release occurs, which is thought to be newly synthesized insulin being released. In type II diabetes, this loss or absence of first-phase insulin release occurs, which is a characteristic feature of type II diabetes.

THERAPEUTIC MODALITIES

METABOLIC CONTROL

In type II diabetes, therapeutic goals are important. For some physicians, rendering a type II diabetic asymptomatic is sufficient, regardless of blood sugar levels. They alleviate the polyuria, polydipsia, and do not worry about the blood sugars. The prevailing opinion, however, is that one should normalize metabolic control (normalize blood sugars) as much as possible because it is thought that if blood sugars can be normalized, perhaps long-term complications of the disease can be prevented.

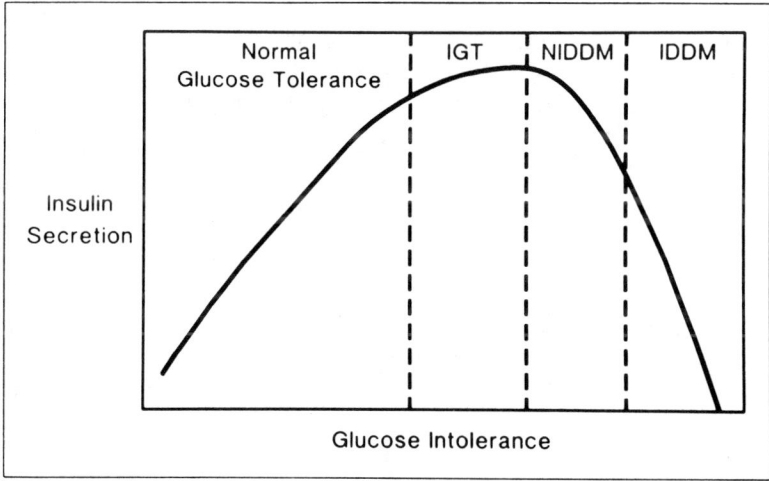

Figure 8-1. Schematic relationship between insulin secretion and insulin resistance in the pathogenesis of noninsulin-dependent diabetes mellitus. IGT = impaired glucose tolerance; NIDDM = noninsulin-dependent diabetes mellitus; IDDM = insulin-dependent diabetes mellitus. (Reproduced with permission of Horton ES: Role of environmental factors in the development of noninsulin-dependent diabetes mellitus. Am J Med 75 (5B):34, 1983)

What is not a foregone conclusion, however, is whether complications can be prevented; this remains a subject of debate. An important question yet to be answered is how normal does diabetic control have to be to prevent complications if complications are, indeed, preventable? This is a controversial question, but one of the generally accepted therapeutic goals is to normalize fasting plasma glucose. Ideally, the 1-hour postprandial plasma glucose should be less than 200 mg/dl. The patient should be rendered aglycosuric. If these three steps are accomplished, then the glycosylated hemoglobin, hemoglobin A_1C, should be normal.

DIET AND WEIGHT CONTROL

Probably the most important, yet most difficult, task to accomplish is control of body weight, which should be as near normal as possible. The weight should be as close as possible to ideal weight for that particular person's height. Losing weight is extremely important for type II diabetics, because the vast majority of these patients are overweight. I submit that if one could get type II diabetic patients to ideal body weight, the diabetes would remit.

Figure 8-2 is from a report by Sims and co-workers, who studied prisoners in a Vermont State Prison about 20 years ago.[11] Their study comprised normal, otherwise healthy volunteers, who had no predilection for diabetes, no previous history of diabetes or glucose tolerance, and no family history of diabetes mellitus. The subjects were force-fed to gain weight, and the question of what would happen to their metabolic control, or blood sugars, as a result was addressed. This was an all-encompassing study. They not only reviewed insulin and blood sugar levels, and glucose tolerance, but other hormonal components as well.

For the sake of this discussion, the findings in terms of insulin and glucose dynamics will be reviewed. Figure 8-2 shows the results of one of the nine participants. It was a year-long study divided into three major segments. During the first segment of the study, the volunteers were fed fairly high-caloric diets, about 4000 calories in three meals per day, and exercise was increased. Afterwards, exercise was limited, and they were force-fed diets as high as 7000 calories per day. A fourth meal was added and continued for a period of several months, during which a steady rise in weight was observed. In many of the subjects, weight increased by as much as 25%. When maximum weight was achieved (no further weight gain was possible), the volunteers were told they could exercise and eat ad lib, and were allowed to exercise. They self-

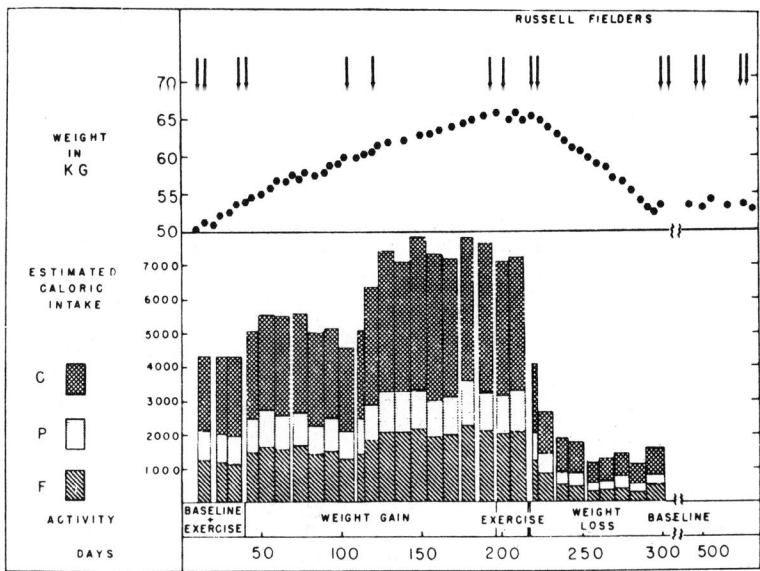

Figure 8-2. Protocol of a typical individual study. The height of the columns indicates the total caloric intake; subdivisions of the columns represent the proportional composition of the diet *by weight*. The pairs of arrows indicate the batteries of tests performed to bracket the experimental periods. (Reproduced with permission of Sims EAH, Goldman RF, Gluck CM et al.: Experimental obesity in man. Trans Assoc Am Phys 81:153–170, 1968)

imposed low-calorie diets, as low as 1000 calories per day, and as a consequence, a rapid weight loss occurred.

Valuable information was derived from this study. With the weight gain, a significant increase in fasting serum insulin levels was seen, which decreased as the subjects were allowed to lose weight. The insulin–glucose ratio increased, but it did not increase as much as one would have expected with the given hyperinsulinemia. This points to the fact that insulin resistance was emerging, confirming that obesity is associated with insulin resistance.

With weight gain, a significant decrease in the glucose disappearance rate (K) occurred. The K value is calculated in the course of doing intravenous tolerance tests (*i.e.*, glucose tolerance worsened, but not to the point of diabetes). A K value of less than one is considered diabetic; above one is not. Although they were not considered diabetic, their glucose tolerance worsened, and with allowance of weight loss, a rise later back to baseline occurred.

The conclusion of this segment of the study, therefore, was

that weight gain as a consequence of excessive intake of calories is diabetogenic. In other words, a state of insulin resistance can be induced, with hyperinsulinemia developing, and a relative glucose intolerance can be created. A study done like this, in a person prone to diabetes (*i.e.*, one who has a history of glucose intolerance or a family history of diabetes, or both), would magnify what is occurring in an otherwise normal host. This study clarifies the problem in type II diabetic patients, in that they eat too much, gain weight, and develop diabetes.

The importance of diet in treatment of type II diabetes cannot be overemphasized. A physician's primary goal should be to advise and help type II diabetic patients lose weight. The most important advice to give type II diabetic patients is to restrict calories across the board, which includes carbohydrates, proteins, and fats in proportion. The exchange list system, while not perfect, allows for prescribing a calculated calorically defined diet with proper portions of food. It is important to structure a calorically defined diet that can be maintained indefinitely. The problem with semistarvation and liquid protein diets is that, although they are effective and the patient loses weight, and in a diabetic situation blood sugars are reduced, these diets cannot be maintained indefinitely. All too familiar is that people lose weight, but often regain what they have lost. Patients, therefore, need to learn to eat normal kinds of foods and limit the portions through self-control.

As mentioned previously, the exchange list system is not perfect, and this has been brought out particularly by the glycemic index. The glycemic index is designed in such a way that, for isocaloric quantities of food, the blood sugar response to ingestion of these different food stuffs is rated, and the scale is set arbitrarily, with a piece of white bread beginning at 100. If isocaloric amounts of food cause a glycemic response of less than 100, this means that they do not cause as high a rise in blood sugar; those that cause a response over 100 have a glycemic response greater than white bread. The glycemic response to an equivalent amount of calories of different types of bread varies, presumably because it is the fiber content of the food stuff that one is ingesting. Other factors are also probably involved.

Addition of fiber in the recommended amount, about 50 g per day, is not totally innocuous; it does cause bloatiness and gastrointestinal gas, which can be uncomfortable. Some have expressed the possibility, although it is not widespread, that there can be mineral and vitamin depletion, which can be taken care of easily by prescribing a multipurpose vitamin or mineral supplement. The prevailing opinion is that increasing the fiber in one's diet goes a long way in reducing the hyperglycemia; however, I again emphasize that caloric restriction alone is the most important thing to impart to patients.

EXERCISE

Another important factor is exercise. Because type II diabetics tend to be older and not as active as when they were younger, the thought of exercise is not appealing. Moreover, as mentioned previously, the vast majority of patients with type II diabetes are overweight. People who are overweight tend to be less active, but whether being overweight begets inactivity or inactivity begets being overweight is a subject of debate. It can probably work either way; nonetheless, exercise need not be what one might expect. A person does not have to be totally breathless, sweaty, in pain, and worried about a heart attack to be doing adequate physical activity and exercise. What is necessary is that one do aerobic physical activity, using the long muscles of the arms and legs. This physical activity can include walking or cycling for the legs, a rowing machine for the arms, or tennis or racquetball for the arms and legs. The general feeling is that, unlike the prescription for cardiovascular training in which one should exercise three to four times a week, a person with type II diabetes should exercise daily for 30 minutes. To induce the habit, it should probably be done at the same time every day. There should be a 5-minute warm-up and 5-minute cool-down period to avoid aggravating any arthritic problems a patient may have.

The question of the rate of exercise has always been a difficult one to answer. The practical answer is that if one gets breathless and cannot carry on a conversation while exercising, that is probably the person's limit and is as fast as he should go. With time he will be able to do more, and carry on a conversation as he is better conditioned.

What are the benefits of exercise? It has been shown that insulin sensitivity increases with physical activity (*e.g.*, the effectiveness of insulin is improved upon and insulin resistance is reduced). Exercise lowers serum lipids, cholesterol particularly. Cholesterol is a risk factor for coronary artery, peripheral vascular, and cerebrovascular disease. Moreover, exercise improves the high-density lipoprotein to low-density lipoprotein ratio. It appears to reduce one's risk for vascular disease.

Exercise also increases muscle tone and endurance, and decreases boredom and depression. These somewhat nonspecific benefits from exercise are extremely important. Increased endurance is important because it reduces the impact of diabetes. If the patient is depressed or bored, one is not likely to get good dietary compliance, if at all, and probably not any compliance with prescribed treatments, whether it be diabetic pills or otherwise.

Obviously, if one is going to initiate a physical exercise program in an older person, precipitating angina and coronary artery disease should be considered. As mentioned previously, however, exercise need not be strenuous, so this concern can be somewhat minimized. Another benefit of exercise to the type II diabetic patient is weight reduction, which is low on the list for good reason; a lot of exercise is required to lose weight and burn up calories. It is not realistic to think the patient can continue to eat the same amounts of food and only exercise more and lose weight. Losing weight requires not only an increase of physical activity, but reduction of calorie intake as well.

SULFONYLUREA AGENTS

Administration of oral sulfonylureas is a further option in the treatment of type II diabetes. Although blood sugars can be normalized (or nearly normalized) 100% of the time with weight reduction and exercise, most people cannot get their weight down to ideal body weight. For this reason sulfonylureas are used commonly. Figure 8-3 shows some of these sulfonylureas: tolbutamide, chlorpropamide, glyburide, and glipizide; the last two being the newer second-generation sulfonylurea agents.[6] The hypoglycemic activity of these agents resides on the amide linkage shown in Figure 8-3. It is common to all of the hypoglycemic agents and is the substitution of the amino group and benzene ring that imparts different properties to these various sulfonylurea agents. In terms of glyburide and glipizide, these are nonpolar substitutions in the amino group and also on the benzene ring, in contradistinction to the first-generation agents, tolbutamide and chlorpropamide, where there are more polar side-chain linkages, as well as substitution with chloride on the benzene ring in chlorpropamide. Of importance is that in rendering the newer agents nonpolar, they are more lipid soluble. This is important in the sense that the adverse effects of sulfonylurea agents, the drug-to-drug interactions that can occur with sulfonylurea agents, are minimized with the second-generation sulfonylureas. They simply do not bind to albumin, whereas the first-generation sulfonylureas do bind to albumin, and any medications that also bind to albumin can cause a drug-to-drug interaction. These problems, therefore, are minimized with the second-generation sulfonylureas.

The sulfonylurea agents work by increasing insulin secretion; they have specific extrapancreatic effects. Sulfonylureas help ameliorate some of the postreceptor deficits that occur in type II diabetes, and as a consequence, lower insulin levels, and can eventually cause upgrading of receptors in insulin-responsive tissue.

Debate continues regarding the most important effect of sulfonylureas. Is it the extrapancreatic effects, in correcting the receptor and postreceptor defects, or is it in enhancing endogenous insulin secretion? The prevailing opinion is that extrapancreatic effects of sulfonylureas predominate. The insulin secretory effect, however, is extremely important, because without some residual beta cell secretory activity (*i.e.*, unless some insulin secretion is occurring in a patient), no extrapancreatic effects will be seen. There is a prerequisite, therefore, of having some endogenous insulin secretion for the sulfonylureas to perform in the periphery. An advantage with the second-generation sulfonylureas is that in contrast to the first-generation sulfonylureas, where this insulin

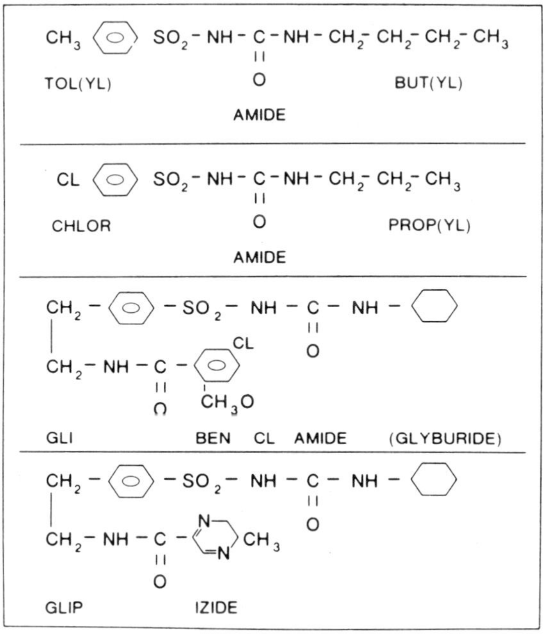

Figure 8-3. Structural formulas of two first-generation (top two boxes) and two second-generation (bottom two boxes) sulfonylureas. (Reproduced with permission of Melander A, Wahlin–Boll E: Clinical pharmacology of glipizide. Am J Med 75(5B): 42, 1983)

secretory effect wanes after several months of treatment, glipizide and glyburide enhance insulin secretion long-term.

Glucose disposal rate is a reflection of insulin resistance in insulin-responsive tissues of muscle and fat. With the use of glyburide, this insulin resistance can be improved after a period of 3 months. While the improvement is significant, it is important to realize that one does not normalize the glucose disposal rate (*i.e.,* one does not completely ameliorate the insulin resistance). Importantly, it has been recognized that the fasting plasma glucose is a reflection of hepatic glucose output. A number of studies have shown that in an untreated, noninsulin-dependent diabetic, the hepatic glucose output is much higher than occurs in normal circumstances (Fig. 8-4).[5] When one treats with glyburide over a 3-month period, a significant drop in hepatic glucose output

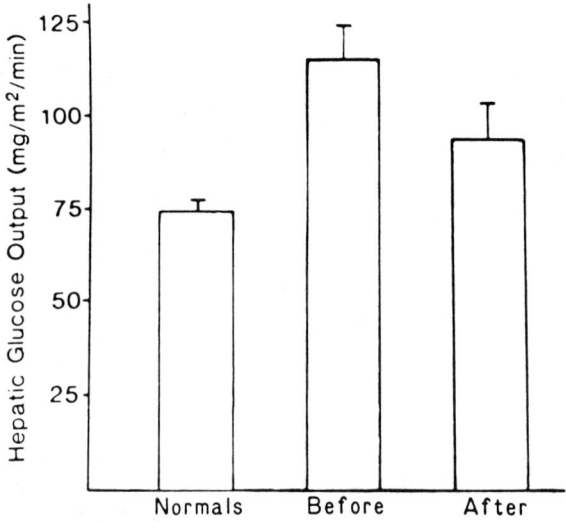

Figure 8-4. Mean steady-state glucose disposal rates for control subjects and nine type II diabetic subjects before and after glyburide therapy for 3 months. The results are from euglycemic glucose clamp studies performed at an insulin infusion rate of 120 mU/M^2/min and are plotted as the mean ±SE. (Reproduced with permission of Kotterman OG, Olefsky JM: The impact of sulfonylurea treatment upon the mechanisms responsible for the insulin resistance in type II diabetes. Diabetes Care [Suppl 1] 17:86, 1984)

occurs, but not nearly what occurs in normals. This is probably how the sulfonylureas reduce fasting plasma glucose (*i.e.*, by reducing hepatic glucose output). If one does an oral glucose tolerance test in untreated type II diabetics, a curve that looks fairly representative is seen (Fig. 8-5).[1] If the glucose tolerance test is repeated after 3 months of glyburide, a decrease in the curve occurs. This decrease in the curve, however, is a consequence of the lowering of the fasting plasma glucose. In other words, it went down from 200 to 100, and as a result, all of the other points on the curve are decreased similarly. Glyburide, in the strictest sense, does not improve glucose tolerance, nor do any of the other sulfonylureas.

In certain circumstances there is some suggestion that oral sulfonylureas (*e.g.*, glyburide) can improve glucose tolerance in the strictest sense. Figure 8-6, in contradistinction to Figure 8-5, shows three plotted intravenous glucose tolerance tests in consecutive order in type II diabetes. In a recent study, we reviewed the response of type II diabetic patients to this triple intravenous glucose tolerance testing.[7] In a normal nondiabetic person, when three consecutive glucose tolerance tests are given hourly, the slope

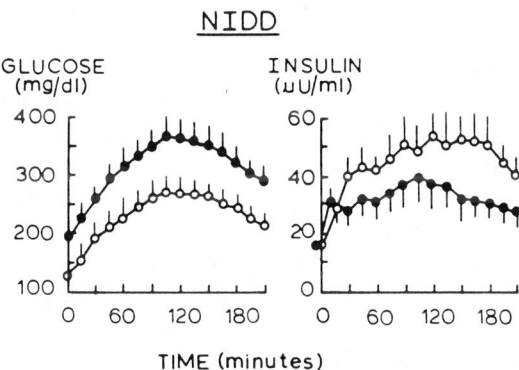

Figure 8-5. Plasma glucose and insulin concentrations during the oral glucose tolerance test in noninsulin-dependent diabetes patients before and 3 months after glyburide treatment; (0—0), preglyburide; (0—0), 3 months postglyburide. (Reproduced with permission of Defronfo RA, Simonson DC: Oral sulfonylurea agents suppress hepatic glucose production in noninsulin-dependent diabetic individuals. Diabetes Care [Suppl I] 17:76, 1984)

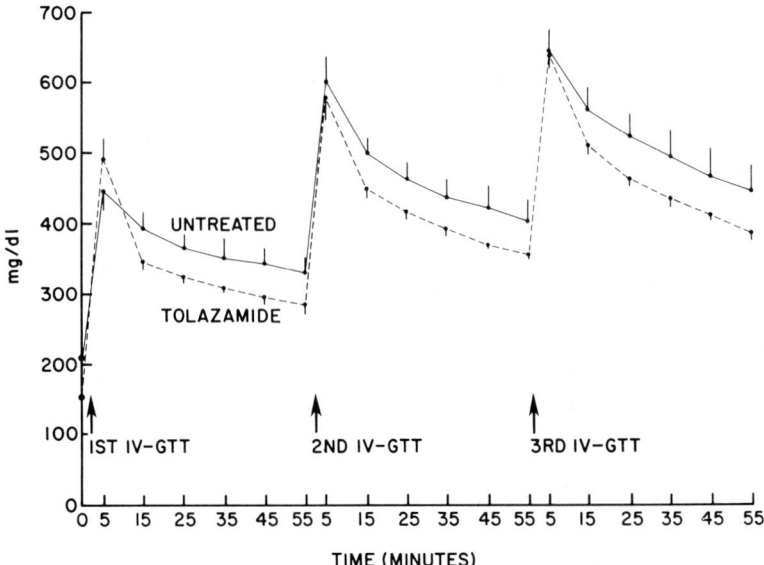

Figure 8-6. Intravenous glucose tolerance tests in type II diabetic patients.

begins to steepen; in other words, the disappearance rate improves. In diabetes, the disappearance rate does not improve. After treatment with one of the first-generation sulfonylureas, the slopes of the curves stay the same; they are superimposable.

Soneru and Abraira substituted glyburide for tolazamide and glucose tolerance improved; again, the disappearance rates improved.[12] This has not been shown for any of the first-generation sulfonylureas.

The different characteristics of the sulfonylureas are shown in Tables 8-1 and 8-2.[2,10] Tolbutamide has been around the longest time. It was first on the market in 1956, followed soon by chlorpropamide, and then by the other first-generation sulfonylureas. The second-generation sulfonylureas have been around for quite a while, glyburide since 1969 and glipizide since 1973. They were first introduced in Europe, and the United States Food and Drug Administration did not approve them until 1984. The experience in Europe was extensive before they become available in the United States.

In terms of maximum dose, the amount of the second-generation agents used is much less than one would have used with

Table 8-1
Relationship Among Sulfonylureas: Metabolism, Potency, Activity, and Side-Effects of Hyperglycemic Drugs

Name and Year It Became Available	Maximum Dose (mg/day)	Rate of Hepatic Metabolism	Duration of Activity (hr)	Percentage in Urine	Equivalent Therapeutic Dose (mg)	Side-Effects (%)
First-Generation Agents						
Tolbutamide (1956)	300	Rapid	6–8	100*	100	3.2, 2.1†
Chlorpropamide (1957)	750	Slow	36‡	96‡	250	6.2, 8.5
Acetohexamide (1963)	1500	Intermediate	12–18	60*	500	2.0
Tolazamide (1966)	1000	Intermediate	24	85*	250	2.9, 4.6†
Second-Generation Agents						
Glyburide (1969)	20	Intermediate	24	50‡	5	1.5, 3.6†
Glipizide (1973)	40	Intermediate	12	89‡	10	1.6

*Excreted as parent compound or metabolites by 24 hours.
†Upjohn-sponsored studies in the United States.
‡Excreted as parent compound or metabolites by 48 to 72 hours.
Reproduced by permission from Feldman JM: Glyburide: A second-generation sulfonylurea hypoglycemic agent. Pharmacotherapy 5:49, 1985

Table 8–2
Comparison of Therapy with the Sulfonylureas

Drug	Tablet Size (mg)	Maximum Total Daily Dose (mg)	Doses/Day	Cost/Day*
First-Generation				
Acetohexamide	250, 500	1500	1 or 2	$0.75
Chlorpropamide	100, 250	500	1	$0.68[†]
Tolazamide	100, 250, 500	1000	1 or 2	$1.12[†]
Tolbutamide	250, 500	3000	2 or 3	$1.02[†]
Second-Generation				
Glipizide	5, 10	40	1 or 2	$1.40
Glyburide	1, 25, 2.5, 5	20	1	$1.12–$1.36

*Wholesale cost to pharmacist of maximal daily dose; cost to patient will generally be higher.
[†]Less expensive generic preparations are available.
Reproduced by permission from Simonson DC: The second-generation sulfonylureas: Mechanisms of action and therapeutic indications. Internal Medicine for the Specialist 6:60, 1985

the first-generation sulfonylureas. This has to do with the fact that for an equivalent therapeutic dose, the second-generation sulfonylureas are about 100-fold more potent than tolbutamide.

Regarding some of the other characteristics of sulfonylureas, the long duration of action, which is somewhat advantageous, occurs with the second-generation sulfonylureas, but not nearly so long as chlorpropamide. This has a drawback—it is such a long duration of activity that in susceptible subjects, a prolonged hypoglycemia can be induced. Other problems occur with chlorpropamide; it decreases free water clearance so that some peripheral edema occurs, as well as hyponatremia. Also, problems of alcohol inducing a disulfiram-like reaction can occur. The side-effect rate seen for chlorpropamide, therefore, is substantially higher than for the second-generation sulfonylurea agents.

The second-generation sulfonylureas are more potent; therefore, the maximum daily recommended dose is much less than one would have used with the first-generation sulfonylureas. Glyburide is probably slightly more potent than glipizide in terms of the amount used, and as a consequence, glyburide can be used as a once-daily dose, whereas glipizide sometimes has to be given as a twice-daily dose. The cost, however, is comparable.

INSULIN

The last area of therapy is the use of insulin in treatment of noninsulin-dependent diabetes. In type I diabetes, where no insulin secretion occurs, a hormone that is lacking is being replaced. In type II diabetes, significant amounts of insulin are in circulation, or at least there appears to be some insulin secretion occurring, but an insufficient amount exists. In type II diabetes, therefore, one is supplementing the insulin that is already being produced in the circulation endogenously.

Using insulin in type II diabetes has several drawbacks. One of the major drawbacks is that it does not meet with much patient acceptance. All physicians have had the circumstance of an overweight type II diabetic patient on a maximum dose of sulfonylureas who does not lose weight, does not like to exercise, and runs consistent blood sugar levels of 300. Patients have difficulty understanding why they must take insulin, because they do not feel like they are sick. Often a type II diabetic has no symptoms; it is difficult to convince someone who feels well he is going to feel better or complications may be reduced if he takes a shot.

There are other reasons for reluctance to using insulin in type II diabetes. One is that if these patients have some residual endogenous insulin secretion, why not maximize that with the use of sulfonylureas? In other words, one should try to induce as much physiologic insulin release as possible. Sulfonylureas increase insulin secretion from the beta cells; insulin then goes, in a physiologic manner, by way of the portal vein to the liver, where insulin is so instrumental in reducing hepatic glucose output. Insulin is being administered in an unphysiologic manner when given exogenously. It is being given systemically and, consequently, to get the same effect on the liver, a larger dose will have to be given than if a little more insulin had been secreted from the pancreas with an oral sulfonylurea.

What happens frequently if insulin is used in type II overweight patients is that a state of insulin resistance emerges. Large doses of insulin are required, which are well beyond what would normally be used in an insulin-dependent type I diabetic, usually something like 40 to 60 units. It is not unheard of to use 80 or more units of insulin a day in overweight type II patients.

The question is, are physicians doing patients harm by overinsulinizing and causing hyperinsulinemia? Current epidemiologic data indicate, in fact, that harm does occur to patients being given these enormous amounts of insulin.[13] In addition, it has been established in *in vitro* studies that insulin, being an anabolic hormone, causes lipid deposition in the endothelial cells of arterial walls.[3] It promotes smooth muscle proliferation, so that plaque formation may, in part, be a consequence of hyperinsulinemia.

In recent years, no less than 12 different studies have been cited in abstract form at the last three national diabetes meetings, attesting to the fact that a combination of insulin and oral sulfonylureas can reduce insulin requirements. All of these studies show the same results, a reduction in insulin requirements and an improvement in metabolic control. The most popular regimen to emerge is the use of bedtime insulin and daytime sulfonylurea.[9] Certainly, one does not normalize blood sugars. In fact, one could argue whether bringing blood sugar levels down from 350 to 240 is significant, but nonetheless it does occur and the adverse reactions and effects have been minimal. One thing not mentioned by these studies, but which becomes obvious, is that the use of combined insulin and glyburide treatment over a long period of time can become expensive.

NORMALIZING POSTPRANDIAL BLOOD SUGARS

My colleagues and I have reviewed combined insulin–glyburide treatment from a different vantage point.[8] We realized the next most difficult task in our therapeutic goals, after trying to get overweight type II diabetic patients to lose weight, is trying to normalize postprandial blood sugars. That is often a difficult clinical problem, and we thought perhaps this combined therapy, using insulin and glyburide together, could reduce postprandial hyperglycemia. In our study 20 volunteers were treated with intermediate insulin and seen for 6 weeks to try to maximize fasting blood sugar. When this was accomplished, the patients were hospitalized and randomly started either on insulin plus glyburide or insulin and placebo. After discharge, they were followed up at monthly intervals for 4 months. The results were that the glycosylated hemoglobin worsened in the placebo group over 4 months, whereas it stayed the same in the glyburide group. Importantly, however, the 2-hour post-breakfast blood sugar worsened in the placebo group, but did not in the glyburide group; granted, it remained around the 250 range. We had hoped to improve the range, but did not in terms of the post-breakfast glucose. A rather marked improvement was seen in the 2-hour post-lunch blood sugar. The 1-hour post-breakfast and 1-hour post-lunch blood sugars did not show any improvement. We concluded from our study that we could not improve postprandial blood sugars with the combination treatment as much as we had hoped; however, as all of the other studies have shown, we were able to decrease insulin requirements. In other words, the glyburide-treated group insulin dose decreased by roughly 50%.

COMBINED INSULIN AND GLYBURIDE THERAPY

I use combined insulin and glyburide therapy in certain circumstances in some patients. One patient, a 62-year-old man who had diabetes for almost 19 years, weighed 245 pounds, was glycosuric, and ran a blood sugar of 290, had a high hemoglobin A_1C (normal being up to 6.1) and was taking 80 units of insulin a day (Fig. 8-7). This type of patient has probably been going to his family physician, and when the blood sugar was high, the insulin was increased by 4 or 6 units. The blood sugar then comes down, and either the patient fears hypoglycemia, or perhaps some increase in appetite from the insulin occurs. For whatever reason, however, the blood sugar goes back up, so the physician increases the insulin an additional 4 or 6 units, and the blood sugar comes down again. In short order, however, the blood sugar is up again, and the patient ends up taking large amounts of insulin. The approach I take with this type of patient is to put him on a 1500 calorie diet and teach him to do self-glucose monitoring. When I am satisfied he can

J.S.	Age:62	Male	Dx 1967			
	12/9/85	12/18	12/26	1/8	2/26	3/26
Diet	1500					
Weight	245	244	241	240	236	237
Ur Gluc	1/2%	N	N	N	N	N
Bl Gluc	290	–	250	160	180	150
Hb A1C	10.4%	–	–	–	–	7.4
Insulin	80L	40L	40L	40	40	40
Glyburide	–	2,5	5	10	10	10

Figure 8-7. Patient management with combined insulin and glyburide therapy.

do it well and he is a compliant, motivated patient, I cut the insulin in half and start him on a small dose of glyburide. Figure 8-7 shows this particular patient did not rigidly follow the diet and did not lose much weight, but importantly, his blood glucoses improved. His hemoglobin A_1C came down nicely, and the past several months he has taken less insulin and is on combination therapy. Whether I am doing him any good is not known, but at least the amount of insulin he is taking is reduced. He is happy and is no longer in a spiral of weight gain, hyperglycemia, and increasing insulin dosage.

SUMMARY

The different therapeutic modalities in type II diabetes have been reviewed. Inasmuch as the vast majority of type II diabetics are overweight, certainly weight reduction and sensible calorie restriction are the mainstays of treatment. Exercise has many beneficial effects in addition to its enhancing insulin sensitivity; exercise, as discussed, need not be strenuous. Advantages of the second-generation sulfonylureas were pointed out, and the potential advantages of using combined insulin-sulfonylurea treatment were discussed.

REFERENCES

1. Defronfo RA, Simonson DC: Oral sulfonylurea agents suppress hepatic glucose in non-insulin-dependent diabetic individuals. Diabetes Care 17(Suppl I):76, 1984
2. Feldman JM: Glyburide: A second-generation sulfonylurea hypoglycemic agent. Pharmacotherapy 5(2):416–419, March/April, 1985
3. Grant N: Insulin and atherosclerosis. N Engl J Med 300:679–680, 1979
4. Horton SE: Role of environmental factors in the development of non-insulin-dependent diabetes mellitus. Am J Med 75(5B):34, 1983
5. Katterman OG, Olefsky JM: The impact of sulfonylurea treatment upon the mechanisms responsible for the insulin resistance in type II diabetes. Diabetes Care 17(Suppl I):86, 1984
6. Melander A, Wahlin-Boll E: Clinical pharmacology of glipizide. Am J Med 75(5B):41–45, 1983
7. Reich AM, Abraira C, Brunker R et al: Potentiation of glucose-stimulated insulin release by tolazamide and paradoxical absence of glucose facilitation (Staub effect) in NIDDM. Metabolism 35:367–370, 1986
8. Reich AM, Abraira C, Lawrence AM: Improved control with combination insulin and glyburide treatment in type II diabetes. Diabetes 34(Suppl I):7A, 1985
9. Riddle MC, Grad T, Hart J: A new regimen for type II diabetes: Bedtime NPH insulin with daytime sulfonylurea. Diabetes 33(Suppl I):182A, 1984
10. Simonson DC: The second-generation sulfonylureas: Mechanisms of action and therapeutic indications. Internal Medicine for the Specialist 6(12):60, 1985
11. Sims EAH, Goldman RF, Gluck CM et al: Experimental obesity in man. Trans Assoc Am Phy 81:153–170, 1968
12. Soneru I, Abraira C: Recovery of Staub effect in NIDDM after glyburide treatment. Clin Res 34:929A, 1986
13. Uusitupa M, Siitonen O, Pyoroal K et al: The relationship of cardiovascular risk factors to the prevalence of coronary heart disease in newly diagnosed type II (non-insulin-dependent) diabetes. Diabetologia 28:653–659, 1985

CHAPTER NINE

New Strategies in the Treatment of Type II Diabetes

James M. Falko*

Human diabetes is classified currently into two general categories: type I or insulin-dependent diabetes, and type II or noninsulin-dependent diabetes. In type I diabetes, an absolute deficiency of insulin secretion exists. In type II diabetes, the abnormal metabolic state is less well understood. Thus, even though Yalow and Berson described the insulin immunoassay in 1960, after 26 years we still do not know if type II diabetes is a disease of impaired insulin secretion or insulin resistance.[19] It is likely they may be linked to each other or share a common basis, or both. The final common pathway, however, is the known heterogeneous constellation of findings associated with hyperglycemia. Figure 9-1 depicts the three major metabolic defects common in type II diabetes that result in hyperglycemia.[8] These include impaired insulin secretion, increased hepatic glucose production, and peripheral insulin resistance to insulin.

IMPAIRED INSULIN SECRETION

In normal subjects, two phases of insulin release occur: (1) an early phase that occurs within the first 10 minutes following glucose stimulation, which probably represents the release of insulin

---

*I wish to thank the following: Ohio State University's Clinical Research Unit and their support staff; the Central Diabetic Association and Women's Diabetes Board; my colleagues; and my former research fellow, Dr. Osei.
 Further, I would also like to acknowledge Professor Victor Wynn at St. Mary's Medical School's metabolic unit in London, England.

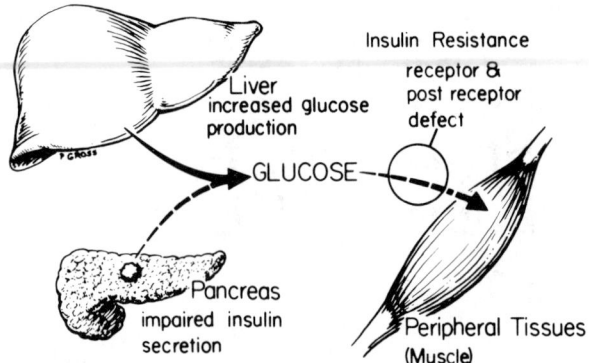

Figure 9-1. Metabolic defects leading to hyperglycemia in Type II diabetes: (1) impaired secretion; (2) increased hepatic glucose production; and (3) peripheral insulin resistance. (Adapted with permission from Olefsky JM: Diabetes mellitus. In Wyngaarden JB, Smith LJ [eds]: Cecil Textbook of Medicine, 17th ed, pp 1320–1339, Philadelphia, WB Saunders, 1985)

stored within the beta cell; and (2) a later phase of insulin secretion that represents newly synthesized insulin. In type II diabetes mellitus, an absence or diminished first phase of insulin secretion occurs. This absent first phase of insulin secretion usually remains in some form despite all forms of antidiabetic therapy. The impairment in early insulin secretion has important physiologic implications. Because the portal vein concentrations of insulin will remain low, basal hepatic glucose production may not be suppressed and continued endogenous output of glucose by the liver supplemented by glucose entering the circulation by food will lead to further hyperglycemia. Eventually, plasma glucose concentration will return to normal, but only at the expense of resultant late hyperinsulinemia. Thus, patients with type II diabetes can have normal or elevated fasting plasma insulin. This postabsorptive hyperinsulinemia reflects an augmented basal rate of insulin secretion, which occurs in response to elevated fasting plasma glucose concentrations. The end result is that all patients with type II diabetes will have a delayed insulin secretory response to glucose with noninsulin-mediated glucose uptake occurring at a higher rate than normal. In general, when the diabetic state becomes severe, the defect in total insulin secretion is greater. In summary, impaired insulin secretion occurs in type II diabetics.

INCREASED HEPATIC PRODUCTION OF GLUCOSE

Figure 9-2 demonstrates the hepatic defect typical of type II diabetes. These studies were performed in our clinical research with the titrated glucose technique. In brief, a prime continuous tracer of titrated glucose is given, followed by a continuous infusion. During the continuous tracer infusion for equilibration and labeling of the glucose pool, two blood samples are obtained for estimation of basal hepatic glucose output. With this single isotope dilution technique in the steady postabsorptive state, glucose entering the circulation is derived predominately from the liver. Thus, the total rate of glucose appearance in the steady state is the same as the basal hepatic glucose output.

Figure 9-2 shows that type II diabetics have an increased production of glucose in the basal state compared with control subjects. The subjects studied were obese, but similar findings occur in nonobese type II diabetics as well.[8,13] Olefsky and colleagues studied this extensively and have shown the importance of this concept by examining the relationship between basal hepatic glucose output and fasting blood sugar in type II diabetics.[8,9,13] They reported a strong correlation between fasting blood sugar and hepatic glucose production. In summary, an increased basal

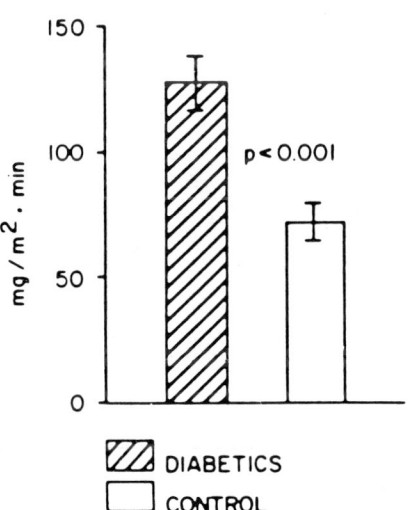

Figure 9-2. Basal hepatic glucose output in Type II diabetics compared with control subjects. (Adapted from Osei K, Falko JM, O'Dorisio TM et al: Gastric inhibitory polypeptide responses and glucose turnover rates after natural meals in type II diabetes. J Clin Endocrinol Metab 62:325–330, 1986)

hepatic production of glucose with insulin inability to suppress hepatic glucose production occurs in type II diabetes.

INSULIN RESISTANCE

It is well established that insulin resistance is present in all patients with type II diabetes. Obesity is frequent in the majority of patients with type II diabetes. Obesity is a known contributing factor; however, obesity does not account for all of the insulin resistance seen in these patients, because nonobese type II diabetics demonstrate insulin resistance also. Insulin exerts a biologic effect by binding to its specific cell receptor; also, cells possess spare receptors. After insulin binding, the insulin-receptor complex is formed and one or more of the insulin actions are generated, which result in insulin's postreceptor effect. Thus, tissue abnormalities in insulin action can be divided into receptor or postreceptor categories. Both abnormalities occur in type II diabetes; therefore, decreased receptors lead to decreased sensitivity to insulin. A pure postreceptor defect in insulin action would lead to a reduction of the biologic effect at all insulin concentrations, producing decreased responsiveness to insulin. If both a receptor and postreceptor defect occurred, insulin resistance would be on the basis of both decreased insulin sensitivity and decreased insulin responsiveness. Olefsky and colleagues demonstrated these concepts using the euglycemic glucose clamp technique, and measuring concomitant 125I insulin binding to monocytes.[8,9,13] The third major defect in type II diabetes, therefore, is peripheral insulin resistance.

MANAGEMENT STRATEGIES

DIET AND EXERCISE

The therapeutic goal in treating type II diabetes is to achieve euglycemia and prevent the complications of diabetes. Diet is the known mainstay of therapy in the 12 million Americans who have type II diabetes, because 80% of the patients are obese. Weight loss even in moderate amounts, however, can achieve improvement in glycemic control in these patients by improving beta cell function, decreasing hepatic glucose production, and improving insulin resistance. Further weight loss may have effects lasting for several weeks, even if weight returns to pretreatment levels. The kind of diets for weight loss and nutritional makeup of the diet for type II diabetes is, however, in a state of controversy concerning which foods and carbohydrates achieve the lowest or highest glycemic index and best long-term result.[1,2] It does appear, however, that incorporation of some simple sugars (in particular, fructose) may not be as detrimental to the diabetic as once thought. In this regard, we evaluated the metabolic effect of moderate supplementation of fructose into the diet of type II diabetics for 8 consecutive weeks and measured glucose and lipoprotein levels. Fructose is sweet, absorbed slowly in the gastrointestinal tract, and metabolized rapidly into triosis.

Figure 9-3 shows that when crystalline fructose (which made up 30% of the carbohydrate energy) was incorporated into the type II diabetics' diet, fasting glucose did not deteriorate after 8 weeks. When fructose was withdrawn, as denoted by the arrow in Figure 9-3, fasting glucose levels rose significantly. Also shown in Figure 9-3 are the glycosylated HbA_1 levels during fructose ingestion, which improved after 8 weeks.

We also measured glucose turnover with the titrated glucose

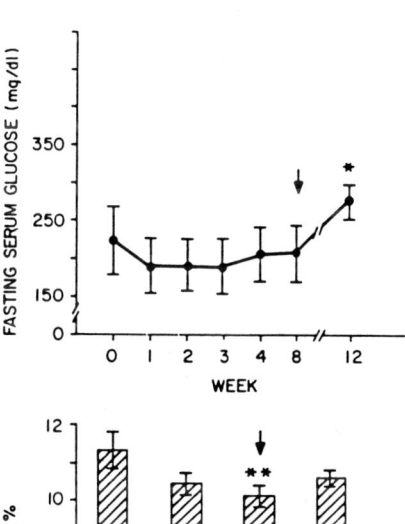

Figure 9-3. Effects of dietary incorporation of fructose on fasting glucose and glycated hemoglobin (HbA_1) in Type II diabetes. The arrow denotes when fructose was withdrawn; asterisks indicate significant differences.

technique under basal conditions and after fructose meals (Fig. 9-4). Basal hepatic glucose production decreased after 8 weeks of fructose ingestion, while the metabolic clearance of glucose did not change after fructose. The metabolic clearance ratio of glucose is calculated by dividing the glucose used by the ambient serum glucose concentration. Of note is that the metabolic clearance ratio does not distinguish between insulin- and noninsulin-mediated glucose uptake and represents both.

Because lipoproteins and apoproteins can be affected in diabetes and altered by fructose, we evaluated several of these measurements as well. Two apoproteins, $ApoA_1$ (the major apoprotein of high-density lipoprotein—the antiatherogenic lipoprotein) and ApoB (the major apoprotein of low-density lipoprotein—the major atherogenic lipoprotein), were measured during this study. These two apoproteins correlate even better with atherosclerosis than high-density lipoprotein-C and low-density lipoprotein-C.

After fructose, the $ApoA_1$/ApoB ratio increased (Fig. 9-5). Thus, fructose did not cause a deterioration in carbohydrate and lipid metabolism, but rather an improvement.[11]

Similar studies using both fructose and sucrose in type II diabetes in a randomized crossover design is shown in Figure 9-6. These studies were done recently in the metabolic unit at St. Mary's Medical School in London, England.[3] With incorporation of either sucrose or fructose supplying one third of the carbohydrate energy in kilocalories, incremental meal glucose areas after sucrose were significantly higher compared with basal levels. After a wash-out

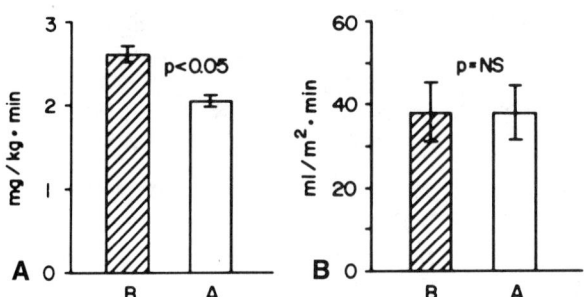

Figure 9-4. (A) Basal hepatic glucose output. (B) Metabolic clearance rate before (B) and after (A) 8 weeks of dietary fructose in Type II diabetes.

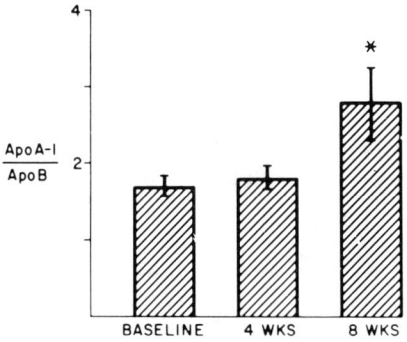

Figure 9-5. ApoA-1/ApoB ratios before and after fructose incorporation in Type II diabetics. Asterisk indicates significant differences.

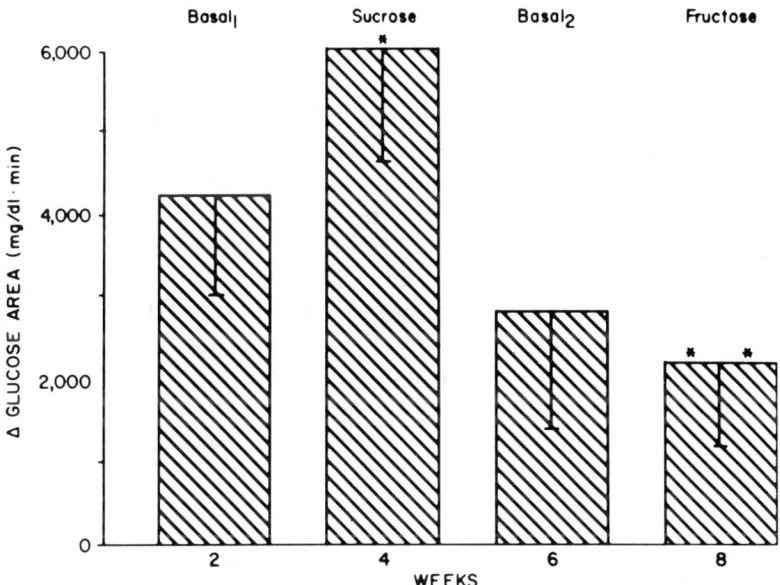

Figure 9-6. Incremental meal glucose responses after physiologic amounts of either sucrose or fructose were incorporated into the diet of Type II diabetes patients. A 2-week "wash-out" period denoted by B_2 (basal period$_2$) occurred before the substitution of each sugar. Single asterisk (*) indicates significant difference between sucrose and each study period. Double asterisks (**) indicate significant difference between fructose and basal period$_1$, and sucrose.

period, fructose was substituted for sucrose and the incremental meal glucose response was significantly lower compared not only with sucrose, but also with basal period glucose responses. Lipoproteins, including the subfractions of high-density lipoprotein, were measured during this study and did not change. Thus, incorporation of fructose and sucrose in physiologic amounts have differential effects on carbohydrate and lipid metabolism in type II diabetics.

With regard to weight-loss diets, the effects of a prolonged 660 Kcal low-calorie liquid diet consisting of 35% protein, 50% carbohydrate in the form of simple sugar, 15% fat on glucose insulin, and C-peptide secretion were also studied in England (John Parr and Professor Victor Wynn, unpublished communication) in both massively obese normal subjects and mild type II diabetics. These patients had dramatic weight losses of 20 kg to 30 kg under close medical supervision, were inpatients for 3 months, and had metabolic balance studies. Both integrated glucose and insulin responses decreased significantly after 3 months of this prolonged treatment, as assessed by a glucose tolerance test. Of interest was that C-peptide, a measure of endogenous insulin secretion by the beta cell, did not change; in fact, it tended to rise. Thus, while insulin levels decreased, beta cell function improved with this diet. Studies such as these need to be evaluated using different dietary approaches to determine the effects of various dietary regimens on glucose metabolism and lipid metabolism in type II diabetes.

In addition to diet and weight loss, exercise is often helpful in the type II diabetic. Moderate amounts of exercise increase glucose use by potentiating the effect of insulin on glucose transport in tissues. In addition, exercise contributes to weight loss, probably improves cardiovascular risk factors, and enriches the quality of life in these patients.

PHARMACOLOGIC THERAPY

Unfortunately, many patients with type II diabetes do not adhere to their diet and weight-loss program and remain hyperglycemic. In these patients, a trial with oral sulfonylurea drugs is warranted because control of hyperglycemia is believed to delay onset and progression of the late complications of diabetes. Patients, particularly in middle age, warrant pharmacologic therapy if they cannot achieve near-normal plasma glucose levels with dietary modification, because they are likely to live long enough to develop late complications.

This is also true because many lipoprotein disarrangements are reserved with improvement in glycemic control.[4] In this regard, oral agents augment beta cell insulin secretion activity and exert an extrapancreatic effect on glucose metabolism. These extrapancreatic effects act on several sites, including the insulin receptor and postreceptor events.

In addition, some oral sulfonylureas reduce basal hepatic glucose production. Thus, sulfonylureas stimulate insulin secretion, potentiate endogenous insulin-mediated glucose uptake, and decrease hepatic glucose production, all of which would help bring fasting and postprandial blood glucose levels to normal. Approximately 60% to 70% of patients with type II diabetes demonstrate an initial satisfactory response to sulfonylurea therapy, 15% to 20% have primary failure, and another 15% to 20% experience secondary failure. The reasons are unclear, but include indiscriminate overeating, advanced beta cell deficiency, or unknown factors.

When secondary or primary failure occurs, administration of insulin is begun. In fact, insulin can be the initial pharmacologic therapy in all type II diabetics and it is theoretically possible for insulin to restore glucose metabolism to normal in all patients with type II diabetes. Thus, Firth and co-workers, in a recent crossover study of eight patients who never received insulin, reported that insulin produced an equivalent glucose lowering, as did sulfonylurea, in mild type II diabetic patients.[5] Chronic insulin, however, may not be the ideal choice because many type II diabetic patients need large doses to overcome the insulin resistance. This usually leads to weight gain, which may be related to lessened glycemia and glycosuria, insulin effect on fat metabolism, or increased appetite. Concern also exists regarding the possible atherogenicity of insulin with the chronically elevated insulin levels.[18] Furthermore, chronic exogenous hyperinsulinism may exacerbate insulin resistance in humans.[17]

In this regard, experienced clinicians know that insulin treatment of patients with type II diabetes is generally disappointing and acknowledge that insulin therapy decreases blood glucose levels toward normal initially; however, patients frequently have increased appetite, eat more, gain more weight, eventually become more insulin-resistant over time, experience higher fasting blood glucose levels, and then require even more insulin. Because of these findings and the large number of patients with type II diabetes, other approaches have been taken in treating patients with type II diabetes whose blood glucose levels have failed to respond to insulin therapy.

It is reasonable, therefore, that a combination of both insulin and sulfonylurea agents may have a theoretic and practical potential in the treatment of type II diabetes. Both forms of therapy can correct the cellular insulin resistance, hepatic defect, and pancreatic defect found in type II diabetes.

We attempted to evaluate this form of therapy in a controlled trial about 2 years ago, because we noted that in several of our type II diabetic patients insulin doses could be reduced if an oral sulfonylurea agent was added to the therapy. Several anecdotal uncontrolled reports appeared in the literature suggesting that combination sulonylurea/insulin therapy may be of benefit in some patients. We, therefore, asked the following questions: Will a combination of insulin/sulfonylurea therapy improve metabolic control in patients who remain poorly controlled on insulin alone? If a response did occur, what would be the clinical or chemical characteristics of the patients who did versus those who did not respond?

We performed this study in a double-blind placebo-controlled manner. Table 9-1 details the clinical characteristics of the patients who were insulin-treated and had poor control. One group of patients received glyburide up to a dose of 20 mg per day in addition to their insulin, and the other group received placebo plus their insulin. Both the placebo and glyburide patients were similar in: age; weight, with the mean ideal body weight being about 130%;

Table 9–1

Characteristics of Type II Diabetes Mellitus Patients Receiving Glyburide or Placebo

Patients	*Glyburide*	*Placebo*
Age (yr)	58.6±2.7	56.3±1.2
Percent IBW*	129.2±6.2	128.4±4.9
Duration of insulin (yr)	8.8±1.3	9.1±2.0
Total daily insulin dose	60.3±7.1	50.27±5.0
FBS[†] (mg/dl)	276.2±27.2	270.1±16
HbA$_1$C[‡] (%)	10.92±0.57	10.37±0.42

No differences were noted between the two groups.
*IBW = Initial body weight.
[†]FBS = Fasting blood sugar.
[‡]HbA$_1$C = Hemoglobin A$_1$C.

duration of insulin therapy; total daily insulin dosage; fasting blood glucose levels; and glycated hemoglobin levels. Both the placebo and glyburide groups of patients were seen frequently to ensure an isocaloric diet. In addition, the dose of insulin was fixed to fully evaluate the addition of the sulfonylurea agent. Dietary patterns, compliance, and weights all remained constant throughout the 16 weeks of study.

Figure 9-7 details the glucose response after a standard 75-g glucose challenge. The placebo-plus-insulin group had no change in their glucose tolerance over the entire 16-week period. At week 4, fasting glucose and glucose tolerance improved significantly in the glyburide-plus-insulin group. By week 16, however, only fasting blood glucose levels remained significantly lower compared with pretreatment values. The glycemic control assessed by glycated hemoglobin showed that hemoglobin A_1C levels decreased significantly by week 4, which persisted to week 16 in the glybu-

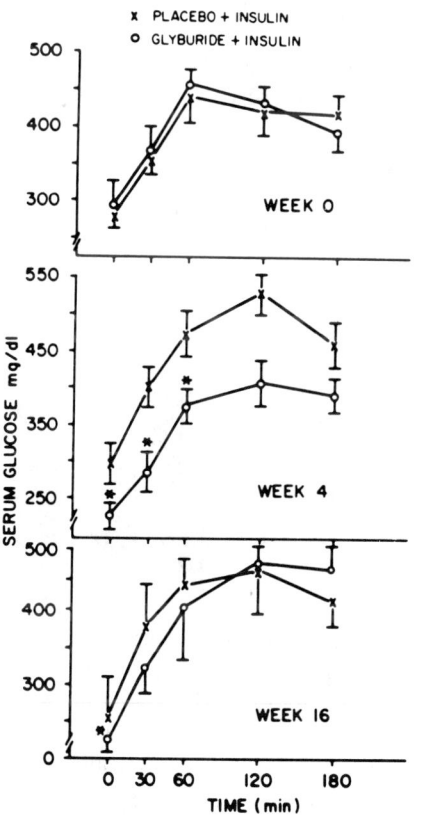

Figure 9-7. Glucose response after a standard glucose tolerance test (75 g) in the placebo-plus-insulin group compared with the glyburide-plus-insulin group. Asterisks indicate significant differences. (Adapted with permission from Osei K, O'Dorisio TM, Falko JM: Concomitant insulin and sulfonylurea therapy in patients with Type II diabetes: Effects on glucoregulation and lipid metabolism. Am J Med 77:1002–1009, 1984)

ride/insulin group. No change occurred in the HbA_1C in the placebo/insulin group.

Figure 9-8 depicts the integrated glucose and C-peptide responses, with C-peptide being an index of endogenous insulin secretion. In the glyburide-plus-insulin group, integrated C-peptide levels were significantly elevated over baseline values at 4 weeks, but decreased at 16 weeks, which matched the improved glucose levels at 4 weeks and deterioration in glucose control at 16 weeks.[14] No change in C-peptide occurred in the placebo-plus-insulin group.

After the code was broken, it appeared that some patients responded well to combination therapy and others did not. We, therefore, divided the patients into responders and nonresponders to combination therapy. Responders were patients who showed a reduction of at least 50 mg/dl from their baseline fasting blood glucose level, or a fasting blood glucose level of >140 mg/dl, which persisted after the first week and lasted for at least 4 consecutive weeks. After the first week of therapy, fasting glucose levels fell significantly in the responders while the nonresponders had no change in their mean fasting blood glucose levels.[10]

Table 9-2 compares the clinical characteristics of the patients

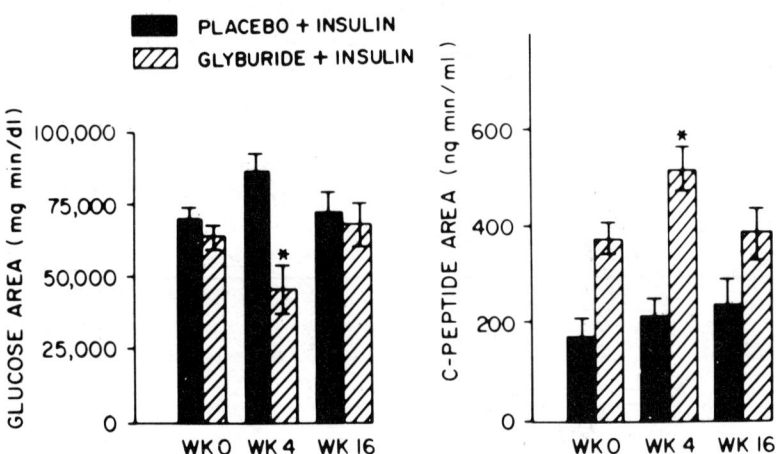

Figure 9-8. Integrated glucose and C-peptide response after a glucose tolerance test in the placebo-plus-insulin group compared with the glyburide-plus-insulin group. Asterisks indicate significant differences. (Reproduced with permission from Osei K, O'Dorisio TM, Falko JM: Concomitant insulin and sulfonylurea therapy in patients with Type II diabetes: Effects on glucoregulation and lipid metabolism. Am J Med 77:1002–1009, 1984)

who responded with those who did not respond. Patients with and without response were similar in mean age, weight, and duration of diabetes. Although not significant, patients with response tended to have been on insulin a shorter period of time and on a slightly smaller dose of insulin.

Figure 9-9 shows glucose and C-peptide levels in the group of patients with response compared to those without response. Mean serum glucose levels in the fasting state and after glucose were similar, as shown in panel A at week zero. After 4 weeks, as shown on panel B, glucose tolerance was improved in the patients who responded to therapy. Panels C and D show the C-peptide responses at weeks zero and 4; mean fasting and stimulated C-peptide levels were higher in the patients with response compared to the patients without response. After oral glucose ingestion, the stimulated C-peptide levels rose significantly at 30 to 180 minutes in the patients with response compared with the blunted C-peptide levels in the patients who were nonresponders to combination therapy.

In summary, the combination of insulin-sulfonylurea therapy improved metabolic control in some type II diabetes mellitus patients. The responders are characterized by a normal fasting serum C-peptide level, which increased significantly after stimulation. The non-responders had low fasting C-peptide levels and blunted responses to stimulation.

Table 9-2

Clinical Characteristics of Type II Diabetes Patients Treated with Combined Insulin and Glyburide

Patients	Responders	Nonresponders
Age (yr)	64±3	55±4
Percent IBW*	132±5	128±14
Duration of diabetes (yr)	10.2±2.6	11.7±1.6
Duration of insulin (yr)	6.6±1.7	10.3±22
Daily insulin (units)	54±10	63±12
FBS[†] (mg/dl)	291±25	246±18
HbA$_1$C[‡] (%)	10.76±0.8	10.16±0.6

*IBW = Initial body weight.
[†]FBS = Fasting blood sugar.
[‡]HbA$_1$C = Hemoglobin A$_1$C.

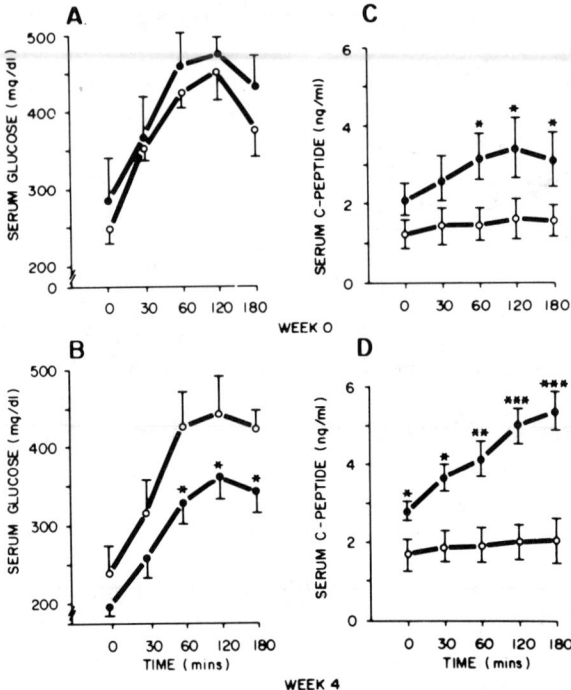

Figure 9-9. Glucose and C-peptide levels in Type II diabetics who responded to combination insulin/sulfonylurea therapy (denoted by closed circles) compared to nonresponders (denoted by open circles) to combination insulin/sulfonylurea therapy. Asterisks indicate significant differences. (Adapted with permission from Osei K, O'Dorisio TM, Falko JM: Concomitant insulin and sulfonylurea therapy in patients with Type II diabetes: Effects on glucoregulation and lipid metabolism. Am J Med 77:1002–1009, 1984)

C-PEPTIDE

Proinsulin splits within the pancreatic islet cell secretory granules to form insulin and connecting or C-peptide. Pancreatic C-peptide and insulin are secreted in equimolar proportions into the portal circulation. While variable hepatic extraction of insulin occurs in both normal and diabetic subjects, C-peptide is minimally extracted. C-peptide is metabolized by the kidney.

Recently, Polonsky and colleagues determined the metabolic clearance rates of biosynthetic C-peptide in dogs, normal subjects, and patients with type I diabetes and reported that peripheral kinetics of C-peptide influence the interpretation of serum C-peptide levels.[15,16] Nevertheless, in the absence of renal insufficiency, serum C-peptide may provide a simple noninvasive clinical modality to estimate endogenous insulin-secreting capacity. For example, in normal subjects, C-peptide can be measured by radioimmunoassay and after glucose a significant increment will occur. In typical insulin-dependent or type I diabetic patients, virtually no C-peptide is present. In typical newly diagnosed obese noninsulin-dependent or type II diabetics, C-peptide is present and an excellent incremental rise will occur after glucose stimulation.

When C-peptide assays became available, more was learned about insulin resistance in obesity and diabetes, and in 1979 the National Diabetes Data Group and World Health Organization tried to solve the problem of the heterogeneity of diabetes by classifying diabetes into two major categories: type I or insulin-dependent diabetes mellitus (IDDM), and type II or noninsulin-dependent diabetes mellitus (NIDDM).[7] It was suggested that patients with type II diabetes did not develop ketosis under ordinary circumstances, although they could require insulin for treatment. The terms, type I and type II diabetes mellitus, are now used in spoken as well as written communication in almost all studies concerning diabetes. This is unfortunate because the clinical descriptive terms, IDDM and NIDDM, equated with the designation type I and type II diabetes, respectively, have strong implications regarding both pathogenesis and therapy. For example, diabetic patients known as type II can become insulin-dependent under normal circumstances. Whether these patients have specific human lymphocyte antigens or islet cell antibodies more typical of type I diabetes, or if they have a more severe form of type II diabetes, is unclear and needs further study. Regardless, we have come to realize that middle-aged obese patients can first appear in diabetic ketoacidosis without any provoking event.

Our studies and those by Hoekstra and co-workers demonstrated these points.[6,12] Depicted in Figure 9-10 are the C-peptide responses after glucagon stimulation in four groups of patients.[6] The top panels illustrate that both nonobese NIDDM (NONIDDM) and obese NIDDM (ONIDDM) patients who were not receiving insulin had good basal amounts of C-peptide that rose after intravenous glucagon was given. The bottom two C-peptide curves represent a group of patients who were receiving insulin. The left lower panel represents young IDDM diabetics who were virtually absent in C-peptide before and after stimulation. The lower right-hand panel represents 16 patients who were middle-aged and obese, developed their diabetes late in life, and were receiving insulin. They are designated OIDDM? (obese IDDM?). The top

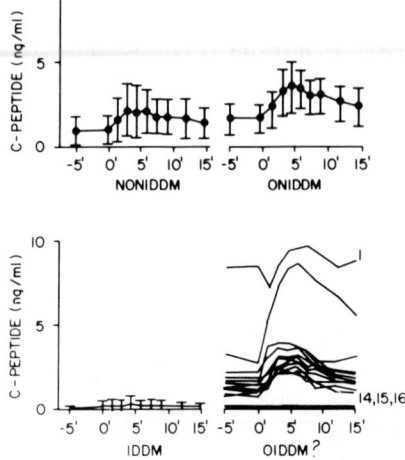

Figure 9-10. C-peptide responses after glucagon stimulation in four groups of patients. (Reproduced with permission from Hoekstra JBL, Van Rijn HJM, Thijssen JHH et al: C-peptide reactivity as a measure of insulin dependency in obese diabetic patients treated with insulin. Diabetes Care 5:585–591, 1982)

patient probably had antibodies to proinsulin. Thirteen of the 16 patients had good C-peptide responses; however, patients 14, 15, and 16 had no C-peptide response. When insulin was stopped in these subjects, beta hydroxy butyric acid rose only in patients 14 and 15. In fact, ketoacidosis ensued and insulin had to be given. These same two subjects had no rise in C-peptide after glucagon (patient 16 did not participate). Thus, in this study it appears that some obese middle-aged diabetics need insulin for prevention of ketoacidosis.

In this regard, we studied the C-peptide responses after glucose in 14 phenotypic type II diabetics treated with insulin. Table 9-3 lists the characteristics of two groups of these patients. One group had spontaneous ketonuria unrelated to stress and the other group did not. Ketones were defined as at least small on an acetest table under basal conditions in the outpatient clinic. Both the ketonuric and nonketonuric groups were similar with regard to age, obesity, duration of diabetes, duration and dose of insulin therapy, and poor glucose control (fasting blood sugars were approximately 300 in both groups).

Figure 9-11 shows C-peptide responses after a glucose challenge. Glucose levels were no different after a glucose tolerance test in the ketonuric group compared with the nonketonuric group, with both indicating poor control. C-peptide responses, however, were low, both in the fasting state and after stimulation in the ketonuric group compared with the nonketonuric group. These data indicate that some type II diabetic patients are insulinopenic and may require insulin for prevention of ketoacidosis, ketosis, and even survival. It is doubtful, however, that C-peptide alone can

Table 9-3

Clinical Characteristics of Obese, Insulin-treated Type II Diabetes Mellitus Patients

Patients	Ketonuric (n = 6)	Nonketonuric (n = 8)
Age (yr)	58±3	62±5
Percent IBW*	133±5	139±5
Duration of diabetes (yr)	11.7±0.5	11.8±1.0
Duration of insulin	8±2	7.7±1.1
Daily insulin (units)	50±5	56±7
FBS† (mg/dl)	320±14	300±20
HbA$_1$C‡ (%)	11.7±0.8	10.5±1.7

Values are $\bar{X}$ + SEM.
*IBW = Initial body weight.
†FBS = Fasting blood sugar.
‡HbA$_1$C = Hemoglobin A$_1$C.

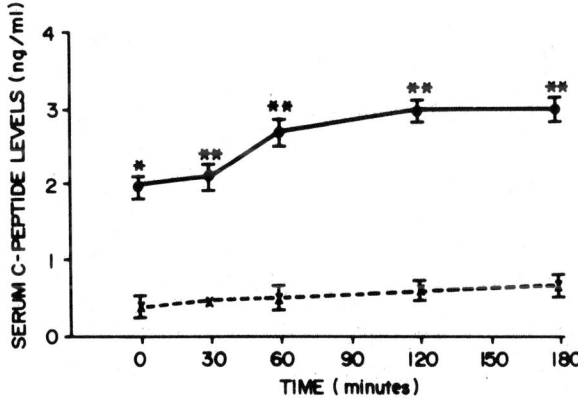

Figure 9-11. C-peptide responses after a glucose tolerance test in "ketonuric" Type II diabetics (denoted by x's) compared with "nonketonuric" Type II diabetes (denoted by closed circles). Asterisks indicate significant differences. Glucose responses were identical in both groups. (Reproduced with permission from Osei K, Falko JM, O'Dorisio TM et al: Significance of spontaneous ketonuria and serum C-peptide levels in obese Type II diabetic patients. Diabetes Care 7:442–447, 1984)

determine which patient will respond to which therapy in type II diabetes. This is, again, because of the heterogeneous nature of the disease and the fact that insulin secretory capacity and insulin resistance are both important determinates of glucose levels and stability. These data, however, indicate that individualization of therapy should be done in all patients diagnosed as type II diabetics.

SUMMARY

Type II diabetes remains a heterogeneous disease with the central common denominator of hyperglycemia. As more is learned about its pathophysiology, better practical management strategies need to be developed. The standard oral agents or insulin may be supplemented by variations of combination therapy. Future directions may include the use of proinsulin or new oral agents with different mechanisms of action such as the newer biguanides, which are currently under investigation.

REFERENCES

1. Bierman EL, Wood FC Jr: Is diet the cornerstone in management of diabetes? N Engl J Med 315:1224–1227, 1986
2. Council on Nutrition of the American Diabetes Association: Glycemic effects of carbohydrates. Diabetes Care 7:607–608, 1984
3. Falko JM, Crook D, McTaggart A et al: Differential effects of physiologic amounts of sucrose and fructose on lipoprotein and carbohydrate metabolism in type II diabetes. Clin Res 34:927A, 1986
4. Falko JM, O'Dorisio TM, Cataland S: Improvement of high density lipoprotein cholesterol levels in ambulatory type I diabetics treated with subcutaneous insulin pump. JAMA 247:37–39, 1982
5. Firth RG, Bell PM, Rizza RA: Effects of tolazamide and exogenous insulin action in patients with noninsulin-dependent diabetes mellitus. N Engl J Med 314:1280–1286, 1986
6. Hoekstra JBL, Van Rijn HJM, Thijssen JHH et al: C-peptide reactivity as a measure of insulin dependency in obese diabetic patients treated with insulin. Diabetes Care 5:585–591, 1982

7. National Diabetes Data Group: Classification and diagnosis of diabetes and other categories of glucose intolerance. Diabetes 28:1039–1057, 1979
8. Olefsky JM: Diabetes mellitus. In Wyngaarden JB, Smith LH (eds): Cecil Textbook of Medicine, 17th ed, pp. 1320–1339. Philadelphia, WB Saunders, 1985
9. Olefsky JM, Ciaraldi TP, Kolterman OB: Mechanisms of insulin resistance in noninsulin-dependent (type II) diabetes. Am J Med 75:12–21, 1985
10. Osei K, Falko M: Serum C-peptide levels determine glycemic responses in type II diabetics treated with combined insulin and sulfonylurea agents. Am J Med Sci 289:148–153, 1985
11. Osei K, Falko JM, Bossetti BM et al: Metabolic effects of fructose as a natural sweetener in the physiologic meals of ambulatory obese type II diabetic patients. Am J Med 83:249–255, 1987
12. Osei K, Falko J, O'Dorisio TM et al: Significance of spontaneous ketonuria and serum C-peptide levels in obese type II diabetic patients. Diabetes Care 7:442–447, 1984
13. Osei K, Falko JM, O'Dorisio TM et al: Gastric inhibitory polypeptide responses and glucose turnover rates after natural meals in type II diabetes. J Clin Endocrinol Metab 62:325–330, 1986
14. Osei K, O'Dorisio TM, Falko JM: Concomitant insulin and sulfonylurea therapy in patients with type II diabetes: Effects on glucoregulation and lipid metabolism. Am J Med 77:1002–1009, 1984
15. Polonsky K, Frank B, Pugh W: The limitation to and valid use of C-peptide as a marker of the secretion of insulin. Diabetes 35:379–386, 1986
16. Polonsky KS, Paixao J, Given BD et al: Use of biosynthetic human C-peptide in the measurement of insulin secretion rates in normal volunteers and type I diabetes patients. J Clin Invest 77:98–105, 1986
17. Rizza RA, Mandarino LJ, Genest J et al: Productions of insulin resistance by hyperinsulinemia in man. Diabetologia 78:70–75, 1985
18. Tzagournis M, Falko JM: Heart disease and cerebrovascular complications in diabetes. In Bleicher SJ, Brodoff BN (eds): Diabetes Mellitus and Obesity, pp. 741–767. Baltimore, Williams & Wilkins, 1982
19. Yalow RS, Berson SA: Immunoassay of endogenous plasma insulin in man. J Clin Invest 39:1157–1166, 1960

CHAPTER TEN
Diabetic Neuropathy
William T. Cefalu
Rex S. Clements, Jr.

The classification of diabetic neuropathies should be based on their presumed pathophysiologic basis. The mononeuropathies multiplex, both the peripheral and cranial neuropathies, are thought to have a vascular etiology. They are presumed to be on an ischemic or localized ischemic basis. In contrast, distal polyneuropathy and the associated autonomic neuropathy are thought to be metabolic neuropathies. Finally, there is the mixed group of vascular and metabolic neuropathies characterized by the clinical condition known as diabetic amyotrophy. Ischemia probably has a dominant role in the mononeuropathies because they occur in older patients with diabetes, are acute in onset, and tend to be reversible within 6 months to a year, suggesting recanalization. In contrast, the metabolic neuropathies are thought to have a different basis.

The major types of neurodegeneration described include axonal degeneration in which the nerve is cut at one point, and has total degeneration distal to this point of transection. Early on it was thought that diabetic neuropathy was a form of segmental demyelination, a toxic type of neuropathy in which areas of loss of the axonal sheath occur and other areas remain relatively intact. Currently, the most popular hypothesis with regard to distal symmetric polyneuropathy is that it may, in fact, be an axonal-type degeneration, closer somewhat to axonal degeneration than segmental demyelination. In this disorder, because of some toxic effect on a nerve, in part determined by the length of the nerve, destruction of the axons occurs as well as degeneration distal to the point of total destruction. This may be caused by focal ischemic episodes culminating in death of an axon distal to a certain location.

PREVALENCE

The prevalence of this disease and its importance in our economy depend somewhat on which definition one chooses for diabetic neuropathy. Diabetic neuropathy consists of signs and symptoms of the disorder; some have stated that it consists of abnormal nerve conduction velocities, others include autonomic dysfunction tests in the definition. If we restrict the diagnosis to patients with typical signs (*i.e.*, loss of distal sensation and, perhaps, ankle jerk), about one quarter of all diabetic patients will have diabetic neuropathy. If we include symptoms with signs, the incidence rate rises to about a third of all patients. If one wishes to define it as abnormal nerve conduction velocities, however, 88% of all diabetic patients will have diabetic neuropathy. No patients with signs and symptoms of the disease will have normal nerve conduction velocities. Nerve conduction velocities, therefore, are not needed to make the diagnosis of diabetic neuropathy. If the patient has signs, symptoms, or both, the nerve conduction velocities will, by definition, be abnormal and will not aid in the diagnosis.

Depending on which definition is used, the prevalence in the United States would be from about 3 to 10 million patients. We prefer to use the signs and symptoms, in combination, to make this diagnosis. Based on this definition, roughly 4 million Americans are currently diagnosed with diabetic neuropathy. In terms of disability, it compares with other debilitating diseases such as rheumatoid arthritis. It is about ten times as prevalent as cystic fibrosis and 100 times as prevalent as multiple sclerosis.

CLINICAL PRESENTATION

The clinical presentation of diabetic neuropathy is familiar. Diabetic feet are easily recognized because of some loss of intertarsal musculature. As a consequence of that loss, a claw toe deformity results. The toes are cocked up; they tend to rub on the upper part of the shoe and cause ulceration at the top of the toes. In addition, the structure of the abnormality caused by the claw toe deformity causes the protective pad to move off of the metatarsal heads. The patient who has little or no feeling in the feet, therefore, is walking on metatarsal heads and will eventually wear a hole through the bottom of the foot. Total destruction of the bony articulations may occur, resulting in a Charcot foot. With extremely severe diabetic neuropathy, involvement of the upper extremities occurs, as well as distal loss of sensation and more proximal diminution of sensation, with obvious distal muscle weakness noted most markedly in the first web space. This patient would tend to drop things, be extremely clumsy with the hands, as well as experience generalized weakness of the hands.

Total absence of sensation occurs until a definite point is reached, reproducible within half a centimeter in any given patient, at which the patient suddenly goes from absence of sensation to diminished sensation. The disease begins with diminished pain and light touch sensation; progresses on to the neuropathic syndrome with burning and tingling, particularly worse at night, keeping the patient awake; and then loss of pain and light touch sensation, decreased vibration sensation, and diminished Achilles reflexes. Frequently, the patient will progress to pain and hyperesthesia, particularly in the lower extremities, and then proceed to absent Achilles reflexes, total loss of vibration sensation, total numbness in the distal extremities, and progressive muscle weakness, ataxia, and eventual formation of neuropathic ulcers. Most physicians do not make the diagnosis of diabetic neuropathy until the patient is well past the preclinical stage of the disease. These patients, therefore, are not referred to the neurologist until the late phases of the disease. Only during the early phases of diabetic neuropathy is this disease potentially preventable or reversible. By the time the patient is experiencing numbness, the physician is dealing with compensatory measures.

A corollary to the presumed natural history scheme is that there may be a threshold phenomenon with regard to neuropathic pain. With the onset of diabetes, nerve function is excellent; however, as diabetes progresses, neurofunction begins to deteriorate and at some point the patient may pass threshold in the bell-shaped portion of the curve. When nerve function deteriorates so that the patient is experiencing numbness, the pain will disappear. If diabetes were treated vigorously and in some way the treatment were to impair nerve function, the patient could go over the pain threshold.

A number of studies have been published regarding the relationship between diabetic control and nerve function. In a study from Brussels, about 4400 patients were reviewed over a period of 25 years; their glycemic control was compared with nerve function and assessed by symptoms and signs.[46] Neuropathy was found to occur in about 10% of the patients who were well controlled (all blood sugar levels under 200 for over 25 years), and did not appear to increase markedly over time. In the patients who were fairly well controlled (about half the blood sugar levels below 200 for over 25 years), about one third developed neuropathy. In patients with poor control, the majority (roughly two thirds) developed signs and symptoms of neuropathy over a period of 25 years, and this was a progressive phenomenon.

Pietri and co-workers[45] reported on a group of type I diabetic patients who were reasonably well controlled by our current standards (blood sugar levels averaged roughly 200 throughout the day, HgA$_1$C approximately 10.5%). Near-normal glucose profile was maintained in these patients with a preprogrammed, continuous, subcutaneous insulin infusion using an insulin pump. This form of therapy normalized the mean 24-hour plasma glucose (approximately 103 ± 8 mg/dl) with a markedly reduced glycated hemoglobin (approximately 6%). They found that the nerve conduction velocities increased significantly with short-term improvement in glycemic control in the median and peritoneal nerves compared to baseline values.

Graf and co-workers[21] addressed somewhat longer-term glycemic control in their 12-month study of a group of type II diabetic patients. A highly statistically significant inverse relationship was found between their blood glucose concentration, assessed with glycated hemoglobin, and nerve function, as measured by nerve conduction velocities.

The current literature cited above suggests a metabolic relationship to distal symmetric polyneuropathy. The question is, how do we study this metabolic phenomenon? Unfortunately, human nerves cannot be biopsied repeatedly, so studies have to be conducted in rats—not an ideal model for diabetic neuropathy, but a reasonable one. A study by Gabby[18] demonstrated when a young rat is made diabetic, the nerve conduction velocities do not increase at the same rate as in the nondiabetic rat. In other words, the normal age-related increase in nerve conduction velocities does not occur in the diabetic rat, but if insulin-therapy is started at 12 weeks of age, nerve conduction velocities can be completely restored to normal. The rat model, however, does not experience the same morphologic changes as do human diabetics. What mechanisms have been elucidated in the diabetic rat model? One mechanism is increased polyol activity, and another is an abnormality in *myo*-inositol metabolism in the nerve. A third potential abnormality is abnormal vascular structure and permeability. A fourth is abnormality in the neural thyroid hormone metabolism. Finally, it is possible that excessive formation of glycated protein products could have a role in the structural aspects of diabetic neuropathy.

POSTULATED MECHANISMS OF NEUROPATHY

Polyol Pathway

A mechanism that has been postulated to have a role in diabetic neuropathy is the polyol pathway. As can be seen in Figure 10-1, glucose is converted to sorbitol and then oxidized to D-fructose.[17] This pathway has been recognized as a constituent of mammalian peripheral nerve for nearly 30 years. The postulate that an abnormality in this pathway may contribute to diabetic complications was made popular by studies in the lens, showing a number of abnormalities in this tissue when sorbitol accumulates within the lens.[56] The mechanism by which this substrate was felt to cause the damage was through an osmotic process. Sorbitol was thought to be osmotically active and, therefore, pull water into the lens. This was postulated to interfere with the ability of the lens to maintain normal concentrations of electrolytes. Over periods of prolonged hyperglycemia, the lens was theoretically felt to swell and develop a mature cataract, the so-called sugar cataract. To apply this mechanism to the peripheral nerve, one first has to demonstrate that the polyol pathway is present in the nerve where the structural damage occurs. It is known that the induction of experimental diabetes in rodents will raise the neural concentrations of sorbitol.[17] By analogy to the lens, it has been proposed that the accumulation of sorbitol within the Schwann cell would result in water accumulation in an osmotic basis, and this osmotic stress could contribute to Schwann cell damage with subsequent demyelination.[17] More recent data have disputed this postulate. Instead of edema of the Schwann cell, the cytoplasm of this cell has been shown to be decreased in hyperglycemic states.[30] In addition, the

$$\text{D-Glucose} + \text{NADPH} + \text{H}^+ \xrightarrow{\text{Aldose Reductase}} \text{Sorbitol} + \text{NADP}^+$$

$$\text{Sorbitol} + \text{NAD}^+ \xrightarrow{\text{Sorbitol Dehydrogenase}} \text{D-Fructose} + \text{NADH} + \text{H}^+$$

Figure 10-1. Pathway of conversion of free glucose to sorbitol and further conversion to fructose. (Adapted from Gabby KH: The sorbitol pathway and the complications of diabetes. N Engl J Med 288(16):831–836, 1973)

water that does accumulate has been shown to be localized to the endoneural space. Because this accumulation of fluid can be prevented with aldose reductase inhibitors, it was felt to be a consequence of increased polyol pathway activity.

Recent studies have demonstrated that an increased sodium content (and pressure) exists in this endoneural space. The hypothesis proposed to explain this observation is that sodium may comigrate with glucose into the endoneural space and the established sodium gradient is maintained by neural metabolism of glucose (or galactose) via the polyol pathway.[44] Because increased polyol pathway activity results in a decrease in nerve sodium-potassium-ATPase activity, it is possible that the nerve exposed to hyperglycemia is unable to pump out sodium at a normal rate.[25]

The osmotic mechanism of diabetic neuropathy has not been substantiated, but mounting evidence exists to state that increased polyol pathway activity is involved in the biochemical abnormalities that lead to nerve damage. This finding is based on studies showing that treatment of the diabetic (or galactosemic) rodent with aldose reductase inhibitors will correct the abnormalities in motor nerve conduction velocities, axoplasmic transport, sodium-potassium-ATPase activity, oxygen uptake, as well as the increased water content and increased endoneural fluid pressure.[25,47,55] Similarly, use of aldose reductase inhibitors has been found to improve nerve conduction velocities slightly in humans with diabetic neuropathy.[16,66] An additional mechanism by which the increased polyol pathway activity may cause nerve damage is by interfering with the neural metabolism of *myo*-inositol phosphoinositides and inositol-phosphates. This has been suggested because virtually all of the functional abnormalities associated with increased polyol pathway activity can be prevented or reversed by dietary *myo*-inositol supplementation.

Inositol Hypothesis

For years it has been recognized that whenever an increase occurs in neural polyol pathway activity, a reciprocal decrease results in concentration of free *myo*-inositol within the peripheral nerve. This was not thought to be of physiologic significance until Green and his colleagues demonstrated that the abnormally lowered sciatic motor nerve conduction velocity of the rat with experimental diabetes could be corrected by dietary *myo*-inositol supplementation.[24] Because improvement in nerve function occurred in the presence of a persistently increased activity of the polyol pathway, and because aldose reductase inhibitors prevented the decrease in nerve *myo*-inositol content, it became clear that the abnormality in nerve *myo*-inositol metabolism was (at least in part) secondary to increased polyol pathway activity.[22,25,55] Currently it is thought that hyperglycemia lowers nerve *myo*-inositol content via two mechanisms. First, glucose competitively inhibits the sodium- and energy-dependent active transport of *myo*-inositol by the nerve.[22] Second, increased polyol pathway activity within the neural cells may induce the loss of *myo*-inositol from those cells.

One consequence of this decrease in cellular *myo*-inositol content is that it may limit the ability of the neurons to synthesize membrane phosphoinositides. It is now recognized that the phosphoinositides serve as reservoirs of potential signal molecules, which can transmit messages across the cell membrane.[39] When hydrolyzed by phosphoinositide-specific phospholipase C's, the phosphoinositides give rise to diacylglycerol and inositol phosphates. Further hydrolysis of diacylglycerol yields arachidonic acid, which can be converted into prostaglandins, thromboxanes, and leukotrienes. The breakdown of phosphoinositides is regulated by membrane lipid constituents (*e.g.*, diacylglycerol), calcium, and guanine nucleotide binding proteins. In response to electrical stimulations of nerve, a rapid hydrolysis of phosphoinositides occurs with production of diacylglycerol and inositol triphosphate.[39] The former stimulates protein kinase C activity, while the latter mobilizes intracellular calcium stores. Both phenomena tend to reinforce the hydrolysis of phosphoinositides and are instrumental in the orchestration of numerous intracellular processes. Obviously, an abnormality in the amount or rate of turnover of membrane phosphoinositides could have adverse effects on peripheral nerve function. That there is, in fact, a defective incorporation of *myo*-inositol into nerve phospholipids has been demonstrated in rats with experimental diabetes.[7]

Another function of the phosphoinositides is that they can serve as boundary- or regulatory-phospholipids for various membrane-associated enzymes. Following the induction of experimental diabetes, nearly a 50% decrease occurs in the activity of sodium-potassium-ATPase, which accounts for a 30% decrease in oxygen uptake by the nerve.[22] These abnormalities (plus the associated slowing of nerve conduction velocity) develop in parallel and are completely corrected in *in vivo* dietary *myo*-inositol supplementation. This suggests (but does not prove) that all of these abnormalities are linked to a defect in membrane phosphoinositide metabolism.

That a decrease is present in the *myo*-inositol and phosphatidylinositol content of human diabetic nerves has been shown by

Mayhew and co-workers.[42] The effect of dietary *myo*-inositol supplementation on peripheral nerve function in patients with diabetic neuropathy has been considerably less impressive than it has been in the rat. Some pilot studies have observed an improvement in peripheral nerve function after inositol feeding,[8,48] while others have not.[27] Additional long-term studies using larger groups of patients are needed before it can be concluded whether inositol feeding is a benefit in diabetic polyneuropathy.

Vascular Hypothesis

Another area of interest has been in the possibility that small ischemic episodes resulting from hyperglycemia could contribute to diabetic neuropathy. This was initially proposed by Fagerberg,[14] who raised the possibility that structural and functional changes involving the vasa nervorum could underlie the development of diabetic polyneuropathy. Light microscopic examination of sural nerve biopsies in patients with clinically obvious diabetic polyneuropathy showed a consistent thickening of the walls of neural arterioles, which was accompanied by an increased staining with the periodic acid Schiff's reagent. With these observations, he proposed that the nerves of patients with diabetic neuropathy may be deprived of nutrients, which leads to neural degeneration. Further, these studies speculated that fluctuations in the permeability of the intraneural vessels might be responsible for the reversible forms of diabetic neuropathy.

Although the vascular hypothesis has been overshadowed by research into metabolic causes of neural degeneration, recent studies using electron microscopy techniques have provided evidence that ischemic microvascular events may have a major role in the genesis of diabetic neural degeneration.[12,13,32] In addition, support for the vascular permeability hypothesis has been provided by studies demonstrating that when new blood vessels develop in a diabetic environment, they demonstrate excessive permeability to radiolabeled albumin.[36,62,64] Similarly, the retina, choroid, and sciatic nerve of the diabetic rat display increased permeability to albumin. These functional changes can be reversed by successful pancreatic islet transplantation and can be prevented with aldose reductase inhibitors, dietary *myo*-inositol supplementation, or castration in the male rat.[8,63] These abnormalities in vascular function can be postulated to lead to nerve damage; however, as yet, the responsible mechanisms have not been identified.

It has also been suggested that extravascular factors, along with phenomena in the lumen, could contribute to the pathogenesis of diabetic neuropathy. This has been suggested by the observation of platelet aggregates within the vasa nervorum of patients with diabetic peripheral neuropathy.[60] Also, as stated above, increased endoneural pressure secondary to increased polyol pathway activity in the rodent can be reversed by administration of aldose reductase inhibitors.[44] An increase in endoneural fluid pressure is thought to decrease nerve blood flow and contribute to nerve fiber damage.[38]

Nonenzymatic Glycation

Another mechanism put forth as a cause for diabetic neuropathy has been that of nonenzymatic glycation. The nonenzymatic glycation reaction can result in sugar-protein adducts, which are described as being early or advanced glycation products. The reaction begins in all cases with glucose attachment to protein amino groups with formation of a Schiff base (Fig. 10-2).[9] The labile Schiff base rearranges and accumulation of a stable, but chemically

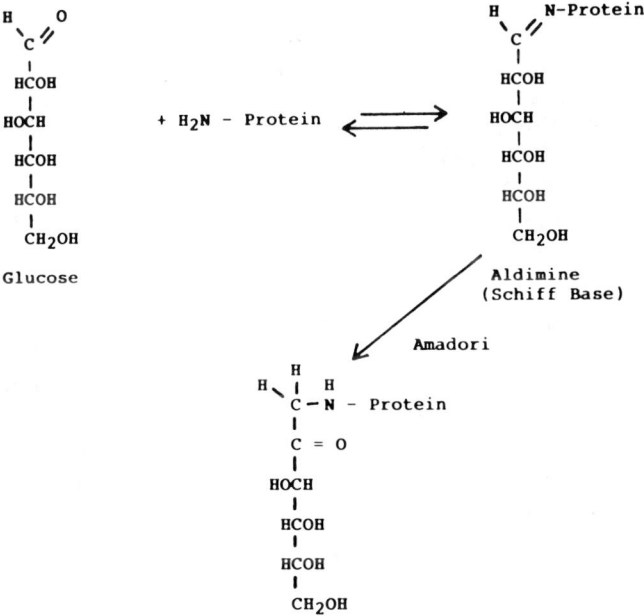

Figure 10-2. Reaction pathway for nonenzymatic glycation of protein. (Adapted from Cohen MP [ed]: Diabetes and Protein Glycosylation: Measurement and Biologic Relevance, p. 6. New York, Springer–Verlag, 1986)

reversible, amadori product occurs. Over weeks, equilibrium is attained, resulting in a constant steady-state level of the measured amadori products. Structural proteins (*i.e.*, myelin), whose half-lives are greater than the time required to reach steady-state amounts of the amadori product, accumulate advanced, or posta-madori, nonenzymatic glycation products. These advanced products participate in protein-protein cross-linkings, which are postulated to contribute to the pathogenesis of diabetic complications.[3]

The role of glycation in the genesis of diabetic neuropathy was felt to revolve around the formation of glycated myelin. Research has demonstrated that in diabetic rats compared to controls a fivefold increase occurs in the amount of glycated myelin.[58] In addition, it has been shown that the glycated myelin may be recognized by specific receptors and endocytosed by macrophages.[57] Importance of the finding has been demonstrated in peripheral nerves of diabetic rodents,[4] and it is postulated that this same process could contribute to the segmental demyelination seen in human diabetic neuropathy.

An additional mechanism implicating nonenzymatic glycation in the pathogenesis of diabetic neuropathy is that of "trapping" soluble proteins such as immunoglobulin G and M by vascular tissue. Because diabetic endoneural capillaries are excessively permeable to plasma proteins,[51] it is not surprising to find increases of 14-fold and 4-fold, respectively, for trapped IgM and IgG on the peripheral nerve myelin of human diabetic subjects.[2] The presence of such trapped immunoglobulin would render the nerve susceptible to classic immunologic attack with resultant cell damage.

A third mechanism related to nonenzymatic glycation and the pathogenesis of diabetic complications relates to the structural and functional consequences on tubulin, a microtubular component participating in neurosecretion and axonal transport. Research has demonstrated that *in vitro* glycation of rat brain tubulin inhibits its GTP-dependent polymerization and renders it insoluble.[61] This excess glycation of tubulin is postulated to occur *in vivo* in hyperglycemic states and result in impaired axonal transport observed in experimental diabetes.

Hormonal Hypothesis

Finally, evidence exists to support the concept of a significant hormonal role in development of diabetic neuropathy—namely, male sex steroids, thyroxine, and insulin. First, castration of male diabetic rats has been shown to prevent the decrease in collagen solubility and increase in vascular permeability normally seen in the diabetic state. Castration, however, was shown to have no effect on nonenzymatic glycation of protein.[65] Thyroid hormone metabolism is linked to diabetic neuropathy in that diabetic and hypothyroid peripheral neuropathies have similar histologic and clinical effects. Also, thyroid hormone treatment was shown to normalize the motor nerve conduction velocities, sodium-potassium-ATPase activity, as well as the free- and lipid-bound inositol concentrations of the streptozotocin-induced diabetic rat.[6] The ideal hormonal manipulation would be use of insulin in an intensive treatment regimen (*i.e.*, multiple daily injections of insulin, or the insulin pump regimen) in an effort to normalize the glucose profile.

We have proposed numerous mechanisms for the pathogenesis of diabetic neuropathy, but all of the proposed mechanisms require a hyperglycemic environment. Establishment of a euglycemic state, therefore, would be postulated to prevent diabetic complications. Because normalizing the glucose profile is not always possible for the brittle diabetic, research into agents that can prevent or reverse this complication offers hope in this area.

TREATMENT

From the above, one can begin to appreciate the role that hyperglycemia has been postulated to have in the genesis of diabetic neuropathy. A goal of euglycemia, therefore, should be the cornerstone of treatment for the diabetic with early peripheral neuropathy. Although ongoing, large-scale studies (*e.g.*, The Diabetes Control and Complication Trial [DCCT])[53] sponsored by the National Institutes of Health will provide much needed direct evidence to answer the questions regarding glycemic control and diabetic neuropathy.

A relationship between the duration of diabetes and improvement in motor nerve conduction velocities after therapy has been established with clinical studies.[26,45,52,59] An intensive insulin regimen (*i.e.*, multiple daily injections of regular insulin or an insulin pump regimen), therefore, would be recommended to normalize the glucose profile. The continuous subcutaneous insulin infusion has been favored because preliminary studies have shown significant improvement in nerve conduction velocities and vibratory thresholds after 8 months of treatment compared to conventional insulin treatment.[50] Regardless of which regimen is used, a useful clinical monitor assessing glycemic status is use of the glycated hemoglobin assay. This assay has become the "gold standard" among physicians caring for diabetics in assessing glycemic control. This assay relies on nonenzymatic glycation of the hemoglobin of the red blood cell. This reaction relies on two factors clinically: degree and duration of the hyperglycemia and the half-life of the protein in question. For the red blood cell with a half-life of 45 days to 90 days, the glycated hemoglobin assay will reflect glycemic control over the previous 2 to 3 months. With this objective test, the ideal goal would be to control the patient such that his glycated hemoglobin is in the normal range, assuring both the patient and physician that a normal glycemic profile has been obtained.

A second aspect of treatment may revolve around use of the aldose reductor inhibitors. Several clinical trials have demonstrated a favorable, although small, response with these agents.[29,34,37] The agents studied thus far are alrestatin, sorbinil, tolrestat, and most recently, statil. These drugs are known to have different potencies, half-lives, and side-effects. Along these lines, the enzyme aldose reductase is present in many tissues not known to be affected by the diabetic state including brain, placenta, muscle, seminal vessels, and erythrocytes[40]; therefore, the long-term effects of these agents in these tissues are unknown. This underscores the tremendous problem in extrapolating animal data to human subjects when discussing aldose reductase effectiveness for peripheral neuropathy.

Alrestatin, the earliest aldose reductase inhibitor, has considerable toxicity and has had conflicting reports regarding its effectiveness.[10,19,28] Sorbinil, a spirohydantoin, has been effective in preventing cataract formation in diabetic animals and has been shown to have some effectiveness in improving motor nerve conduction velocity in diabetic rats. Human studies with use of sorbinil have shown an improvement in subjective symptoms of pain and paresthesia, and in nerve conduction velocities.[33] Other studies have commented on the reported effectiveness of this agent in peripheral neuropathy.[5,15,31,37] Sorbinil, however, is not without reported side effects such as an immune-complex mediated macular-erythematous rash, pancytopenia, and lymphadenopathy, usually appearing 6 days to 14 days after starting therapy and disappearing with drug cessation.[31] Tolrestat, the newest aldose reductase inhibitor, has shown promise in symptomatic diabetic neuropathy with improved nerve conduction.[1,54] It was reported, however, in a recent multicenter study, to have been associated with reversible elevation of liver enzyme levels. It should be noted that, at present, none of the aldose reductase inhibitors are approved for use in the United States.

An area of great interest in the treatment of diabetic neuropathy is dietary myoinositol supplementation; however, the data have been inconclusive.[8,27,48] Nevertheless, studies have demonstrated that significant clinical improvement may occur with these agents in the presence of a minimal change in nerve conduction velocity.[23] Still, more data are needed before recommendations can be made regarding dietary myoinositol supplementation.

All of the interventions addressed above are based on various hypotheses of the cause of neuropathy (*i.e.*, nonenzymatic glycation, inositol hypothesis, polyol pathway). On a clinical level, however, the practicing physician is faced with the treatment for symptomatic painful diabetic neuropathy. This aspect of treatment is probably the most difficult and represents an area of frustration for both the health-care professional and patient. Along these lines, use of a combination of phenothiazines and antidepressants, as widely used in the clinical arena, are not without conflicting reports of effectiveness.[11,20,43] There have been some promising results, however, with use of tricyclic drugs alone. "The beneficial effect of these agents in treating painful diabetic neuropathy has been suggested to be independent of mood elevation."[41] Phenytoin, which has been used clinically, should be discouraged not only because it was found to be of no significant value,[49] but because evidence exists to suggest an inhibitory effect on insulin secretion. A lidocaine infusion (5 mg/kg body weight) given under continuous cardiac monitoring may result in a significant improvement of pain lasting 3 days to 21 days in patients resistant to other treatments.[35]

Finally, narcotic analgesics are the final approach to treatment and should be used with caution because of the inherent problems. The neuropathic pain syndrome, however, is a debilitating aspect of diabetic neuropathy and control of the pain will markedly improve the patient's outcome.

A number of biochemical and structural abnormalities are known to culminate in the development of diabetic neuropathy. If we wish to treat this disorder, it appears rational to approach it early before it has gotten into the structural phase and is still in the reversible metabolic phase. It is hoped that over the next decade there will be an additional half dozen mechanisms we can approach pharmacologically.

REFERENCES

1. Boulton AJ: Effects of Tolrestat, a new aldose reductase inhibitor, on nerve conduction and paresthetic symptoms in neuropathy. Diabetologia 29:521A, 1986
2. Brownlee M, Vlassara H, Cerami A: Trapped immunoglobulins on peripheral nerve myelin from patients with diabetes mellitus. Diabetes 35:999–1003, 1986
3. Brownlee M, Vlassara H, Cerami A: Nonenzymatic glycosylation and the pathogenesis of diabetic complications. Ann Intern Med 101:527–537, 1985
4. Carson KA, Bossen EH, Hanker JS: Peripheral neuropathy in mouse heredity diabetes mellitus. Neuropathol Appl Neurobiol 6:361–374, 1980
5. Christensen JE, Varnek L, Gregersen G: The effect of an aldose reductase inhibitor (Sorbinil) on diabetic neuropathy and neural function of the retina: A double-blind study. Acta Neurol Scand 71:164–167, 1985
6. Clements RS, Kassira W, Garcia AR et al: Thyroid status and nerve function in experimental diabetes. Diabetes 35:105A, 1986
7. Clements RS, Stockard CR: Abnormal sciatic nerve *myo*-inositol metabolism in the streptozotocin-diabetic rat: Effect of insulin treatment. Diabetes 29:227–235, 1980
8. Clements RS Jr, Vourganti B, Kuba T et al: Dietary *myo*-inositol intake and peripheral nerve function in diabetic neuropathy. Metabolism 28(Suppl 1):477–483, 1979
9. Cohen MP (Ed): Diabetes and Protein Glycosylation: Measurement and Biologic Relevance. New York, Springer-Verlag, 1986
10. Culebras A, Alio J, Herrera JL et al: Effect of an aldose reductase inhibitor on diabetic peripheral neuropathy: Preliminary report. Arch Neurol 38:133–134, 1981
11. Davis JL, Lewis SB, Gerich JE et al: Peripheral diabetic neuropathy treated with amitriptyline and fluphenazine. JAMA 238:2291–2292, 1977
12. Dyck PJ, Karnes JL, O'Brien P et al: The spatial distribution of fiber loss in diabetic polyneuropathy suggests ischemia. Ann Neurol 19:440–449, 1986
13. Dyck PJ, Lais A, Karnes JL et al: Fiber loss is primary and multifocal in sural nerves in diabetic polyneuropathy. Ann Neurol

14. Fagerberg SE: Diabetic neuropathy: A clinical and histological study on the significance of vascular affections. Acta Med Scand 164(Suppl 345):1-80, 1959
15. Fagius J, Brattbery A, Jameson S et al: Limited benefit of treatment of diabetic polyneuropathy with an aldose reductase inhibitor: A 24-week controlled trial. Diabetologia 28:323–329, 1985
16. Fagius J, Jameson S: Effects of aldose reductase inhibitor treatment in diabetic polyneuropathy: A clinical and neurophysiological study. J Neurol Neurosurg Psychiatr 44:991–1001, 1981
17. Gabby KH: The sorbitol pathway and the complications of diabetes. N Engl J Med 288(16):831–836, 1973
18. Gabby KH: Role of the sorbitol pathway in neuropathy. In Camerini-Davalos RA, Cole HS (eds): Vascular and Neurological Changes in Early Diabetes, pp 417–424. New York, Academic Press, 1972
19. Gabby KH, Spack N, Loo S et al: Aldose reductase inhibition: Studies with alrestatin. Metabolism 28(4 Suppl 1):471–476, 1979
20. Gomez-Perez FJ, Rull JA, Dies H et al: Nortriptyline and fluphenazine in the symptomatic treatment of diabetic neuropathy: A double-blind cross-over study. Pain 23:395-400, 1985
21. Graf RJ, Halter JB, Pfiefer MA et al: Glycemic control and nerve conduction abnormalities in non-insulin dependent diabetic subjects. Ann Intern Med 94:307–311, 1981
22. Green DA: A sodium-pump defect in diabetic peripheral nerve corrected by sorbinil administration: Relationship to *myo*-inositol and nerve conduction slowing. Metabolism 35(Suppl 1):60–65, 1986
23. Green DA, Brown MJ, Braunstein SN et al: Comparison of clinical course and sequential electrophysiological tests in diabetics with symptomatic polyneuropathy and its implications for clinical trials. Diabetes 30:139–147, 1981
24. Green DA, DeJesus PV, Winegrad AI: Effects of insulin and dietary *myo*-inositol on impaired peripheral motor nerve conduction velocity in acute streptozotocin diabetes. J Clin Invest 55:1326–1336, 1975
25. Green DA, Lattimer SA: Action of sorbinil in diabetic peripheral nerve: Relationship of polyol (sorbitol) pathway to a *myo*-inositol mediated defect in sodium-potassium ATPase activity. Diabetes 33:712–716, 1984

26. Gregersen G: Variations in motor conduction velocity produced by acute changes in metabolic state in diabetic patients. Diabetologia 4:273–277, 1968
27. Gregersen G, Borsting H, Theil P et al: Myoinositol and function of peripheral nerve in human diabetics: A controlled clinical trial. Acta Neurol Scand 58:21–28, 1978
28. Handelsman DJ, Turtle JR: Clinical trial of an aldose reductase inhibitor in diabetic neuropathy. Diabetes 30:459–464, 1981
29. Harati Y, Niakan E, Comstock J et al: Aldose reductase inhibitor (tolrestat) therapy in patients with diabetic peripheral neuropathy. Ann Neurol 22:129(A), 1987
30. Jakobsen J: Axon dwindling in early experimental diabetes: A study of cross-sectioned nerves. Diabetologia 12:539–546, 1976
31. Jaspan JB, Towle LV, Maselli R et al: Clinical studies with an aldose reductase inhibitor in the autonomic and somatic neuropathies of diabetes. Metabolism 35(4 Suppl 1):83–92, 1986
32. Johnson PC, Doll SC, Cromey DW: Pathogenesis of diabetic neuropathy. Ann Neurol 19:450–457, 1986
33. Judzewitsch RG, Jaspan JB, Polonsky KS et al: Aldose reductase inhibition improves nerve conduction velocity in diabetic patients. N Engl J Med 308:119–125, 1983
34. Kador PF, Kinoshita JH, Sharpless E: Aldose reductase inhibitors: A potential new class of agents for the pharmacological control of certain diabetic complications. J Med Chem 28:841–849, 1985
35. Katstrup J, Petersen P, Dejgard A et al: Intravenous lidocaine infusion—a new treatment of chronic painful diabetic neuropathy? Pain 28:69–75, 1987
36. Kilzer P, Chang K, Marvel J et al: Albumin permeation of new vessels is increased in diabetic rats. Diabetes 34:333–336, 1985
37. Lewin IG, O'Brien IA, Morgan MH et al: Clinical neurophysiological studies with the aldose reductase inhibitor, sorbinil, in sympotomatic diabetic neuropathy. Diabetologia 26:445–448, 1984
38. Low PA, Dyck PJ, Schmelzer JD: Chronic elevation of endoneurial pressure is associated with low-grade pathology. Muscle Nerve 5:162–165, 1982
39. Majerus PW, Connolly TM, Deckmyn H et al: The metabolism of phosphoinositide-derived messenger molecules. Science 234:1519–1526, 1986
40. Malone JI, Leavengood H, Peterson MJ et al: Red blood cell sorbitol as an indicator of polyol pathway activity: Inhibition by

sorbinil in insulin-dependent diabetic subjects. Diabetes 33:45–49, 1984
41. Max MD, Culinane M, Schafer SC et al: Amitriptyline relieves diabetic neuropathy pain in patients with normal or depressed mood. Neurology 37:589–596, 1987
42. Mayhew JA, Gillon KRW, Hawthorne JN: Free and lipid inositol, sorbitol and sugars in sciatic nerve obtained post-mortem from diabetic patients and control subjects. Diabetologia 24:13–15, 1983
43. Mendel CM, Klein RF, Chappell DA et al: A trial of amitriptyline and fluphenazine in the treatment of painful diabetic neuropathy. JAMA 255:637–639, 1986
44. Mizisin AP, Powell HC, Meyers RR: Edema and increased endoneurial sodium in galactose neuropathy: Reversal with an aldose reductase inhibitor. J Neurol Sci 74:35–43, 1986
45. Pietri A, Ehle AL, Raskin P: Changes in nerve conduction velocity after six weeks of glucoregulation with portable insulin infusion pumps. Diabetes 29:668–671, 1980
46. Pirart J: Diabetes mellitus and its degenerative complications: Prospective study of 4,400 patients observed between 1948 and 1973. Diabetes Care 1:168–188, 1978
47. Robinson WG: Aldose reductase and diabetic neuropathy. In Cogan DG (Mod): Aldose reductase and complications of diabetes. Ann Intern Med 101:82–91, 1984
48. Salway JG, Whitehead L, Finnegan JA et al: Effect of *myo*-inositol on peripheral-nerve function in diabetes. Lancet 2:1282–1284, 1978
49. Saudek CD, Werns S, Reidenberg MM: Phenytoin in the treatment of diabetic symmetrical polyneuropathy. Clin Pharmacol Ther 22:196–199, 1977
50. Service FJ, Rizza RA, Daube JR et al: Near normoglycemia: Improved nerve conduction and vibration sensation in diabetic neuropathy. Diabetologia 28:722–727, 1985
51. Takekazn O, Poduslo JF, Dyck PJ: Increased endoneurial albumin in diabetic polyneuropathy. Neurology 35:1790–1791, 1985
52. Terkildsen AB, Christensen NJ: Reversible nervous abnormalities in juvenile diabetics with a recently diagnosed diabetes. Diabetologia 7:113–117, 1971
53. The DCCT Research Group: The Diabetes Control and Complications Trial: Design and methodologic considerations for the feasibility phase. Diabetes 35:530–545, 1986
54. The Tolrestat in Painful Neuropathy Study Group: Objective (nerve conduction) and subjective (painful symptom) improve-

ment in diabetic neuropathy following administration of Tolrestat, a new aldose reductase inhibitor. Diabetologia 29:588(A), 1986
55. Tomlinson DR, Holmes PR, Mayer JH: Reversal by treatment with an aldose reductase inhibitor of impaired axonal transport and motor nerve conduction velocity in experimental diabetes mellitus. Neurosci Lett 31:189–193, 1982
56. Van Heyningen R: Formation of polyols by the lens of the rat with "sugar" cataract. Nature (Lond) 184:194–195, 1959
57. Vlassara H, Brownlee M, Cerami A: Recognition and uptake of human diabetic peripheral nerve myelin by macrophages. Diabetes 34:553–557, 1985
58. Vlassara H, Brownlee M, Cerami A: Excessive nonenzymatic glycosylation of peripheral and central nervous system components in diabetic rats. Diabetes 32:670–674, 1983
59. Ward JD, Barnes CG, Fisher DJ et al: Improvement in nerve conduction following treatment in newly diagnosed diabetic patients. Lancet 1:428–431, 1971
60. Williams E, Timperley WR, Ward JD et al: Electron microscopical studies of vessels in diabetic peripheral neuropathy. J Clin Pathol 33:462–470, 1980
61. Williams SK, Howarth NL, Devenny JJ et al: Structural and functional consequences of increased tubulin glycosylation in diabetes mellitus. Proc Natl Acad Sci 79:6546–6550, 1982
62. Williamson JR, Chang K, Rowald E et al: Islet transplants in diabetic Lewis rats prevent and reverse diabetes-induced increases in vascular permeability and prevent but do not reverse collagen solubility changes. Diabetologia 29:392–396, 1986
63. Williamson JR, Chang K, Rowald E et al: Diabetes-induced increases in vascular permeability are prevented by castration and by sorbinil. Diabetes 34:108(A), 1985
64. Williamson JR, Chang K, Rowald E et al: Sorbinil prevents diabetes-induced increases in vascular permeability but does not alter collage cross-linking. Diabetes 34:703–705, 1985
65. Williamson JR, Rowald E, Chang K et al: Sex steroid-dependency of diabetes-induced changes in polyol metabolism, vascular permeability and collagen cross linking. Diabetes 35:20–27, 1986
66. Young RD, Ewing DJ, Clarke BF: A controlled trial of sorbinil, an aldose reductase inhibitor, in chronic painful diabetic neuropathy. Diabetes 32:938–942, 1983

CHAPTER ELEVEN
Drugs That Affect the Hemorrheologic Properties of Blood
Brian W. King

Diabetes is a disease associated with adverse effects throughout the cardiovascular system, including the blood itself. Historically, the effects of diabetes on development of atherosclerosis have long been suspected, while additional problems associated with the microcirculation and blood have only recently been appreciated. This chapter summarizes the interactions between blood and blood vessels in diabetics and reviews the drugs available or under investigation that can alter these interactions.

HEMORRHEOLOGY IN DIABETICS

Hemorrheology is the study of the flow properties of blood. A comprehensive review of hemorrheology in diabetics is contained in Chapter 1.

Diabetes is associated with a number of alterations in the flow of blood and in the interactions between blood components and the vascular endothelium. Whole blood viscosity is increased in diabetics and may be positively correlated to microvascular complications.[3] Most of the factors affecting whole blood viscosity are also altered by diabetes, including an increase in fibrinogen levels and enhanced platelet aggregation.[22,32] Perhaps best-studied are the changes in erythrocytes (red blood cells) that occur in diabetics. Red blood cells from diabetics are less flexible and aggregate more readily, potentially leading to higher whole blood viscosity and reduced microcirculatory flow.[18] Furthermore, diabetic red blood cells have altered cell membranes, which can cause adherence to endothelial cells.[43] The result may be further reduction of microcirculatory flow and, perhaps, an intrinsic role in the pathogenesis of diabetic vascular disease.[44]

DRUGS AFFECTING HEMORRHEOLOGY

A number of compounds have been developed that may alter the hemorrheologic properties of blood. In most cases, the hemorrheologic effect of a drug was discovered only after the compounds had been studied for various cardiovascular disorders. Table 11-1 summarizes the proposed mechanisms of action of the drugs discussed below.

PENTOXIFYLLINE

Pentoxifylline is the only drug currently available in the United States designated as a hemorrheologic drug. Although pentoxifylline is a substituted methylxanthine, its pharmacologic properties are distinctly different from those of the commonly encountered methylxanthines, caffeine and theophylline.[24] Briefly, pentoxifylline shows much less potency in producing "typical" methylxanthine effects, such as smooth muscle relaxation and central nervous system stimulation. The hemorrheologic effects of pentoxifylline in patients with peripheral arterial disease include reduction of elevated plasma fibrinogen levels;[38] decreased platelet aggregation, possibly caused by increased release of prostacyclin from endothelial cells;[34] increased red blood cell flexibility;[38] and reduced whole blood viscosity.[2] Pentoxifylline has recently been found to enhance leukocyte chemotaxis[21] and reduce the adherence of polymorphonucleocytes to endothelial cells.[4]

The precise mechanism of action of pentoxifylline has remained elusive, although the diverse pharmacologic effects of the drug point to an action on a second messenger. It has been suggested that the drug works by inhibition of phosphodiesterase, with a consequent increase in cyclic adenosine monophosphate in red blood cells. The lack of hemorrheologic activity of other known phosphodiesterase inhibitors such as theophylline, however, does not support this view. Recently, studies on the leukocyte effects of pentoxifylline have shown that the compound and certain congeners are modulators of interleukin-1 and tumor necrosis factor, two

Table 11–1
Mediator Blockade by Hemorrheologic Drugs

Drug	Calcium Channel	S-2 Serotonergic	H-1 Histaminergic	Alpha-adrenergic	Interleukin-1	Tumor Necrosis Factor
Pentoxifylline	– –	– –	– –	– –	+	+
Cinnarizine, flunarizine	+	– –	+	– –	– –	– –
Buflomedil	+/–	– –	– –	+	– –	– –
Naftidrofuryl	– –	+	– –	+/–	– –	– –
Ketanserin	– –	+	– –	– –	– –	– –

cytokines with numerous actions.[39] Should this prove to be the ultimate mechanism of action of pentoxifylline, a number of acute uses of the drug may be possible, especially septic and hemorrhagic shock. Animal studies in these areas have been encouraging.[30,45]

Regardless of the precise mechanism of action, pentoxifylline has been shown in double-blind placebo-controlled studies to improve walking distance in 50% to 70% of claudicants with chronic use,[26] and increase the oxygen tension in skeletal muscle affected by peripheral arterial disease.[14] Improved microcirculatory blood flow and, perhaps, increased polymorphonucleocyte chemotaxis, are probably responsible for the ability of pentoxifylline to aid in healing ischemic ulcers.[46] Other studies have shown that pentoxifylline may reduce proteinuria in diabetics and delay the advancement of retinopathy,[36] possibly by an increase in red blood cell flexibility.[33]

CALCIUM CHANNEL BLOCKERS

The calcium channel blockers are a diverse group of drugs that inhibit calcium entry into a variety of cells, often with some tissue specificity. Although some calcium channel blockers, such as nifedipine, have been used in vasospastic disorders, recent research indicates that other calcium channel blockers may have activity as hemorrheologic agents. The two drugs most studied in this regard are cinnarizine and a longer-acting congener, flunarizine. Neither drug is yet available in the United States.

Calcium ions can make red blood cells more rigid by inducing phosphorylation of spectrin, reducing the intracellular adenosine triphosphate concentration, and changing the cell membrane lipids. Although most calcium channel blockers probably have some hemorrheologic activity by way of an effect on red blood cells, cinnarizine and flunarizine are of particular interest because they have relatively little effect on the heart, but are potent in vascular beds and red blood cells.[15] Interestingly, these compounds are also histamine blockers.

Both compounds have been found to increase red blood cell flexibility and reduce whole blood viscosity in patients with peripheral arterial disease.[11] Although blood flow to the calf and walking distance were both improved in claudicants in one study,[29] the selective calcium antagonist nature of these compounds has caused them to be most studied for cerebrovascular disorders, including migraine. It appears unlikely that either drug will be available in the United States as a hemorrheologic agent suitable for use in diabetics with vascular disease in the near future.

BUFLOMEDIL

Buflomedil is a hemorrheologic drug that has some properties similar to pentoxifylline, yet is not a methylxanthine. *In vitro* and *in vivo*, buflomedil has been shown to increase the flexibility of red blood cells in diabetics without macroangiopathy.[10] The drug also causes inhibition of platelet aggregation by a mechanism unrelated to prostacyclin.[35] Although buflomedil does not reduce elevated fibrinogen levels, and hence plasma viscosity, whole blood viscosity is lowered because of the drug's actions on red blood cells and platelets in diabetic patients.[10]

The precise mechanism of action of buflomedil has not been elucidated. It is known that the drug is a rather weak alpha adrenoceptor antagonist,[42] which can, by an unknown mechanism, increase intracellular cyclic adenosine monophosphate and adenosine triphosphate in erythrocytes.[6] Of particular interest is the finding that, although oxygen metabolism is not affected by buflomedil in various tissues *in vitro*,[25] oxygen uptake is reduced significantly in dogs *in vivo*.[9] Further studies are required to determine if these observations signal a beneficial drug effect or an unwanted toxic effect.

One clinical study has demonstrated that buflomedil can increase walking distance in diabetic patients with intermittent claudication.[40] The efficacy of buflomedil in intermittent claudication appears to be comparable to that of pentoxifylline and better than naftidrofuryl.

NAFTIDROFURYL

Naftidrofuryl may have hemorrheologic properties, in addition to being a serotonin receptor blocker. A recent study of ten healthy women showed that the drug can increase red blood cell flexibility and blood flow in the carotid and femoral arteries, but no studies have been done to confirm this.[19] *In vitro*, naftidrofuryl is a competitive inhibitor of S2 serotonergic receptors and may also have some calcium channel blocking activity.[47] Clinically, naftidrofuryl has produced an increase in distance walked in the patient with claudication in a double-blind, placebo-controlled study.[1] The drug has not been investigated clinically in diabetic patients with vascular disease, however, and its ultimate clinical use in this patient group remains unknown.

KETANSERIN

Dormandy has suggested that serotonin released from platelets can reduce red blood cell flexibility, increase leukocyte "stickiness," and increase vascular permeability, resulting in impaired microcirculatory blood flow.[13] His hypothesis is based mostly on the fact that competitive serotonin inhibitors, such as naftidrofuryl and ketanserin, are able to affect the rheology of blood.

Ketanserin is a drug that has been most studied as an antihypertensive and a laboratory tool to block serotonergic receptors. From a hemorrheologic standpoint, however, ketanserin blocks serotonin-induced platelet aggregation and increases red blood cell flexibility.[17,48] Clinically, the drug has been found to produce large increases in blood flow to the feet of diabetic patients when given intravenously, an effect measured with a pulse volume plethysmograph.[31] The authors concluded that serotonin is a primary factor in reducing blood flow to the diabetic foot.

In patients with peripheral arterial disease, ketanserin has produced mixed reports in terms of increasing claudication distance. Double-blind, placebo-controlled trials have shown ketanserin to be better than,[12] equal to,[8] or worse than[5] placebo in improving claudication distance on a treadmill. It is possible that a reduction in perfusion pressure caused by the hypotensive action of ketanserin can overcome the beneficial hemorrheologic effect. While ketanserin shows promise for treatment of Raynaud's phenomenon[27] and hypertension,[16] its usefulness in treating the vascular complications of diabetes remains unproven.

FISH OIL

Recent interest in the possible ability of fish oil supplements to reduce serum lipids has also led to a number of investigations on the hemorrheologic changes induced by eicosapentaenoic acid, a component of fish oil. Clinical studies have shown that fish oil causes increased red blood cell flexibility, even in normal subjects,[28] and a reduction in whole blood viscosity in both normals and diabetics.[23] Results on platelet aggregation have been variable, but it seems likely that fish oil has little inhibitory effect.[20] Nevertheless, capillary blood flow velocity is increased.[7]

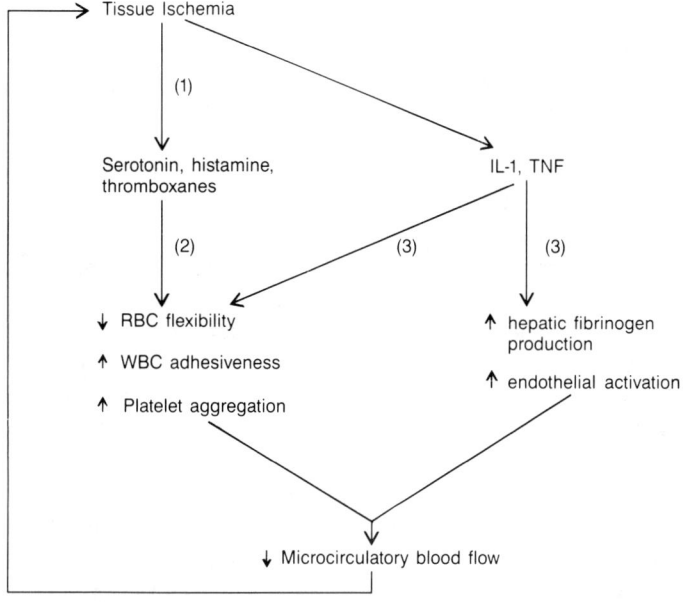

(1) Modulated by calcium channel blockers

(2) Modulated by buflomedil, naftidrofuryl, ketanserin

(3) Modulated by pentoxifylline

Figure 11-1. Flow chart showing possible sites of action of hemorrheologic drugs.

In rats, fish oil has been found to prevent insulin resistance induced by feeding a high-fat diet, an effect that, on the surface at least, would seem to make fish oil an attractive hemorrheologic treatment in diabetics.[37] Unfortunately, fish oil has also been found to cause hypercholesterolemia in type I diabetics, a result that severely limits the usefulness of this form of therapy in diabetics with vascular disease.[41]

SUMMARY

The drugs reviewed in this chapter have diverse mechanisms of action, which are seemingly unrelated. Vascular injury and ischemia, however, are associated with the release of cytokines and autocoids, which have profound effects on the cellular components of blood as well as on the vasculature. With the exception of fish oil, each of the hemorrheologic agents reviewed above is able to block one or more of the chemical mediators released by an ischemic event.

Figure 11-1 illustrates one possible mechanism by which this diverse group of hemorrheologic drugs could reduce tissue ischemia. In the absence of any drug, tissue ischemia produced by exercise or an acute thrombotic event might set up a vicious cycle in which the release of endogenous mediators in response to ischemia results in decreased erythrocyte flexibility; increased "stickiness" of white blood cells; platelet aggregation; increased hepatic fibrinogen production; and activation of the endothelium, which, in turn, inhibits microcirculatory blood flow, resulting in further tissue ischemia. Obviously, some gradation of response must be present to prevent ischemia from progressing immediately to microvascular stasis and tissue necrosis. In this scheme, calcium channel blockers could slow the cycle by diminishing release of the mediators (step 1), while the other drugs could block the effects of the released mediators.

Hemorrheologic drugs should provide definitive treatment in diabetic patients with vascular disease in whom surgery is contraindicated, or adjunctive therapy in the operated patient. Additional research in this area is aimed at further characterizing the precise mechanism of action of these drugs to select candidates for hemorrheologic therapy more appropriately.

REFERENCES

1. Adhoute G, Bacourt F, Barral M et al: Naftidrofuryl in chronic arterial disease. Results of a six month controlled multicenter study using naftidrofuryl tablets 200 mg. Angiology 37(3, Pt 1):160–167, 1986
2. Angelkort B, Spurk P, Habbaba A et al: Blood flow properties and walking performance in chronic arterial occlusive disease. Angiology 36:285–292, 1985
3. Barnes AJ, Locke P, Scudder PR et al: Is hyperviscosity a treatable component of diabetic microcirculatory disease? Lancet 2:789–791, 1977
4. Bertocchi F, Proserpio P, Dejana E: The effect of pentoxifylline on polymorphonuclear cell adhesion to cultured endothelial cells. A preliminary report. In Mandell GL, Novick WJ Jr (eds):

Pentoxifylline and Leukocyte Function. Somerville, NJ, Hoechst-Roussel Pharmaceuticals, 1988
5. Bounameaux H, Holditch T, Hellemans H et al. Placebo-controlled, double-blind, two-centre trial of ketanserin in intermittent claudication. Lancet 2(8467):1268–1271, 1985
6. Briguglio F, di Marco V, Circosta C et al: Metabolic effects of buflomedil hydrochloride. J Int Med Res 13:131–138, 1985
7. Bruckner G, Webb P, Greenwell L et al: Fish oil increases peripheral capillary blood cell velocity in humans. Atherosclerosis 66(3):237–245, 1987
8. Clement DL, Duprez D: Effect of ketanserin in the treatment of patients with intermittent claudication: Results from 13 placebo-controlled parallel group studies. J Cardiovasc Pharmacol 10(Suppl 3):S89–S95, 1987
9. Clissold SP, Lynch S, Sorkin EM: Buflomedil—A review of its pharmacodynamic and pharmacokinetic properties, and therapeutic efficacy in peripheral and cerebral vascular diseases. Drugs 33:430–460, 1987
10. Coccheri S, Palareti G, Poggi M et al: Improvements in the rheologic properties of blood induced by medium-term treatment with buflomedil in diabetic patients. J Int Med Res 10:394–398, 1982
11. De Cree J, De Cock W, Geukers H et al: The rheological effects of cinnarizine and flunarizine in normal and pathologic conditions. Angiology 30:505–515, 1979
12. De Cree J, Leempoels J, Geukers H et al: Placebo-controlled double-blind trial of ketanserin in treatment of intermittent claudication. Lancet 2(8406):775–779, 1984
13. Dormandy JA: Serotonin and haemorheology. Int J Cardiol 14:213–219, 1987
14. Ehrly AM: The effect of pentoxifylline on the muscle tissue oxygen pressure of claudicants after pedoergometic exercise. Angiology 37:398, 1986
15. Godfraind T: Classification of calcium antagonists. Am J Cardiol 59(3):11B–23B, 1987
16. Hansson L, Hedner T: The rationale for ketanserin therapy in hypertension. J Carviovasc Pharmacol 10(Suppl 3):S39–S44, 1987
17. Houston DS, Vanhoutte PM: Serotonin and the vascular system. Role in health and disease, and implications for therapy. Drugs 31(2):149–163, 1986
18. Jones RL, Peterson CM: Hematologic alterations in diabetes mellitus. Am J Med 70:339–352, 1981
19. Jung F, Kiesewetter H, Mrowietz C et al: Hemorrheological,

micro- and macrocirculatory effects of naftidrofuryl in an acute study: A randomized, placebo-controlled, double-blind individual comparison. Int J Clin Pharmacol 25(9):507–514, 1987

20. Knapp HR, Reilly IA, Alessandrini P et al: *In vivo* indexes of platelet and vascular function during fish-oil administration in patients with atherosclerosis. N Engl J Med 314(15):937–942, 1986
21. Krause PJ, Kristie J, Wang WP et al: Pentoxifylline enhancement of defective neutrophil function and host defense in neonatal mice. Am J Pathol 129(2):217–222, 1987
22. Lowe GDO, Lowe JM, Drummond MM et al: Blood viscosity in young male diabetics with and without retinopathy. Diabetologia 18:359–363, 1980
23. Miller ME, Anagnostou AA, Ley B et al: Effect of fish oil concentrates on hemorrheological and hemostatic aspects of diabetes mellitus: A preliminary study. Thromb Res 47(2):201–214, 1987
24. Muller R: Pentoxifylline—A biomedical profile. J Med 10:307–329, 1979
25. Paggi MG, Santis RD, Martino CD et al: Studies on buflomedil. J Exp Clin Cancer Res 3:29–37, 1984
26. Porter JM, Cutler BC, Lee BY et al: Pentoxifylline efficacy in the treatment of intermittent claudication: Multicenter controlled double-blind trial with objective assessment of chronic occlusive arterial disease patients. Am Heart J 104:66–72, 1982
27. Roald OK, Seem E: Treatment of Raynaud's phenomenon with ketanserin in patients with connective tissue disorders. Br Med J 289(6445):577–579, 1984
28. Rogers S, James KS, Butland BK et al: Effects of a fish oil supplement on serum lipids, blood pressure, bleeding time, haemostatic and rheologic variables. A double-blind randomized controlled trial in healthy volunteers. Atherosclerosis 63(2–3):137–143, 1987
29. Rudofsky G, Brock FE, Ulrich M et al: Clinical evaluation of flunarizine: Walking distance, ergometric performance and hemodynamic and biochemical effects. Angiology 30:470–479, 1979
30. Schade UF, Van Der Bosch J, Schonharting MM: Increase of survival rate by pentoxifylline in endotoxic shock. In Mandell GL, Novick WJ Jr (eds): Pentoxifylline and Leukocyte Function. Somerville, NJ, Hoechst-Roussel Pharmaceuticals, 1988
31. Schneider SH, Tendler M, Apelian A et al: Effects of ketan-

serin, a 5-HT2-receptor antagonist, on the blood flow response to temperature changes in the diabetic foot. J Clin Pharmacol 25(6):413–417, 1985
32. Sharma SC: Platelet adhesiveness, plasma fibrinogen, and fibrinolytic activity in juvenile-onset and maturity-onset diabetes mellitus. J Clin Pathol 34(5):501–503, 1981
33. Simpson LO: Intrinsic stiffening of red blood cells as the fundamental cause of diabetic nephropathy and microangiopathy: A new hypothesis. Nephron 39:344–351, 1985
34. Sinzinger H: Pentoxifylline enhances formation of prostacyclin from rat vascular and renal tissue. Prostaglandins Leukotrienes Med 12:217–226, 1983
35. Sinzinger H, Wirthumer-Hoche C: *In vitro* effects of buflomedil on parameters regulating hemostatic balance via the prostaglandin system. Vasa 14:71–73, 1985
36. Solerte SB, Ferrari E: Diabetic retinal vascular complications and erythrocyte filterability: Results of a 2-year follow-up study with pentoxifylline. Pharmatherapeutica 4:341–350, 1985
37. Storlien LH, Kraegen EW, Chisholm DJ et al: Fish oil prevents insulin resistance induced by high-fat feeding in rats. Science 237(4817):885–888, 1987
38. Strano A, Davi G, Avellone G et al: Double-blind, crossover study of the clinical efficacy and the hemorrheological effects of pentoxifylline in patients with occlusive arterial disease of the lower limbs. Angiology 35:439–446, 1984
39. Sullivan GW, Carper HT, Novick WJ et al: Pentoxifylline inhibits the inflammatory effects of endotoxin and endotoxin induced cytokines on neutrophil function. In Mandell GL, Novick WJ Jr (eds): Pentoxifylline and Leukocyte Function. Somerville, NJ, Hoechst-Roussel Pharmaceuticals, 1988
40. Trubestein G, Balzer K, Bisler H et al: Buflomedil in arterial occlusive disease: Results of a controlled multicenter study. Angiology 35(8):500–505, 1984
41. Vandongen R, Mori TA, Codde JP et al: Hypercholesterolaemic effect of fish oil in insulin-dependent diabetic patients. Med J Aust 148(3):141–143, 1988
42. Vanhoutte PM, Aarhus LL, Coen E et al: Effects of buflomedil on the responsiveness of canine vascular smooth muscle. J Pharmacol Exp Ther 227:613–620, 1983
43. Wali RK, Jaffe S, Kumar D et al: Alterations in organization of phospholipids in erythrocytes as factor in adherence to endothelial cells in diabetes mellitus. Diabetes 37:104–111, 1988

44. Wautier JL, Paton RC, Wautier MP et al: Increased adhesion of erythrocytes to endothelial cells in diabetes mellitus and its relation to vascular complications. N Engl J Med 305(5):237–242, 1981
45. Waxman K: Pentoxifylline and hemorrhagic shock: Experimental studies. In Mandell GL, Novick WJ Jr (eds): Pentoxifylline and Leukocyte Function. Somerville, NJ, Hoechst-Roussel Pharmaceuticals, 1988
46. Weitgasser H: The use of pentoxifylline (Trental 400) in the treatment of leg ulcers: Results of a double-blind trial. Pharmatherapeutica 3(Suppl 1):143–151, 1983
47. Zander JF, Aarhus LL, Katusic ZS et al: Effects of naftidrofuryl on adrenergic nerves, endothelium and smooth muscle in isolated canine blood vessels. J Pharmacol Exp Ther 239(3):760–767, 1986
48. Zannad F, Voisin P, Pointel JP et al: Effects of ketanserin on platelet function and red cell filterability in hypertension and peripheral vascular disease. J Cardiovasc Pharmacol 7(Suppl 7):S32–S34, 1985

CHAPTER TWELVE
Medical Management of the Diabetic Foot
Marvin E. Levin

In the United States, there are 11 million diabetics with a total of 110 million diabetic toes. In a lifetime, these diabetics walk nearly 100,000 miles, approximately four times around the earth. If they are overweight, as most diabetics are, additional pressure is applied to the feet. In many diabetics, the situation is compounded by development of peripheral vascular disease and peripheral neuropathy. These complications can ultimately lead to amputation. Eight percent of type II diabetics have evidence of peripheral vascular disease at the time of diagnosis. Forty-five percent have peripheral vascular disease after 20 years of the disease.[16] In one series, 22% had calcification of the peripheral arteries at diagnosis after 13 years, 61% of the men and 32% of the women had evidence of calcification of the lower-extremity arteries.[11] Peripheral neuropathy leads to the insensitive foot, in which painless trauma leads to ulceration. Fifteen percent of diabetics will develop diabetic foot ulcers.[16]

Amputation rates are 15 times more common in the diabetic than in the nondiabetic. There are approximately 50,000 amputations in diabetics every year in the United States. The amputation rate is estimated to be six per 1000 diabetics each year.[16] Fifty percent of all the nontraumatic amputations in the United States occur in diabetics. The hospital cost for an amputation is approximately $25,000, which does not include loss of time from work, possible loss of job, cost of prosthesis, rehabilitation, or disability payments.

In patients who undergo amputation, 42% lose the contralateral leg within 3 years and 56% within 3 to 5 years for two main reasons. First, the same process, peripheral neuropathy and peripheral vascular disease, is present in the opposite leg. Second, the remaining leg is now subjected to additional stress when increased pressures are shifted to this leg. Neuropathy and the resulting insensitive foot are the major causes of diabetic foot problems. Three times as many patients are admitted to the hospital with neuropathic lesions, compared to those experiencing ischemic pain.[10] Because of the insensitive foot, the physician who treats diabetic patients must try to prevent lesions caused by painless trauma. This can only be accomplished through patient education, foot care, and the use of special shoes when indicated.

DIABETIC PERIPHERAL VASCULAR DISEASE

The atherosclerotic process in the diabetic is not qualitatively different from that in the nondiabetic. In both groups, the stenotic plaque consists of cholesterol, lipids, calcium, smooth muscle cells, and platelets. There are, however, important differences (Table 12-

Table 12–1

Differences in Diabetic and Nondiabetic Peripheral Vascular Disease

Degree of Peripheral Vascular Disease	*Diabetic*	*Nondiabetic*
Clinical	More common	Less common
	Younger patient	Older patient
	More rapid	Less rapid
Male:female	2:1	30:1
Occlusion	Multisegmental	Single segment
Vessels adjacent to occlusion	Involved	Not involved
Lower extremities	Both	Unilateral
Vessels involved	Tibials	Aortic
	Peroneals	Iliac
	Small vessel	Femoral
	Arterioles	
Gangrene	Patchy areas of foot and toes	Extensive
In-hospital mortality with amputation	approximately 3%	Significantly less

(Adapted from Levin ME: Medical evaluation and treatment. In Levin ME, O'Neal LW [eds]: The Diabetic Foot, 4th ed. St Louis, CV Mosby, 1988)

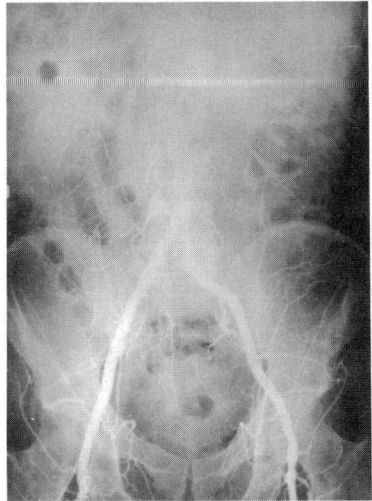
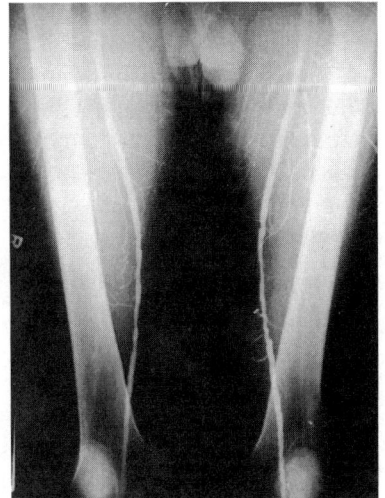
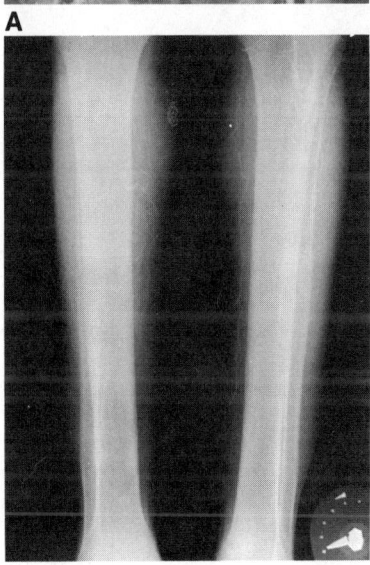

Figure 12-1. A single arteriogram from a patient with diabetic vascular disease. (A) Pelvic vessels showing minimal atheromatous involvement. (B) Thigh vessels in the same arteriogram showing moderate arteriosclerosis. (C) Branches of the popliteal artery in the same arteriogram showing diffuse severe occlusive vascular disease. (Reproduced with permission from Staple TW: Radiology of the diabetic foot. In Levin ME, O'Neal LW [eds]: The Diabetic Foot, 4th ed. St. Louis, CV Mosby, 1988)

1). In the diabetic, the atherosclerotic process occurs at an earlier age and progresses more rapidly. Diabetic men and women have almost the same incidence of peripheral vascular disease. In the nondiabetic, however, men have a much greater incidence of peripheral vascular disease than women. One of the important differences between the two groups is which vessels are involved. Figure 12-1 demonstrates an angiogram in a diabetic. This patient, typical of most diabetic patients, has a normal aorta and excellent iliac and femoral vessels; however, below the knee there is evidence of marked peripheral vascular disease. The vessels most often involved in the diabetic are those below the knee, the peroneal and tibial vessels. The disease tends to be bilateral and diffuse, not involving just a single segment as in the nondiabetic. Involvement of the smaller vessels makes vascular surgery more difficult in the diabetic; the most common type of peripheral vascular surgery in these patients consists of tibioperoneal bypass (Fig. 12-2). The signs and symptoms of peripheral vascular disease in the lower extremity are listed below.[13]

> Intermittent claudication
> Cold feet
> Nocturnal pain
> Rest pain
> Nocturnal and rest pain relieved with dependency
> Absent pulses
> Blanching on elevation
> Delayed venous filling after elevation
> Dependent rubor
> Atrophy of subcutaneous fatty tissues

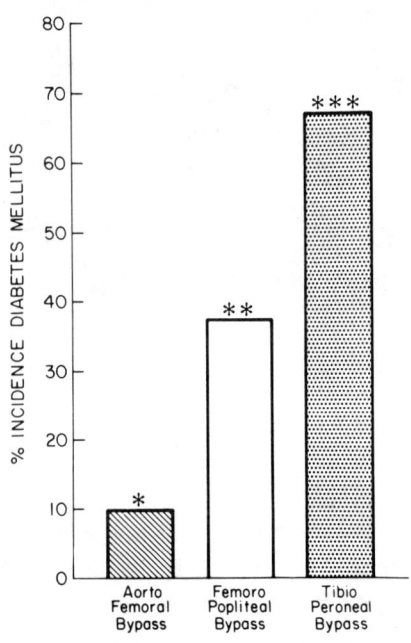

Figure 12-2. Percentage of types of peripheral vascular surgery performed on diabetics. (Reproduced with permission from Sicard GA, Walker WB, Anderson CB: Vascular surgery. In Levin ME, O'Neal LW [eds]: The Diabetic Foot, 4th ed. St. Louis, CV Mosby, 1988)

Shiny appearance of skin
Loss of hair on foot and toes
Thickened nails, often with fungus infection
Gangrene
Miscellaneous: Blue toe syndrome
  Acute vascular occlusion

Intermittent claudication, rest pain, and nocturnal pain are the major problems. It should be noted that all patients who experience leg pain or discomfort when walking do not necessarily have intermittent claudication and vascular insufficiency. They may have so-called pseudoclaudication caused either by arthritis, disk disease, compression on the cauda equina, thrombophlebitis, anemia, and even myxedema. In myxedema, infiltration of mucopolysaccharides into the muscle causes pain when walking. A differentiation between pseudoclaudication and intermittent claudication can be made by the patient's history. The patient with intermittent claudication needs only to stop and rest for a moment or two and the pain or discomfort, usually in the calf, will subside and they can resume walking. Patients with pseudoclaudication usually need to sit down and rest for 15 minutes to 20 minutes before the symptoms will abate. The vascular laboratory can be important in helping to evaluate the location of the stenosis and degree of peripheral vascular disease. Using the photoplethysmograph, toe pressures can also be measured. The pressure used most commonly is at the ankle, which should be the same as in the brachial artery. The ratio of the ankle:arm pressure index gives a numerical evaluation of the vascular disease. This index should be 0.9 or greater. The lower the ratio, the greater the degree of peripheral vascular disease.

Recently, there has been a great deal of debate about the existence of small vessel disease in the diabetic foot.[15] Microvascular disease leads to retinopathy and nephropathy; however, microvascular disease does not appear to have a significant role in the pathogenesis of diabetic foot lesions.[15] Nevertheless, small vessel disease, such as the vessels in the toes, is more common. Figure 12-3 shows Doppler pressures and waveforms in a 60-year-old insulin-requiring woman who had evidence of vascular problems in her toes. The blood pressure at the ankles was exactly the same as at the arm—an index of one. The pressure in her toe on the right, however, was only 60 mmHg, with an index of 0.44. Figure 12-4 shows the blunted waveforms in the left great toe of this patient compared with waveforms in a normal left great toe. This demon-

DIABETES AND VASCULAR DISEASE

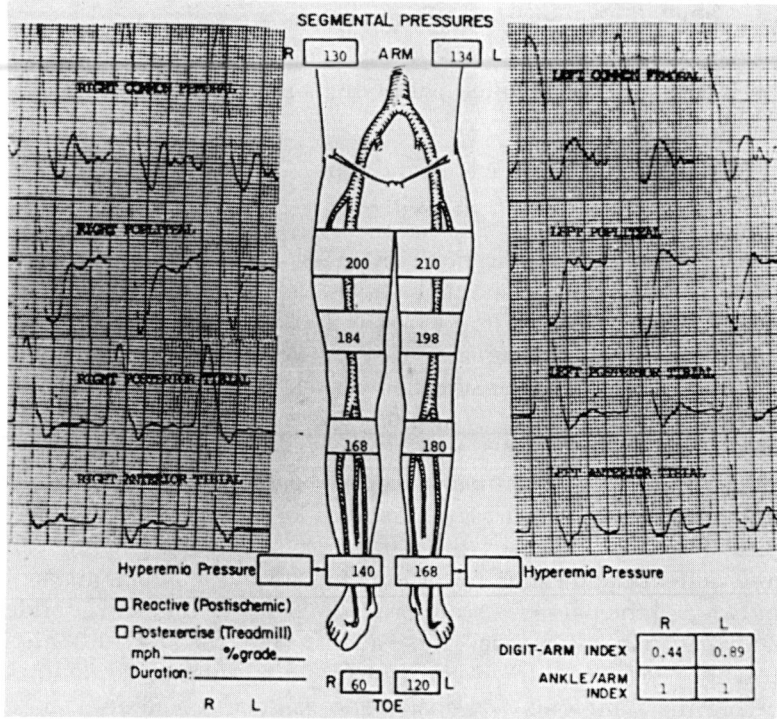

Figure 12-3. Doppler waveforms in the lower extremity of a 60-year-old woman with Type II diabetes, who had ischemic changes in the right great toe. Note normal ankle:arm indices, but low pressure in the right great toe. Low toe pressure and normal ankle pressure are confirmatory evidence of small vessel disease of the great toe. (Reproduced with permission from Levin ME: The diabetic foot: Pathophysiology, evaluation, and treatment. In Levin ME, O'Neal LW [eds]: The Diabetic Foot, 4th ed. St. Louis, CV Mosby, 1988)

strates that while the pressures at the ankle and dorsalis pedis and posterior tibial pulses may be normal, there may be significant vascular disease in the toes confirming the presence of small vessel disease.

Thus, the noninvasive vascular laboratory is important in peripheral vascular disease evaluation. It should be used in conjunction with the clinical history and physical examination.

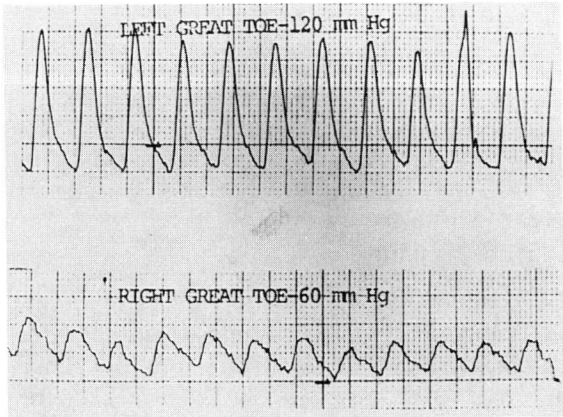

Figure 12-4. Doppler pressures in the right and left great toes of the patient depicted in *Figure 12-3*. Note normal waveforms and normal pressures in the left great toe, but blunted waveforms and lower pressure in the right great toe. (Reproduced with permission from Levin ME: The diabetic foot: Pathophysiology, evaluation, and treatment. In Levin ME, O'Neal LW [eds]: The Diabetic Foot, 4th ed. St. Louis, CV Mosby, 1988)

DIABETIC PERIPHERAL NEUROPATHY

The signs and symptoms of diabetic peripheral neuropathy in the diabetic foot and leg are listed below.[13]

Paresthesia

Hyperesthesia

Hypoesthesia

Radicular pain

Loss of deep tendon reflexes

Loss of vibratory and position sense

Anhydrosis

Heavy callus formation over pressure points

Trophic ulcers

Infection complicating trophic ulcers

Foot drop

Changes in shape of foot produced by:
  A. Muscle atrophy
  B. Changes in bone and joints
Radiographic signs:
  A. Demineralization
  B. Osteolysis
  C. Charcot's joint

The insensitive foot, a common problem in the diabetic, becomes vulnerable to repeated painless trauma, which may be mechanical, chemical, or thermal. In fact, most hospital admissions for diabetic foot problems are secondary to neuropathically induced lesions (*e.g.*, infected plantar ulcers). It is the peripheral vascular disease, however, that prevents the delivery of oxygen, leukocytes, and antibiotics to these lesions and impairs healing. The classic neuropathic ulcer develops over a pressure point. The most common pressure areas are over the first and fifth metatarsal heads and on the plantar surface of the big toe. Ulcerations that occur along the sides of the foot are indicative of ill-fitting shoes. The body attempts to protect the area subjected to increased pressure and repetitive stress with callous build-up. The callouses ultimately break down and ulcerate. Infections in these ulcers lead to progressive microthrombi, gangrene, and the final catastrophic event, amputation.

The heel of the diabetic is prone to injury, particularly when the patient is confined to bed for a prolonged period of time (*e.g.*, because of hip fracture, myocardial infarction, or surgery). These patients have no feeling in their heels and, therefore, fail to change the position of their feet. The heel remains in a constant position and may undergo pressure necrosis; therefore, diabetic patients, hospitalized or at bedrest for any period of time, should wear heel protectors and the heels must be inspected daily.

Diabetic foot and toe deformities, hammer toes, and cocked-up toes secondary to peripheral neuropathy are common. These deformed feet and toes will not fit into ordinary shoes; the result is ulcerations on the top and tip of their toes (Fig. 12-5). The patients should be encouraged to undergo prophylactic surgery to correct these deformities while the circulation is still good, and avoid the possibility of future ulceration, infection, and amputation. If the toes are not straightened, then the shoe should have a large toe box to accommodate this deformity.

Figure 12-6 depicts the ultimate in the deformed foot, the Charcot's foot. Fragmentation and collapse of the distal ends of the

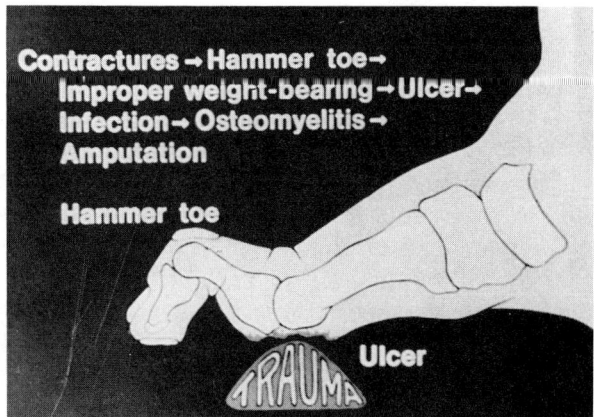

Figure 12-5. Progression of contractures leading to hammer toes, improper weight-bearing, ulceration, infection, and osteomyelitis. Because ulcerations then can occur at the top of the toe, I have referred to this as the *tip-top-toe syndrome*. (Copyright 1983. The University of Michigan. Reprinted with permission from the Michigan Diabetes Research and Training Center. Photo reproduced with permission from Levin ME: The diabetic foot: Pathophysiology, evaluation, and treatment. In Levin ME, O'Neal LW [eds]: The Diabetic Foot, 4th ed. St. Louis, CV Mosby, 1988)

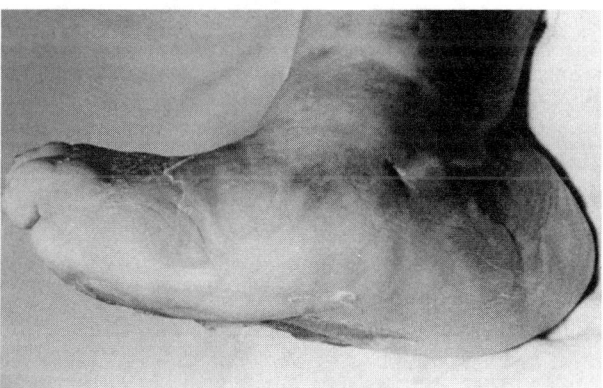

Figure 12-6. A club-foot appearance of patient with Charcot's foot with collapse of the metatarsal joints. (Reproduced with permission from Levin ME: The diabetic foot: Pathophysiology, evaluation, and treatment. In Levin ME, O'Neal LW [eds]: The Diabetic Foot, 4th ed. St. Louis, CV Mosby, 1988)

metatarsals may occur and the tarso–metatarsal joint is usually involved in the bony and joint collapse. The foot shortens, the arch ultimately collapses, and the foot takes on a rocker-bottom appearance. All of the pressure is now on the plantar surface of the arch. The increased pressure can lead to massive ulcerations in this area (Fig. 12-7).The patient with new onset Charcot's foot is found on examination to have a foot resembling cellulitis. It is red, swollen, warm, and moderately painful, making the differential diagnosis of cellulitis difficult. If cellulitis is present, a break in the skin is usually found for the entrance of bacteria; however, cellulitis can occur without an obvious portal of entry. The Charcot's foot, as noted, has excellent circulation with bounding pulses. An x-ray examination shows no calcification of the interosseous vessels. An increase in arteriovenous shunts may be the explanation for the increase in circulation that, in turn, can remove calcium from bones resulting in dissolution and fragmentation of the metatarsals.[3]

Diabetics also lose their autonomic nerve function. The result is decrease in perspiration and dry scaly skin, which tends to crack and serves as a portal of entry for bacteria. The treatment is to return moisture to the foot. After bathing and wiping the foot, some moisture remains, which should be sealed in with bland lubricating lotions or creams, such as plain petroleum jelly, non-scented hand lotions, or aqueous lanolin. Only a thin coating

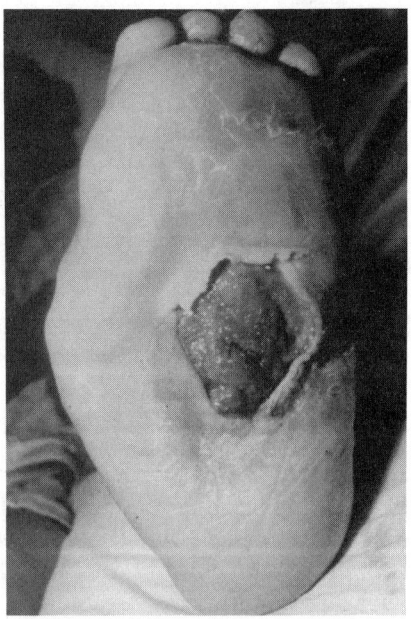

Figure 12-7. A massive ulcer on the plantar surface of the arch in the patient with Charcot's foot depicted in *Figure 12-6*. (Reproduced with permission from Levin ME: Pathophysiology of diabetic foot lesions. In Davidson JK [ed]: Clinical Diabetes Mellitus: A Problem Oriented Approach. New York, Thieme–Stratton, 1986)

should be used. Lubricants should never be used between the toes, because this can lead to maceration and subsequent infection.

The diabetic with the insensitive foot does not complain. The patient does complain, however, and often bitterly, when the peripheral neuropathy causes pain and paresthesias. A wide variety of therapeutic approaches has been used, including Tegretol and Dilantin. In my opinion, they are not specifically helpful for painful neuropathy. Reports of their success probably stem from the fact that painful neuropathy is self-limiting and the pain ultimately goes away on its own, although this may take weeks, months, and sometimes years. Tegretol and Dilantin, however, may have serious side effects. A variety of vitamins, including B_{12} injections and megavitamins, have been advocated and are of no help. The tricyclics appear to be helpful in some patients.[8] When these work, the benefit is seen within a few days to a week. I do not feel this to be a psychogenic effect, because that takes several weeks to achieve. These drugs also have side effects, such as the anticholinergic effects, which can cause urinary retention in men with prostate problems. Prolixin has been suggested as an adjunct with the use of tricyclics, but it can cause parkinsonism in some patients.[8] Tricyclics in relatively low doses do not appear to have a major cardiac effect; as a matter of fact, they have been demonstrated to have an antiarrhythmic effect.[20] Every diabetic with peripheral neuropathy does not necessarily have this on the basis of diabetes. Some causes of peripheral neuropathy are listed below.[13]

Diabetes mellitus	Pernicious anemia
Alcoholism	Malignancy
Herniated nucleus pulposus	Pressure neuropathy
	Uremia
Heavy metals	Porphyria
Vitamin deficiencies	Leprosy
Collagen disease	Drugs

One of the newest treatments for peripheral neuropathy under clinical investigation is the use of aldose reductase inhibitors. Glucose enters the nerve without the need for insulin; it is converted by the enzyme, aldose reductase, to sorbitol and then to fructose. These polyols pull water into the nerve by osmosis, the nerve swells, and nerve function decreases. High levels of these polyols or glucose itself may interfere with the production of *myo*-inositol, an important substance in nerve metabolism and function. The use of aldose reductase inhibitors has been demonstrated to improve motor nerve conduction velocity; however, to date the Federal Drug Administration has not approved these drugs.

SAVING THE DIABETIC FOOT

One of the primary goals of treating diabetics is to save the diabetic foot. This can be accomplished by:

1. Correction of vascular risk factors
2. Improved circulation
3. Proper treatment of diabetic foot ulcers
4. Teamwork
5. Most importantly, patient education in foot care

CORRECTION OF VASCULAR RISK FACTORS

The vascular risk factors listed in Table 12-2 (heredity, age, and duration of diabetes) cannot be treated; however, cessation of smoking, control of hypertension, and lowering of cholesterol, triglycerides, and hyperglycemia can be accomplished.[13] Hyperinsu-

Table 12–2

Risk Factors for Diabetes Macrovascular Disease

Nontreatable	*Treatable*	*Miscellaneous*
Genetic	Smoking	Inotropic drugs
Age	Hypertension:	Beta blockers
Diabetes	systolic	
Duration of diabetes	diastolic	
	Hypercholesterolemia	
	Hypertriglyceridemia	
	Hyperglycemia	

(Adapted from Levin ME: Medical evaluation and treatment. In Levin ME, O'Neal LW (eds): The Diabetic Foot, 4th ed. St Louis, CV Mosby, 1988)

linemia may, in itself, be a risk factor. Insulin can do two things, which may relate to its role in atherosclerosis. First, it can stimulate the deposition of fat into macrophages or foam cells that form part of the stenotic plaque. Insulin is also a growth hormone-like factor and may be partially responsible for stimulating the mitotic division and growth of smooth muscle cells from the media into the plaque.

IMPROVED CIRCULATION

In addition to the correction of risk factors, what else can be done to improve circulation? Certainly, exercise is important in helping to build up collaterals. Vasodilators have been widely advertised; however, they have little or no benefit in diabetic peripheral vascular disease.[4] Diabetes is not a vasospastic disease, so there will only be a limited amount of dilatation possible. Also, a questionable "steal effect" of vasodilators exists. When vessel dilatation is possible, it is the healthy vessels that will dilate and these may, at least theoretically, steal blood away from the ischemic areas and worsen the condition. Because of the increased role of platelets in the pathogenesis of diabetic peripheral vascular disease, Colwell and co-workers, in a cooperative clinical Veterans Administration Hospital study, conducted a double-blind study using the antiplatelet drugs, aspirin and Persantin.[6] In their study, the incidence of gangrene and amputation was not decreased.

Diabetes is a hypercoagulable state in which an increase in fibrinogen, Von Willebrand's factor, platelet aggregation, and adherence occurs. In addition, the red cells and, perhaps, white cells may also be involved. The red blood cell measures approximately 7.4 μ, the capillary about 5 μ. Obviously, the red cell has to change its shape to pass through these narrowed areas. Evidence indicates that the red cells in diabetics may have lost some ability to change their shape. Their ability to be flexible has been decreased. Recently, a new medication, pentoxyfylline (Trental), has become available, which can increase red cell flexibility, thus increasing blood flow and decreasing blood viscosity.[12,17,19] The Federal Drug Administration has approved this drug for the treatment of intermittent claudication and it is helpful in approximately 50% of these patients.

Figure 12-8 depicts the classic diabetic foot. The skin is atrophic with loss of hair on the dorsum of the foot. Note the cocked-up toes, interosseous atrophy, and atrophy of the subcutaneous tissue. The skin appears to be pulled tightly around the foot because of the loss of the subcutaneous fatty tissue. The atrophic skin is

Figure 12-8. Classic diabetic foot with ischemic skin changes: atrophy of the subcutaneous tissues, loss of hair on the dorsum of the foot, thickening of the nails, atrophy of the interosseous muscles resulting in cocked-up toes and the commonly seen superficial skin ulcerations. (Courtesy of John F. Fairbairn II, M.D., Mayo Clinic, Rochester, Minnesota, and The Upjohn Company, Kalamazoo, Michigan)

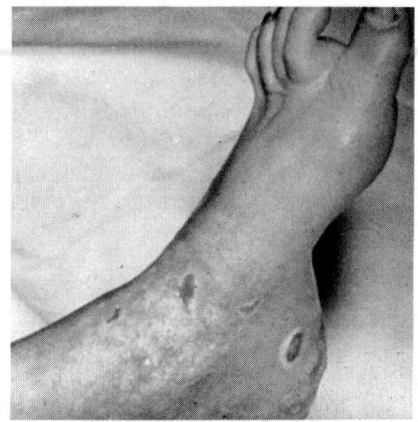

vulnerable to minimal trauma. These ischemic feet may not yet require vascular surgery. Anecdotal reports have suggested that these superficial ulcers have been improved with the use of Trental. To achieve the effects of Trental, either on intermittent claudication or the possible healing of superficial ulcers, may require 2 to 3 months or longer. Trental is not the treatment for neuropathic plantar ulcers.

Rest pain and night pain in the legs are ominous signs. These patients are in danger of losing their legs unless vascular surgery is performed. Many of these diabetic patients, however, do not complain of night and rest pain despite severe ischemic feet and legs, because neuropathy has destroyed the ability to pick up the pain sensation. These patients have a serious problem, even though they have no pain. The physician, therefore, must use the experienced hand and eye and examine extremities of all diabetic patients at every visit.

Nocturnal pain may also occur with diabetic peripheral neuropathy. The differential diagnosis between ischemic pain and neuropathic pain can be done by history. Patients with ischemic night or rest pain will sit up in a chair all night and let their legs dangle down, frequently with the development of edema. By dangling their legs, they benefit from the use of gravity and some motion to improve the circulation. They may even walk a few feet, but any extended walking or elevation of the legs causes increased pain. The patient with painful nocturnal neuropathic pain will get up and do a great deal of walking. By history, one can help to differentiate the etiology of the night pain.

Ulcers that will not heal, infections resistant to treatment, and incipient gangrene are all indications for vascular surgery. Before the surgeon can perform vascular surgery, angiography is necessary to establish the location of the block and operability. Angiography is not without its risks. Patients may have hemorrhage and thrombus formation at the site of injection of the contract material and may develop peripheral emboli. One of the major concerns is renal shutdown following the use of contrast material. The exact etiology for this is not clear, but keeping the patient well-hydrated with excellent urine volume helps to prevent renal shutdown. Nevertheless, any diabetic with creatinine values of 2 to 2.5 mg/dl or over should be followed closely for renal shutdown after the injection of contrast material. This follow-up should be done for 2 to 3 days after the procedure.

TREATMENT OF DIABETIC FOOT ULCERS

The treatment of infected diabetic foot ulcers is a difficult problem and can be divided into two major categories, the primary and secondary approach.

The primary approach in the treatment of foot ulcers consists of nine steps:

1. *Evaluation:* Clinical appearance, establishment of depth, and radiology to establish the possible presence of osteomyelitis or foreign objects.
2. *Metabolic control:* Leukocytes do not function well when blood sugars are high.
3. *Culture:* The ulcers must be cultured both aerobically and anaerobically. Anaerobic cultures require special techniques and cannot be achieved by simply taking a culture from the surface of the ulcer.
4. *Antibiotic therapy:* Begin at once and then adjust antibiotics when the cultures are returned. Consultation with an expert in infectious disease is frequently indicated. Antibiotics should be administered parenterally. These patients, as noted, have poor circulation and it is difficult to deliver high concentrations of antibiotics by the oral route. In addition, many of the newer antibiotics can only be given parenterally.
5. *Daily debridement:* Removal of necrotic tissue is necessary.
6. *Do not soak the feet:* Soaking the feet contributes little to the treatment program.[14] In addition, soaking in

chemical solutions can result in chemical burns. Hot soaks to insensitive feet can result in severe blistering and gangrene.

7. *Non-weight-bearing:* This is critical to healing the ulcer. These patients, with their insensitive feet, feel no pain despite large ulcers and will continue to walk, adding to the pressure necrosis and pushing bacteria deeper into the tissues. Absolute non-weight-bearing includes not even allowing the patient to walk to the bathroom. One of the newer techniques for providing ambulation and non-weight-bearing is the use of contact casts.[2] These casts protect the ulcer, decrease edema, and redistribute the pressures so that the patient is ambulatory and non-weight-bearing at the same time. These casts must be applied with special techniques and only by experts trained in their use. The casts are contraindicated in patients with severe peripheral vascular disease, obesity, osteomyelitis, ataxia, and blindness, and in the aged.

8. *Vascular surgery:* If an ulcer is not responding to the intensive therapy described above, vascular surgery should always be considered.

9. *Posthealing treatment:* Patient education is important in management of the foot after healing. The healed ulcer area is vulnerable and subject to breakdown again and recurrence of the ulcer. In addition, scar tissue beneath the healed ulcer is vulnerable to the stress forces of walking. These patients must be educated to reduce the amount of walking they do and to take shorter steps. They may need to change jobs, particularly if the job entails being on their feet or requires a great deal of walking.

Special therapeutic shoes are frequently necessary for these patients. A recent series by Edmond and co-workers showed only a 19% recurrence in patients who had healed ulcers and used special shoes.[9] A 91% recurrence was noted in patients who returned to wearing their regular dress shoes. Many of these patients frequently go back to wearing their ordinary shoes because they have insensitive feet and feel no pain; however, this is a dangerous practice.

The secondary approach to foot ulcer therapy is the use of a variety of topical preparations, which include proteolytic enzymes, antibacterials, such as Silvadene, povidone-iodine, and resins. These may be useful adjuncts, but if they are used as the first line of treatment, valuable time may be lost in treating these foot ulcers vigorously. The use of hyperbaric oxygen may be helpful, but is still experimental.

TEAM APPROACH

Care of the diabetic foot is a complicated task and requires the teamwork of a variety of medical disciplines, which includes podiatrists, orthopedists, physical therapists, vascular surgeons, radiologists, infectious disease experts, and nurse educators. All of these specialists, when indicated, should be under the orchestration of the primary physician.

PATIENT EDUCATION

Until peripheral vascular disease and diabetic neuropathy can be prevented, the most important thing the physician can do is educate the patient in foot care. Unfortunately, foot inspection is often neglected.[1,5] This should be done at every visit. The physician should remove the patient's shoes and stockings and examine the feet and in between the toes carefully at each visit. The patient instructions for the care of the diabetic foot listed below should be repeated at every visit.[13]

>   Do not smoke.
>   Inspect toes and between toes daily for blisters, cuts, and scratches; use of a mirror can aid in seeing the bottom of the feet.
>   Wash feet daily; dry carefully, especially between the toes.
>   Avoid extremes of temperatures; test water before bathing.
>   If feet feel cold at night, wear socks; do not apply hot water bottles or heating pads.
>   Do not use chemical agents for removal of corns and calluses.
>   Inspect inside of shoes daily for foreign objects, nail points, and torn linings.
>   Wear properly fitted stockings, do not wear mended stockings, avoid stockings with seams, change stockings daily.

Do not wear garters.

Shoes should be comfortable at the time of purchase; do not depend on them to "stretch out."

Do not wear shoes without stockings.

Do not wear sandals with thongs between the toes.

Do not walk barefooted, and never on hot surfaces such as sandy beaches or around swimming pools.

Cut nails straight across.

Do not cut corns and calluses: follow special instructions from your physician or podiatrist.

See your physician regularly and be sure the feet are examined at each visit.

If vision is impaired, have a family member inspect feet daily and trim nails and buff down calluses.

Be sure to inform your podiatrist that you are a diabetic.

Even at the risk of repetition, it is critically important to remind the patient not to smoke. Smoking a single cigarette can cause vasospasm for an hour and sometimes for many hours. The patient should be instructed to examine the feet daily. Many of these patients either have arthritis, are obese, or have impaired vision and cannot examine their feet properly. This should be done by a family member. Patients should be cautioned not to soak their feet.[14] Because of poor circulation, these patients frequently have cold feet. With little or no nerve function, if they put their feet into hot water to warm them—the result is severe burns and not infrequently this leads to amputation. The use of lubricants on dry skin has already been discussed. Patients should be cautioned not to use chemical agents for removing calluses and corns; this can result in chemical burns. They should inspect the inside of their shoes daily for foreign objects, nail points, and torn linings. The importance of special shoes has been emphasized. The shoes should be comfortable at the time of purchase, and one should not be talked into buying a shoe that is too tight by a salesperson who claims they will stretch out. Normally, shoes should be made of leather, because leather tends to expand and breathe; however, there is evidence that running shoes will cut down on the rapidity of callous build-up and can be considered useful in selected patients.[18] Patients should not wear sandals with thongs between the toes. The patients should be instructed not to walk barefooted, not only because of trauma, but especially on areas such as hot sandy beaches or on the hot cement around swimming pools. This activity has resulted in severe burns to insensitive feet. The patients must not cut corns and calluses. After proper instruction from the physician or podiatrist, they may be taught to handle calluses properly. Difficult calluses should be treated by the physician or podiatrist. Patients should be cautioned not to try and cut out their own ingrown toenails. This will almost invariably result in infection and frequently the loss of a toe and foot. Patients should also be cautioned to inform the physician treating their feet that they have diabetes.

Do patient education, foot inspection, and special shoes help? The answer is an emphatic yes. Davidson and co-workers, at Emory University, conducted a 3-year study at a diabetic foot center.[7] He and his team, by using the approaches described in this chapter and by prescribing special shoes, were able to decrease the amputation rate by 50% each year.

SUMMARY

Every primary physician who treats diabetic patients will, on many occasions, be faced with problems of the diabetic foot. If the physician understands the pathophysiology of diabetic peripheral vascular disease and neuropathy, corrects (as best possible) vascular risk factors, improves the circulation (when indicated), treats diabetic foot ulcers vigorously, uses consultation, inspects the patient's feet at every hospital visit, and provides detailed patient education, it is reasonable to expect that the amputation rate can be reduced by 50%. Every physician owes the diabetic patient good foot care.

REFERENCES

1. Bailey TS, Yu HM, Rayfield EJ: Patterns of foot examination in a diabetes clinic. Am J Med 78:371–374, 1985
2. Boulton AJM, Bowker JH, Gadia M et al: Use of plaster casts in the management of diabetic neuropathic foot ulcers. Diabetes Care 9:149–152, 1986
3. Boulton AJM, Scarpello JHB, Ward JD: Venous oxygenation in the diabetic neuropathic foot. Evidence of arterial venous shunting. Diabetologia 22:6–8, 1981
4. Coffman JD: Vasodilator drugs in peripheral vascular disease. N Engl J Med 300:713–717, 1979
5. Cohen SJ: Potential barriers to diabetes care. Diabetes Care 6:499–500, 1983

6. Colwell JA, Bingham SF, Abriara C et al: Veterans Administration cooperative study on antiplatelet agents in diabetic patients after amputation for gangrene: II. Effects of aspirin and dipyridamole on atherosclerotic vascular disease rates. Diabetes Care 9(2):140–148, 1986
7. Davidson JK, Alonga M, Goldsmith M et al: Assessment of program effectiveness at Grady Memorial Hospital—Atlanta. In Steiner G, Lawrence PA (eds): Educating Diabetic Patients, pp 329–361. New York, Springer-Verlag 1981
8. Davis JL, Lewis SB, Gerich JE et al: Peripheral diabetic neuropathy treated with amitriptyline and fluphenazine. JAMA 238:2291–2292, 1977
9. Edmonds ME, Blundell MP, Morris ME et al: Improved survival of the diabetic foot: The role of a specialized foot clinic. Q J Med 60(232):763–771, 1986
10. Jauw-Tjen L, Brown AL Jr: Normal structure of the vascular system and general reactive changes of the arteries. In Fairbairn JF, Juergens JL, Spittell JA (eds): Peripheral Vascular Diseases, pp 45–61. Philadelphia, WB Saunders, 1972
11. Krienes K, Johnson E, Albrink M et al: The course of peripheral vascular disease in non-insulin dependent diabetes. Diabetes Care 8(3):23S, 1985
12. Lee BY, Berkowitz P, Savitsky JP et al: Pentoxifylline treatment of moderate to severe chronic occlusive arterial disease. Clin Cardiol 8:161–165, 1985
13. Levin ME: Medical evaluation and treatment. In Levin ME, O'Neal LW (eds): The Diabetic Foot, 3rd ed. St Louis, CV Mosby, 1983
14. Levin ME, Spratt IL: To soak or not to soak. Clin Diabetes 4:44–45, 1986
15. LoGerfo FW, Coffman JO: Vascular and microvascular disease of the foot in diabetes. N Engl J Med 311:1615–1619, 1984
16. Palumbo PJ, Melton LJ III: Peripheral vascular disease and diabetes. In Harris MI, Hamman RF (eds): Diabetes in America. Bethesda, MD: The National Diabetes Data Group, NIADDK, U.S. Department of Health and Human Services, Public Health Services National Institutes of Health, National Institute of Arthritis, Diabetes and Digestive and Kidney Disease, NIH Publication No. 85-1468, vol. XVI, pp 1–21, 1985
17. Porter JM, Cutler BS, Lee BY et al: Pentoxifylline efficacy in the treatment of intermittent claudication: Multicenter controlled double-blind trial with objective assessment of chronic occlusive arterial disease patients. Am Heart J 104:66–72, 1982

18. Soulier SM: The use of running shoes in the prevention of plantar diabetic ulcers. J Am Podiatr Med Assoc 76:395–400, 1986
19. Taylor LM Jr, Porter JM: Drug treatment of claudication: vasodilators, hemorrheologic agents, and antiserotonin drugs. J Vasc Surg 3:374–381, 1986
20. Veith RC, Raskind MA, Caldwell JH et al: Cardiovascular effects of tricyclic antidepressants in depressed patients with chronic heart disease. N Engl J Med 306:954–959, 1982

CHAPTER THIRTEEN

Nonoperative Treatment of Intermittent Claudication*

John M. Porter
Eric I. Friedman

PERSPECTIVE

Intermittent claudication defines a pain syndrome resulting from inadequate blood supply to meet the metabolic demands of exercising muscle. The majority of patients with intermittent claudication have fixed arterial obstructions in the large arteries proximal to the exercising muscle. Interestingly, identical symptoms may occur with normal blood flow in the presence of profound hypoxemia or anemia, thus validating the definition of inadequate blood supply to meet metabolic demands.

Most patients with intermittent claudication have diminished or absent peripheral pulses, although this is not essential for the diagnosis. The critical evaluation required to quantitate the functional significance of intermittent claudication is the postexercise vascular laboratory evaluation. Sumner and Strandness showed the relationship of the severity of claudication to the drop in ankle:brachial pressure index after exercise.[22] The amount of pressure drop after exercise and time required for recovery of the ankle:brachial pressure index after exercise allow quantitative assessment of not only the magnitude of arterial blockage, but also the amount of collateralization around the blockage. Without question, the behavior of the ankle:brachial pressure index after exercise (or reactive hyperemia) is the most important test in evaluating the objective status of patients with intermittent claudication.

---

*Supported in part by Grant RR00334 from the General Clinical Research Center Branch, Division of Research Resources, National Institutes of Health.

LACK OF EXERCISE AND SMOKING AS LIMITING FACTORS

The two most widely used nonoperative treatments of intermittent claudication are exercise and cessation of smoking. Occasional patients clearly benefit from pharmacologic treatment. Data from a large group of patients indicate that 70% to 80% of patients with intermittent claudication who exercise and stop smoking will stabilize or improve their walking distance without the need for arterial reconstruction; 10% to 15% will ultimately require arterial surgery; and only 5% to 10% will require amputation for limb ischemia. These numbers appear to reflect accurately the general population. Cronenwatt and associates reported their experience from a Veterans Administration Hospital population and found a less optimistic outcome in patients with intermittent claudication in whom arterial reconstruction surgery was not performed.[8] Thus, in selected population groups, the optimistic data presented above may not apply precisely.

A large majority of patients with intermittent claudication will show a marked improvement in walking distance after a lower-extremity exercise program. It is a completely unsubstantiated hypothesis, however, that such exercise stimulates the development of collateral blood circulation. Considerable recent evidence indicates that exercise induces adaptive changes in muscle enzymes, permitting the more efficient extraction of oxygen. Following a program of regular exercise, patients with intermittent claudication develop a considerable widening of the arteriovenous oxygen difference at the femoral level.[21] The patient with intermittent claudication who exercises will extract oxygen from the arterial circulation more efficiently and, thereby, walk further. Strain-gauge plethysmography and venous occlusion plethysmography have shown no consistent differences in limb blood flow following an exercise program.

PHARMACOLOGIC MANIPULATION

Following is a partial listing of the pharmacologic agents proposed in the past several decades for the treatment of intermittent claudication:

Anticoagulants

Vasodilators

Antiplatelet agents

Prostaglandins E_1 (PGE$_1$) and I_2 (PGI$_2$)
Thromboxane synthetase inhibitors
Metabolic enhancers (naftidrofuryl)
Hemorrheologic agents
Antiserotonin agents
Calcium channel blocking agents

The efficacy of anticoagulants has never been proved and they are not currently being widely used, if at all, in the treatment of intermittent claudication. Vasodilators have constituted the foundation of the pharmacologic treatment of intermittent claudication for almost 50 years. Some of the agents used frequently over the years include phenoxybenzamine, tolazoline, isoxsuprine, and cyclandelate.

Vasodilators were proposed originally based on the assumption that vasoconstriction existed in ischemic areas. It is easy to understand how this error was made. The early clinicians, seeing the blanched feet of patients with intermittent claudication, assumed intuitively that vasospasm and vasoconstriction must occur in the legs of these patients. It is now known that this blanching is the result of a selective redistribution of a limited amount of blood entering the limb to the dilated arterial circulation in the proximal muscle mass, and is not related to vasoconstriction. In fact, the ischemic limb is already near-maximally vasodilated, apparently caused by a local accumulation of the products of anaerobic metabolism.[7] Vasodilators may result in the "steal" of blood away from ischemic areas. No vasodilator however been shown to increase the blood flow to exercising muscle, and none has ever been classified as effective by the Federal Drug Administration. Two of the oldest vasodilators, however, cyclandelate and isoxsuprine, have been subjected to controlled clinical trials (unpublished data). These small-volume trials show interesting small benefits in favor of the drugs, and the drugs are currently being re-examined by the Federal Drug Administration. The observed benefit may be secondary to their hemorrheologic properties and not secondary to the vasodilating action.

ANTIPLATELET AGENTS

Antiplatelet drugs, especially aspirin, are probably the most common pharmacologic agents prescribed for patients with peripheral vascular disease. There appears to be a small, but real, benefit of aspirin in the treatment of patients with transient ischemic attacks.[14] It is uncertain whether aspirin may beneficially diminish fibrointimal hyperplasia. Clowes and co-workers reported that the platelet-derived growth factor is probably operative only in the early phases, 7 days to 14 days, after a new anastomosis.[5] Subsequently, the endothelial cell-derived growth factor or other substances may be more important in initiating and sustaining cell proliferation.

Aspirin has been shown clearly to have an important role in decreasing early vein graft occlusion. Chesebro and associates have shown clear-cut improvement in the early and intermediate patency rates of aorta-coronary grafts in patients treated with aspirin compared with placebo.[4]

The efficacy, if any, of antiplatelet agents in the treatment of intermittent claudication has never been convincingly demonstrated. A recent study by Hess and co-workers, however, showed a decrease in the progression of occlusive arterial disease in the legs as measured by sequential arteriography before, and 2 years after, antiplatelet drug treatment.[16] The reduction of progression was greatest in the aspirin-dipyridamole-treated group. Unfortunately, no assessment was made of the patients' symptoms in any of the treatment groups. This area obviously warrants further careful study.

The encouraging results of multiple clinical studies of cerebral and coronary vascular disease, as well as the overwhelming weight of experimental evidence, lead us to treat unoperated as well as postoperative patients with peripheral vascular disease with antiplatelet drugs. The dose required for the optimal beneficial effects is not known. Our current recommendation is for 325 mg of aspirin daily.

PROSTAGLANDINS

Prostaglandins are a fascinating family of drugs, which unfortunately have no clearly established role in the treatment of peripheral vascular disease. The two most frequently used prostaglandins in peripheral vascular disease are prostaglandin E_1 (PGE_1) and prostaglandin I_2 (PGI_2). Neither of these prostaglandins is new; both have been investigated for more than a decade. They have anecdotally appeared beneficial in intermittent claudication as well as in the healing of arterial ischemic ulcers. Unfortunately, they both have a half-life of only several seconds and, therefore, require intravenous administration. Additionally, they possess significant side effects. Recent prospective randomized studies have failed to show any benefit of these drugs in the healing of arterial ischemic ulcers.[9,20]

Despite the enthusiastic early anecdotal reports of benefit from prostaglandins, when the requisite randomized placebo-controlled trials were performed, no benefit was noted. Sadly, these results were predictable. Insofar as prostaglandins function as vasodilators, their use will likely be as futile as that of any other vasodilator proposed for the treatment of peripheral arterial disease. Their potent antiplatelet action may confer some benefit; however, with a half-life of only several seconds, it is difficult to envision any effects persisting for a reasonable length of time following parenteral administration.

Thromboxane A_2 (TxA_2) synthetase inhibitors are another interesting family of drugs being investigated for use in the treatment of intermittent claudication. There may be some critical balance between platelet TxA_2 and endothelial PGI_2. Some simple and well-tolerated pharmacologic agents will totally block TxA_2 synthetase. If this enzyme is blocked, the metabolism of arachidonic acid is shifted preferentially toward the formation of PGI_2. This should result, theoretically, in net vasodilation and a platelet anti-aggregatory effect. Preliminary anecdotal results have suggested some benefit with these drugs in the treatment of intermittent claudication.[11]

While the thromboxane synthetase inhibitors may appear to be promising theoretically and anecdotally, randomized double-blind studies are essential to permit an accurate assessment of their clinical usefulness in treatment of intermittent claudication. The optimal antiplatelet therapy in the future may consist of a combination of a thromboxane synthetase inhibitor and low-dose aspirin.[1]

OTHER PHARMACOLOGIC MODALITIES

Naftidrofuryl was a relatively important drug in Europe for a brief period of time; however, it was never popular in the United States. It stimulates the entry of carbohydrate into the Krebs' cycle, and theoretically stimulates the production of additional adenosine triphosphate in ischemic muscle. Similar to many other agents, it had a promising mechanism of action and early, anecdotally beneficial results. When double-blind control studies were conducted, however, no benefit resulted from the drug.[6]

Recently, interest has again been devoted to the microcirculation and its potential importance in patients with intermittent claudication. This was first suggested in the early 1960s with reports from Scandinavia concerning the use of dextran.[15] Dextrans have three properties that make them potentially clinically useful: plasma volume expansion, antithrombotic effects, and microcirculatory blood flow enhancement.

Dextrans are potent intravascular hydrophilic agents that cause rapid volume expansion. This appears to be the major cause of the microcirculatory flow enhancement, because a decrease in blood viscosity occurs during plasma volume expansion.

Dextrans appear useful in selected areas of vascular surgery. They appear as effective as low-dose heparin in the prevention of venous thrombosis in selected patients and may be especially valuable in preventing pulmonary emboli. Both experimental and clinical evidence exists that dextran may improve the patency of small artery and vein anastomoses.[19] Unfortunately, despite early anecdotal reports of benefit in the treatment of severe limb ischemia, no randomized, controlled study demonstrates the usefulness of dextrans in this setting. They are used infrequently in the United States as a primary agent in treatment of severe limb ischemia.

An important component of metabolic substrate and oxygen delivery occurs in the microcirculation at the precapillary and capillary levels. The volume of fluid passing through a conduit is inversely proportional to the viscosity. Whole blood viscosity is enormously complex and is the end-product of multiple factors including the red blood cell count, red blood cell deformability, red blood cell aggregation, and plasma viscosity. In the early 1970s, several investigators noted a slight increase in whole blood viscosity in patients with severe intermittent claudication.[13,18] These same patients appeared to have a significant decrease in red blood cell deformability, as measured by constant suction of red blood cells across polycarbonate membranes with specific pore sizes.

PHARMACOLOGIC AGENT(S) AND RED BLOOD CELL DEFORMABILITY

Red blood cell deformability is of considerable physiologic importance, because 8-μ red blood cells must routinely pass through 4-μ to 6-μ capillaries. Normal red blood cells become considerably elongated during passage through the capillaries. If these cells become rigid and nondeformable, a microcirculatory impediment to the extraction of oxygen in the ischemic tissue would occur. Observers have suggested that hyperosmolarity and decreased pH, such as occurs in areas of ischemia associated with anaerobic metabolism, contribute to red blood cell rigidity.[13,18] Decreased red blood cell deformability has been associated with decreased red blood cell adenosine triphosphate, which has been found in patients with intermittent claudication.

Pentoxifylline is a drug first formulated in the 1930s as a vasodilator; however, it appeared to have no use as a vasodilator and was not further investigated until the 1960s. It is a xanthine derivative and is structurally simple. Pentoxifylline increases red blood cell adenosine triphosphate and cyclic adenosine monophosphate by phosphodiesterase inhibition. Early studies suggested this may increase red blood cell deformability and slightly decrease blood viscosity.[3] The drug also has a minor effect on decreasing platelet aggregation.

Ehrly, in Germany, found that the use of pentoxifylline in patients with severe intermittent claudication increases the diminished muscle oxygen tensions of claudicants to near normal, as determined by micropipette technique.[12] This is the only drug that has been shown to do this. To date, however, this important observation has never been confirmed independently.

Pentoxifylline appeared beneficial in the treatment of intermittent claudication in clinical trials in Europe.[2] A multicenter trial, therefore, was carried out in the United States.[17] The study was a prospective, randomized, double-blind evaluation of pentoxifylline versus placebo in patients with intermittent claudication. All patients in the study had intermittent claudication for at least 6 months, and all had to be able to walk on a treadmill for at least 50 m. The primary responses were recorded for initial and absolute claudication distances—the distance at which the patient first complained of intermittent claudication or lower-extremity pain and the point at which the patient stopped walking because of pain. The drug was analyzed with the intention to treat; therefore, no patients were dropped from analysis after they were entered into the study. This is important, statistically.

During the 24-week observation period of 127 patients from seven centers, an initial claudication distance benefit of 38% was apparent in favor of the drug-treated group (Fig. 13-1).[17] The benefit became maximum at approximately 10 weeks. There was a similar benefit (22%) in the absolute claudication distance in favor of the drug-treated group (Fig. 13-2). The placebo-treated patients were also observed to improve, which represented the well-described effects of conditioning and training. Results of this study indicate a significant improvement of 30% in favor of drug over placebo. This improvement was sufficient for Federal Drug Admin-

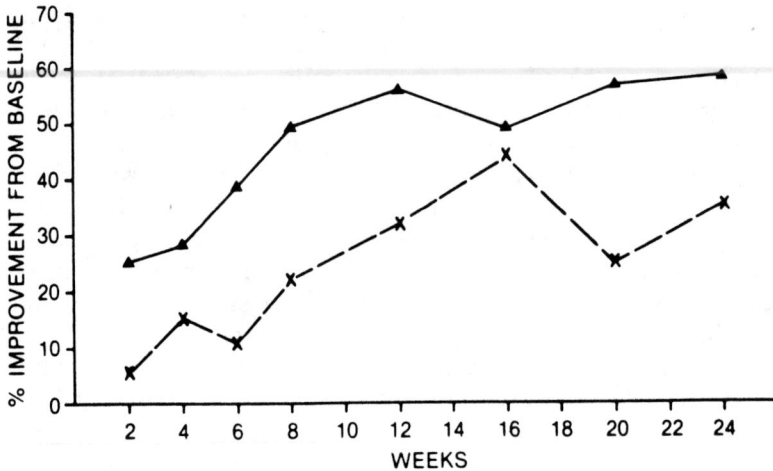

Figure 13-1. Initial claudication distance (ICD). Percent change from baseline on treadmill testing (weeks 2 through 24). The treatment group (pentoxifylline) is the upper line; the placebo group is the lower line. (Reproduced with permission from Porter JM, Cutler BS, Lee BY et al: Pentoxifylline efficacy in the treatment of intermittent claudication: Multicenter controlled double-blind trial with objective assessment of chronic occlusive arterial disease patients. Am Heart J 104:66–72, 1982)

istration approval of the drug. Currently, it is the only drug approved for treatment of patients with intermittent claudication. This 30% improvement, however, is so small that it will probably not be appreciated by either the patient or physician.

Individual responses to the drug may vary remarkably for unknown reasons. Of the pentoxifylline-treated patients, 31% improved in excess of 100%, compared with 9% of the placebo group (Table 13-1). This amount of improvement, a doubling of the walking distance, is likely to be clinically apparent.

Since the initial study, approximately 800 patients have been randomly assigned to either placebo or pentoxifylline with generally confirmed results.[23] Side effects of the drug have been minimal, primarily gastrointestinal.

While pentoxifylline may represent an important advance, it should not constitute first-line therapy for intermittent claudication. Our current position is to exhaust the nonpharmacologic modalities of exercise and cessation of smoking before considering pentoxifylline. Additionally, the physician must realize that individual responses are highly variable and the maximal drug benefit may not occur for up to 10 weeks to 12 weeks.

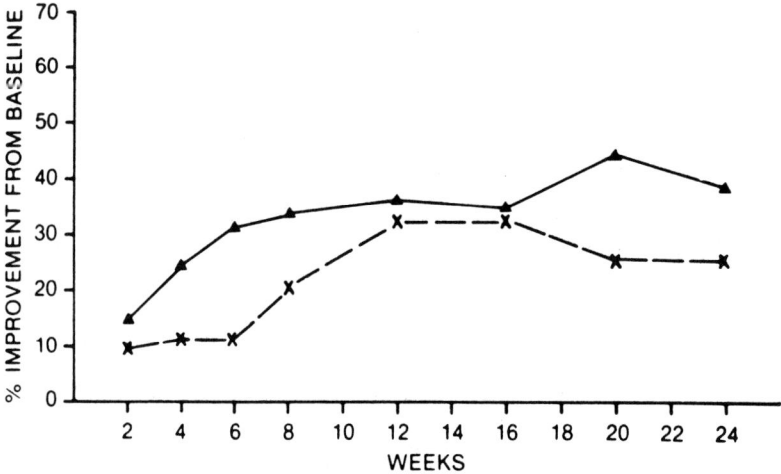

Figure 13-2. Absolute claudication distance (ACD). Percent change from baseline on treadmill testing (weeks 2 through 24). The treatment group (pentoxifylline) is the upper line; the placebo group is the lower line. (Reproduced by permission from Porter JM, Cutler BS, Lee BY et al: Pentoxifylline efficacy in the treatment of intermittent claudication: Multicenter controlled double-blind trial with objective assessment of chronic occlusive arterial disease patients. Am Heart J 104:66–72, 1982)

SEROTONIN-RELATED AGENTS

Other drugs are currently receiving active consideration. Serotonin has experienced a resurgence of interest in the field of vascular surgery. Serotonin is a powerful vasoconstrictor, which stimulates platelet aggregation and mediates the inflammatory response. Serotonin is particularly abundant in platelets.

Ketanserin, a serotonin antagonist, is an S_2 serotonin receptor blocker, which antagonizes vasoconstriction and platelet aggregation. Interestingly, it also promotes red blood cell deformability. The drug has undergone prospective, randomized, controlled studies and was found to be beneficial in the treatment of intermittent claudication.[10] The benefit realized is similar to that noted with pentoxifylline. This drug is not currently available in the United States. Curiously, it was noted that the patients in the drug-treated arm of the trial had a low rate of myocardial infarctions and strokes, while the placebo group had the anticipated number for age and risk group. This finding suggests the possibility that, in addition to the benefit in intermittent claudication, ketanserin may exert a "protective" effect against morbid cardiovascular events. Cur-

Table 13–1
Improvement in Initial Claudication Distance/Absolute Claudication Distance (ICD/ACD) at Week 24, Number of Patients Improved, Percentage Improvement

Variable	Treatment	N	<25%	25% to 49%	50% to 100%	>100%	p Value
ICD	Pentoxifylline	42	16	4	9	13	0.053
	Placebo	40	20	6	8	6	
ACD	Pentoxifylline	42	16	5	12	9	0.047
	Placebo	40	25	3	6	6	

(Porter JM, Cutler BS, Lee BY et al: Pentoxifylline efficacy in treatment of intermittent claudication: Multicenter controlled double-blind trial with objective assessment of chronic occlusive arterial disease patients. Am Heart J 104:66–72, 1982)

rently, an international, multicenter trial is underway evaluating ketanserin in the prevention of sudden death, myocardial infarction, stroke, and transient ischemic attacks in patients with peripheral vascular disease.

Calcium channel blockers are powerful vasodilators. Occasionally, patients have anecdotally reported improvement in their intermittent claudication while taking one of the calcium channel blockers for another reason. Dazadopine is a dihydropyridine derivative that may selectively dilate arteries in skeletal muscle, a property shared with no other calcium channel blocker. A multicenter, randomized, clinical trial is currently underway to evaluate this drug in the treatment of intermittent claudication.

SUMMARY

Several drugs hold promise of modest benefit in the treatment of intermittent claudication. Pentoxifylline is the only drug approved and available currently in the United States. The hemorrheology of patients with intermittent claudication is currently under intense investigation. The first real advance in the pharmacologic treatment of intermittent claudication may be at hand.

REFERENCES

1. Bertele V, Flanaga A, Tomasiak MA et al: Platelet thromboxane synthetase inhibitors with low dose aspirin: Possible resolution of the "aspirin dilemma." Science 220:517–519, 1983
2. Bollinger A, Frei C: Double-blind study of pentoxifylline against placebo in patients with intermittent claudication. Pharmatherapeutica 1:557–562, 1977
3. Braasch D: Red cell deformability and capillary blood flow. Physiol Rev 51:679–701, 1979
4. Chesebro JH, Clements IP, Fuster V et al: A platelet inhibitor-drug trial in coronary artery bypass operations. Benefit of perioperative dipyridamole and aspirin on early postoperative vein-graft patency. N Engl J Med 307:73–78, 1982
5. Clowes AW, Reidy MA, Clowes NM: Mechanisms of stenosis after arterial injury. Lab Invest 49:208–215, 1983
6. Clyne CAC, Galland RB, Fox RJ et al: A controlled trial of naftidrofuryl (Praxilene) in the treatment of intermittent claudication. Br J Surg 67:347–348, 1980

7. Coffman JD: Vasodilator drugs in peripheral vascular disease. N Engl J Med 300:713–717, 1979
8. Cronenwatt JL, Warner KG, Zelenock GB et al: Intermittent claudication. Current results of nonoperative management. Arch Surg 119:430–436, 1984
9. Cronenwett JL, Zelenock GB, Whitehouse WM Jr et al: Prostacyclin treatment of ischemic ulcers and rest pain in unreconstructable peripheral arterial occlusive disease. Surgery 100:369–375, 1986
10. DeCree J, Leempoels J, Geukens H et al: Placebo-controlled double-blind trial of ketanserin in treatment of intermittent claudication. Lancet 2:775–778, 1984
11. Ehrly AM.: Influence of a thromboxane synthesis inhibitor on the muscle tissue microcirculation of patients with intermittent claudication. Br J Clin Pharmacol 15(Suppl 1):117s–118s, 1983
12. Ehrly AM: The effect of pentoxifylline on the deformability of erythrocytes on the muscular oxygen pressure in patients with chronic arterial disease. J Med 10:331–338, 1979
13. Ehrly MA, Kohler HJ: Altered deformability of erythrocytes from patients with chronic occlusive arterial disease. Vasa 5:319–322, 1976
14. Fields WS, Lemak NA, Frankowski RF et al: Controlled trial of aspirin in cerebral ischemia. Stroke 8:301–315, 1977
15. Gelin LE: Influence of low viscosity dextran on peripheral circulation in man. Acta Chir Scand 122:303–308, 1961
16. Hess H, Mietaschk A, Dichesel G: Drug-induced inhibition of platelet function delays progression of peripheral occlusive arterial disease. Lancet 1:415–421, 1985
17. Porter JM, Cutler BS, Lee BY et al: Pentoxyifylline efficacy in the treatment of intermittent claudication: Multicenter controlled double-blind trial with objective assessment of chronic occlusive arterial disease patients. Am Heart J 104:66–72, 1982
18. Reid HL, Dormandy JA, Barnes AJ et al: Impaired red cell deformability in peripheral vascular disease. Lancet 1:666–667, 1976
19. Rutherford RB, Jones DN, Bergentz SE et al: The efficacy of dextran 40 in preventing early postoperative thrombosis following difficult lower extremity bypass. J Vasc Surg 1:765–773, 1984
20. Schuler JJ, Flanigan DP, Holcroft JW et al: Efficacy of prostaglandin E_1 in the treatment of lower extremity ischemic ulcers secondary to peripheral vascular disease. J Vasc Surg 1:160–170, 1984

21. Sorlie D, Myhre K: Effects of physical training in intermittent claudication. Scand J Clin Lab Invest 38:217–222, 1978
22. Sumner DS, Strandness DE Jr. The relationship between calf blood flow and ankle blood pressure in patients with intermittent claudication. Surgery 65:763–771, 1969
23. Taylor LM Jr, Porter JM: Drug treatment of claudication: Vasodilators, hemorrheologic agents, and antiserotonin drugs. J Vasc Surg 3:374–381, 1986

CHAPTER FOURTEEN
Medical and Surgical Management of Peripheral Vascular Disease in the Diabetic Patient
John S. Kirkland

This chapter addresses the pathophysiology of atherosclerosis, diagnosis of peripheral vascular occlusive disease, and medical and surgical management in the diabetic patient. There are approximately ten million diabetics in the United States, with numerous new diabetics diagnosed every year. Approximately 85% of diabetics will have some problem with peripheral vascular disease if they live 20 years or more after the diagnosis is made.[12] In a setting of vascular disease, the cost of hospitalization for a person who develops a diabetic foot ulceration is at least $20,000.

PATHOPHYSIOLOGY OF ATHEROSCLEROSIS

Table 14-1 shows the risk factors in the pathogenesis of atherosclerosis. Antiplatelet drugs may prevent atherosclerosis by preventing the deposition of platelets over an area of denuded endothelium. Platelets tend to stimulate smooth muscle ingrowth and infiltration and may have an important role in development of the atherosclerotic plaque. We are aware of the importance of cigarette smoking in the pathogenesis and complications of atherosclerosis. Hypertension has an important role. Obviously, diabetes is important, and hyperlipidemia, stress with release of epinephrine, and diet have a role in terms of managing hyperlipidemia and

Table 14–1

Risk Factors for Atherosclerosis

Nonmodifiable Risk Factors	*Modifiable Risk Factors*
Age	Smoking
Sex	Hyperlipidemia
Heredity	Diabetes
	Hypertension
	(Lifestyle)

diabetes. A recent study by Strandness reviewed patients with peripheral vascular occlusive disease with and without diabetes mellitus.[13] Arm:ankle:brachial indexes were measured to determine evidence of progression. Using a drop of 0.15 in the index as evidence of progression, it was found that over 2 years only about 1% of the controlled patients had progression of peripheral vascular disease, whereas 17% of the diabetic patients had a significant progression. In reviewing the natural history of atherosclerosis in diabetic and nondiabetic patients, the death rate in 10 years in diabetic patients is almost two and one-half times that of nondiabetics (17% versus 38%, respectively). In 15 years the nondiabetic patient death rate from atherosclerosis has risen to 33% and the diabetic death rate to 69%.[11] It is a devastating disease in the diabetic and requires a team approach to manage it.

The prevalence rate of the various types of peripheral vascular disease in diabetic carotid artery disease is approximately eight times more common in the type II diabetic than in the general controlled population. Peripheral vascular occlusive disease is about 20 times more common in the type II diabetic than in the matched control population without diabetes.

SMOKING

The risk of sudden death from coronary disease in smokers less than 65 years of age is twice the rate of that in nonsmokers. Most of these are caused by ventricular arrhythmias. The risk of claudication developing in men over 45 years of age who smoke over 15 cigarettes a day is nine times the risk of nonsmokers. In claudicators with established claudication followed over 5 years, nonsmokers—those who stopped smoking, exercised, lost weight, and followed a conservative regimen—lost no legs in recent study. Over a 5-year period, 11.4% of smokers had an amputation.[3]

Early studies have been equivocal about whether cigarette smoking has a direct correlation with carotid artery disease.[6] A study done in Hawaii followed a large number of men, both smokers and nonsmokers.[1] The risk of stroke in male smokers was felt to be two to three times that of nonsmokers. Symptomatic subjects who continued to smoke during follow-up had a four to six times increased risk of cerebrovascular accident, and smokers who stopped smoking had a greater than 50% reduction in cerebrovascular accident risk.

Patients who stop smoking after about 5 years return to 50% of their previous risk.[1] In terms of cardiovascular disease, after about 10 years it is as if they had never smoked.[3] Patients who undergo arterial reconstructions need to understand that if they continue to smoke after their arterial reconstruction, there is a good chance the operation will fail.

DIAGNOSIS OF PERIPHERAL VASCULAR OCCLUSIVE DISEASE

Making the diagnosis of peripheral vascular disease in the diabetic patient is no different than in any other patient. The exception is the question of whether they will experience rest pain; they may have so much neuropathy that they are insensitive. Obviously, skin color, temperature, hair distribution, presence of atrophic changes, pulses, presence of bruits, aneurysms, and evidence of peripheral emboli are all important factors in peripheral vascular disease.

Careful inspection of the foot is a necessity. In a patient who has a foot that is cold, pale on elevation, and ruborous when it is dependent, with the typical atrophic changes of shiny skin, loss of nails, and loss of hair, all of these signs are suspicious for peripheral arterial disease in both the diabetic and nondiabetic.

One cannot always palpate a foot pulse; it is symmetrically absent to palpation in 15% of women and 5% of men. Edema may further compound the inability to feel a pulse.

Careful examination and listening for bruits are important because many of these patients, although they have primarily distal arterial disease, will have a femoral artery bruit, a reflection of more proximal disease. Bruits elsewhere in the body can be an indication of a significant problem. A recent study pointed out that the carotid bruit is a significant marker for coronary artery disease.[2] This study confirmed that the death rate over 5 years from coronary artery disease was considerably higher than the death rate from stroke.

Careful palpation of the abdominal, femoral, and popliteal

areas for aneurysms is important. A patient with a femoral artery aneurysm has about a 40% chance of also having an abdominal aortic aneurysm. Patients who have bilateral femoral aneurysms have a 92% chance of having an abdominal aneurysm. Detecting aneurysms on physical examination, therefore, can be important, particularly in an obese patient.

The vascular diagnostic laboratory can be of assistance in determining whether the patient has peripheral arterial disease. The segmental arterial pressures are useful in identifying large vessel disease primarily. The arterial pulse wave analysis, or so-called arterial flow study, allows one to review the character and quality of the pulse wave. If a bruit is present, spectral analysis will assist in determining percentage of stenosis. Photoplethymyosgraphy can be used to determine the presence of small vessel disease in the distal vasculature of the toes and feet.

The graduated treadmill exercise test continues to have an important role in detecting a stenosis in the large vessel that has not yet reached the point where the patient has a decrease in resting ankle pressure. With exercise, the patient will claudicate and a decrease in pressure can be demonstrated. Normally, the ankle:brachial index is 1; when it falls to approximately 0.65, the patient begins to develop intermittent claudication. The diabetic patient may develop intermittent claudication at a slightly higher ankle:brachial index. Any ankle:brachial index of <0.9 is abnormal. The patient with an ankle:brachial index in the range of 0.3 will begin to develop signs of tissue ischemia and rest pain; in those with an ankle:brachial index of <0.2, tissue loss and gangrene are noted frequently. Figure 14-1 shows an arterial flow study indicating the typical findings in a patient with large vessel disease, normal triphasic arterial waveform in the femoral area, normal triphasic waveform in the dorsalis pedis and posterior tibial, with an ankle pressure of 120. Occlusion of the iliac artery results in an attenuation of the waveform with a biphasic waveform and a pressure of 80 all the way down. It is important to note that patients can have significant disease even with a normal ankle pressure.

Arteriography is essential in defining whether a given lesion is reconstructable. A few years ago it was thought that digital angiography would replace conventional angiography, but conventional angiography was found to be more useful than the digital intravenous mode. Digital angiography can be more useful in the arterial mode, where a catheter is introduced into the area to be filmed, a smaller amount of dye is injected, and the digital computerized technique is used to enhance the quality of the angiogram.

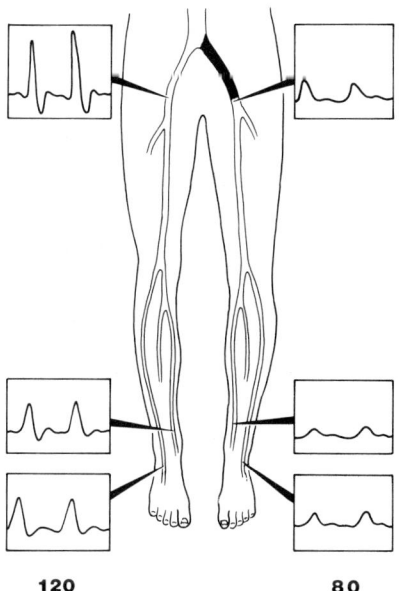

Figure 14-1. Segmental pressure and waveform alterations associated with left iliac occlusion.

INTERMITTENT CLAUDICATION

Intermittent claudication can sometimes be difficult to diagnose. The distribution of pain is related to location of the arterial blockage. Patients experience cramplike pain in the legs; their legs tire easily and feel weak. Many patients have more difficulty going up stairs and hills and limit their activity because of the disability.

Intermittent claudication is caused by occlusion or stenosis in an artery proximal to the affected muscles, with a decrease in blood flow and increase in viscosity. The red blood cells tend to aggregate, and a further decrease in blood flow occurs. The typical sequential signs of the patient with intermittent claudication are: exercise, insufficient blood supply, calf pain, rest, experience relief, and go on again. In contrast, the patient who has ischemic rest pain will have a fixed blockage, usually at two levels; it generally takes more than one level of occlusion to produce ischemic rest pain. Exercise is not necessary to produce these symptoms.

MEDICAL MANAGEMENT

An exercise program is important in medical management of peripheral vascular disease. Patients are advised to begin walking and to set a goal for distance. If they claudicate after they walk one block, they should walk that block and a little further each time. They are advised to walk until they experience pain in the calf or thigh, then walk through the claudication.

There is no doubt that an exercise program in a patient whose only symptom is claudication will result in improvement in the claudication in a significant number of people.

Smoking abstinence is important in the management of peripheral vascular disease, as stated previously.

Control of diabetes is essential. A lipid profile should be done on all patients seen initially to determine their lipid status.[5]

Weight reduction is important, because a person carrying an additional 50 lb may claudicate. If a patient loses 50 lb, or even 15 lb or 20 lb, the claudication will disappear because of the decreased metabolic demand of weighing less.

Foot care is extremely important. (See Chap. 12 for specific information on care and medical treatment of the diabetic foot.)

DRUG THERAPY

Administration of anticoagulants, vasodilators, hemorrheologic agents, and aspirin may reduce blood viscosity. These drugs do not have any effect on red cell flexibility; they do result in some increased risk of bleeding or hemorrhage.

Coumadin has a place in the treatment of patients with peripheral arterial disease in some instances; in particular, patients who have small bypasses or following re-do small vessel distal reconstructions.

In the early postoperative period, evidence also exists to indicate that use of antiplatelet drugs may reduce the deposition of platelets at the junction between the prosthetic graft and distal artery. Most prosthetic grafts tend to fail because of intimal hyperplasia at the distal anastomosis. The intimal hyperplasia develops initially because of platelet aggregation; if the platelet aggregation can be limited, so can the intimal hyperplasia. Antiplatelet drugs are, therefore, used in patients with peripheral arterial disease, but not necessarily in an attempt to treat claudication.

Peripheral vasodilators are not particularly useful in treatment of patients with intermittent claudication. Collateral vessels tend to dilate more than muscular vessels and in patients treated with oral vasodilators, the ischemic limb is probably already maximally vasodilated. In the diabetic it may be autosympathectomized and a potent vasodilator may reduce the blood pressure and cause a decrease of blood flow to the limb.

Several hemorrheologic agents tend to change the viscosity of the blood. Prostacyclin, although it has not been released for clinical use, affects platelet aggregation. Reducing the level of fibrinogen may also change the viscosity of the blood. Pentoxifylline (Trental) changes the erythrocyte flexibility and does not have a vasodilator effect. It is effective orally and indicated only for treatment of patients with intermittent claudication. The ischemic red cell is not as flexible as the normal red cell, resulting in the roleaux formation and increased viscosity of the blood. Tissue oxygen in skeletal muscle has been shown to increase after treatment with Trental in claudicating subjects.[4] In a multicenter study reported by Porter and co-workers in 1982, Trental was used for 6 months.[8] The patients on placebo who exercised, stopped smoking, and did not take the drug had a considerable improvement; those who took the drug had about 20% improvement in walking distance from baseline values. One can expect with pentoxifylline that roughly 60% of patients are able to walk 20% further. Eight to 12 weeks are required for a appreciable effect.

SURGICAL MANAGEMENT

Some of the indications for operative reconstruction in patients are ischemic rest pain, ischemic ulceration, peripheral embolization, threatened limb loss, and the rare indication of disabling claudication. Arterial reconstruction is difficult to justify in patients when that reconstruction may result in loss of a limb, if they were not already at risk for limb loss. Patients whose only symptom is intermittent claudication have about a 1% amputation rate per year. Diabetics have a higher amputation rate, but should be assessed more carefully. Life- or limb-threatening aneurysms, popliteal aneurysms in particular, are sometimes ignored because they do not produce symptoms. The first symptom may be distal embolization of atheromatous material from the popliteal aneurysm and the loss of a limb. Most of those limbs are not retrievable if the popliteal aneurysm thromboses and embolizes.

RECONSTRUCTIVE TECHNIQUES

PERCUTANEOUS TRANSLUMINAL ANGIOPLASTY

What role does percutaneous transluminal angioplasty play in arterial reconstruction today? A number of the centers previously in favor of aggressive balloon angioplasty are no longer as liberal in the use of this procedure, primarily because of the restenosis rate and peripheral embolization. It is useful in certain clinical settings; the patient with an isolated iliac artery stenosis is an excellent candidate for balloon angioplasty because the large vessel lesion can be dilated with a high degree of success and without significant risk of distal embolization. In patients who have multiple or long-segment, superficial femoral artery stenosis, successful long-term recanalization with balloon angioplasty is difficult. Distal stenoses are even less amenable to angioplasty.

LOCAL ENDARTERECTOMY

Local endarterectomy was a popular technique 20 to 25 years ago, but fell into disuse in favor of bypass grafting. Local endarterectomy may be useful in certain areas, especially in the iliac vessels where there is a large vessel with a short area of stenosis, particularly after a failed angioplasty. Sometimes one can use a less traumatic retroperitoneal approach to the iliac artery. A vein patch angioplasty may avoid the use of synthetic graft material.

CONVENTIONAL BYPASS RECONSTRUCTION

In the diabetic patient, arterial disease tends to be more distal; it occurs frequently in the vessels below the knee, and bypass reconstruction techniques are more difficult and less successful. Using an autogenous saphenous vein bypass has been the standard technique for treating these patients for a number of years. In this technique the vein is harvested from the leg and reversed, resulting in flow in the opposite direction so that the flow is not obstructed by patent venous valves or used *in situ* with a device to remove the venous valves. There are disadvantages with the reverse vein technique. When the vein is removed and reversed, a certain amount of trauma occurs to the vein, and the adventitial blood supply of the vein has been interrupted. The other problem is strictly geometric. The distal graft is frequently two to four times as large as the artery to which it is being anastomosed and can result in disturbed-flow velocities, turbulence, and subsequent thrombosis.

IN SITU VEIN GRAFT TECHNIQUE

The *in situ* vein graft technique has been used by our group for about 5 years. A recent review of our results showed a 89.3% early patency rate and an 80% 2-year patency rate in tibial arterial reconstruction; the historical development of the technique and results of other investigators are also summarized elsewhere.[9] In this technique, the vein is left in place in the leg. The valves are removed mechanically with instruments specially designed for this purpose. The result is a small distal vein to anastomose to a small distal artery, with a better size match in the groin between the proximal saphenous vein and femoral artery. The adventitia of the vein is not interrupted; therefore, the blood supply is better preserved. Electron microscopic studies indicate that the endothelium of the vein is well preserved with the *in situ* technique, and the early patency rate, in particular, tends to be better with this technique.[9]

ANGIOSCOPY

Angioscopy is an exciting field only recently coming into use. This technique involves using a fiberoptic scope introduced into the blood vessel to allow the lumen of the vessel to be viewed directly. The angioscope is similar to any other fiberoptic scope (bronchoscope, gastroscope, esophagoscope), only smaller. It is 2.5 mm in diameter and consists of a catheter with a cuff at the end, which can be inflated; a fiberoptic fiber for illumination; a channel for inflating the cuff; a fiberoptic viewing channel; and a channel for irrigation. The angioscope is introduced through a small incision in the artery. The scope is passed down to the area to be viewed, and the cuff is inflated. The irrigation fluid flushes the blood out of the artery to permit the lumen to be visualized. In most atherosclerotic patients with poor distal collaterals, one can insert the scope and look directly at the lumen and visualize the atherosclerotic plaques.[7]

In comparison, angiography provides only a two-dimensional picture of the vessel. It denotes the severity and approximate location, but does not allow as accurate identification of the morphologic nature of the underlying disease process.

LASER ANGIOPLASTY

Laser angioplasty will become more common in the next few years. Most of the initial studies have used a bare laser fiber introduced into the vessel. The bare laser fiber was used to apply laser energy to the plaque to blast away or burn a hole through the plaque. This technique has certain obvious disadvantages in that the energy is not focused, causing damage to the arterial wall.

A new technology has been developed called a hot tip catheter, which is a laser fiberoptic catheter tipped with a small olive-shaped metal ball about 2 mm in diameter.[10] The ball is heated by the laser energy and creates the channel. Early results with the laser catheter are promising, and extensive reconstruction of below-knee-level vessels may be possible with further refinements.

SUMMARY

The risk factors of hyperlipidemia, smoking, and hypertension all contribute to the pathophysiology of peripheral vascular disease. Critical evaluation of the extremity; accurate history and physical assessment; and noninvasive vascular diagnostic laboratory, including Doppler ultrasound, photoplethysmography, graduated treadmill exercise testing, and following arteriography, aid in diagnosis and independent assessment of the disease process. Medical management, of course, means controlling all of the adverse metabolic factors; it can include exercise and possibly some drug therapy. Surgical management is for rest pain and tissue breakdown or claudication interfering with one's lifestyle. Claudication is not a direct threat to limb loss, although rest pain and tissue breakdown are. Current interventional techniques include percutaneous transluminal angioplasty, laser angioplasty, endarterectomy, and bypass surgery. There are unlimited future opportunities in the field of surgical reconstruction; the number of diabetics with vascular disease is ever increasing.

REFERENCES

1. Abbott RD, Yin Yin MA, Reed DM, Katsuhiko Y: Risk of stroke in male cigarette smokers. N Engl J Med 315:717–720, 1986
2. Chambers BR, Norris JW: Outcome of patients with asymptomatic neck bruits. N Engl J Med 315:860–865, 1986
3. Couch NP: On the arterial consequences of smoking. J Vasc Surg 3:807–812, 1986
4. Ehrly AM: Effects of orally administered pentoxifylline on muscular oxygen pressure in patients with intermittent claudication. IRCS Med SC 10:401–402, 1982
5. Garrison RJ, Feinleib M, Castelli WP et al: Cigarette smoking as a confounder of the relationship between relative weight and long-term mortality, the Framingham study. JAMA 249:2199–2203, 1983

6. Herman B, Leyten ACM, Van Luijk et al: An evaluation of risk factors for stroke in a Dutch community. Stroke 13:334–339, 1982
7. Litvack F, Grundfest WS, Lee ME et al: Angioscopic visualization of blood vessel interior in animals and humans. Clin Cardiol 8:65–70, 1985
8. Porter JM, Cutler BS, Lee BY et al: Pentoxifylline in the treatment of intermittent claudication: Multicenter controlled double-blind trial with objective assessment of chronic occlusive arterial disease patients. Am Heart J 104:66–72, 1982
9. Rogers DM, Rhodes EL, Kirkland JS: *In situ* saphenous vein bypass for occlusive disease in the lower extremity. Surg Clin North Am 66:319–331, 1986
10. Sanborn TA, Faxon DP, Haudenschild CC et al: Experimental angioplasty: Circumferential distribution of laser thermal energy with a laser probe. JACC 5:934–938, 1985
11. Silbert S, Zazeela H: Prognosis in arteriosclerotic peripheral vascular disease. JAMA 166:1816–1821, 1958
12. Stemmen EA: Vascular complications of diabetes mellitus. In Moore WW (ed): Vascular Surgery, a Comprehensive Review. New York, Grune & Stratton, 1983
13. Strandness DE: Natural history of peripheral arterial disease. Presented at Tulane University Symposium on Peripheral Arterial Disease, New Orleans, Louisiana, 1986

CHAPTER FIFTEEN
Peripheral Vascular Disease and the Diabetic Patient

Donald L. Akers
Gordon Cohen
Morris D. Kerstein

Evaluation and management of patients with peripheral vascular disease are often complex, difficult to achieve, and confusing; the situation is further worsened when peripheral vascular disease is combined with diabetes. Diabetes can confuse the presentation of the symptoms, evaluation of the disease, and definitive management of the disease process. Diabetes also hastens progression of the disease. In the Tulane University Medical Center, progression of vascular disease was dramatically accelerated in the diabetic versus nondiabetic population. The incidence of limb loss increased significantly in the diabetic population. The combination of poor vascular supply and diabetic derangement of the tissue can defeat even the most aggressive surgeon or conscientious patient.

PATHOPHYSIOLOGY

Progressive tissue loss and destruction of peripheral vascular disease in the diabetic extremity involves two primary mechanisms: increased neuropathy and decreased vascular perfusion. The neuropathy is a reflection of a sensory deficit, motor loss, and autonomic dysfunction. Decreased perfusion is usually a result of atherosclerosis of the large vessel, which is often bilateral, multilevel, and multisegmented in the diabetic. Frequently, the atherosclerotic process is most severe in the blood vessels below the knee.[48] The disease process of the diabetic patient also involves the microvasculature, resulting in increased thickness in capillary basement membranes.[31] This condition also contributes to local tissue damage by hypoxia. A combination of mechanisms, therefore, contributes to the accelerated rate of peripheral vascular disease in the diabetic patient.

The mechanism of the development of neuropathy is shown in Figure 15-1. Sorbitol, a sugar alcohol, is formed from glucose by the enzyme, aldose reductase.[17] This enzyme is present in highest concentrations in tissue where glucose transport is independent of insulin, such as lens epithelium, kidney papillae, and Schwann cells of peripheral nerves. Because the Michaelis-Menton constant (Km) of aldose reductase for glucose is high, sorbitol is only formed in significant amounts when glucose levels are elevated. Because of poor membrane transport mechanisms, the majority of sorbitol will remain intracellular. The major mechanism for cellular metabolism

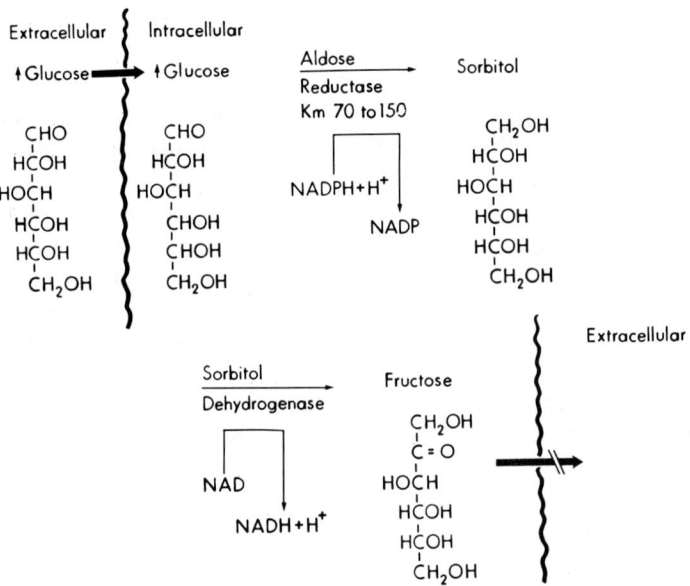

Figure 15-1. Sorbitol pathway—under normal circumstances little formation of sorbitol exists because the enzyme aldose reductase has a low affinity for glucose and galactose (70 to 150 km). In the diabetic population, however, the elevated glucose results in increased production of sorbitol and fructose. These sugar alcohols accumulate in the cell, causing degeneration and destruction of the peripheral nerves.

of sorbitol is its conversion to fructose, a five-carbon sugar (Fig. 15-1). The enzyme also has a high Km for sorbitol; thus, a slow conversion results. Subsequently, sorbitol will accumulate, which results in intracellular hyperosmolarity. This increased osmolarity has severe consequences, especially pronounced in the lens, kidneys, and peripheral nerves. While lens and kidney effects of sorbitol are important, the development of neuropathy is a critical factor in the rapid progression of peripheral vascular disease in the diabetic patient.[14,35,50]

Peripheral neuropathy involves somatic, autonomic, and motor fibers. Small fibers are usually the initial deficit in development of the neuropathy, and small fiber dysfunction results in the loss of pain and thermal sensation.[22] Small fiber loss can also result in a sympathetic denervation, characteristic of the warm and dry diabetic foot. The neuropathy will usually progress to involve the large myelinated fibers, which results in a corresponding loss of touch, vibration, and proprioception. This condition will continue to progress, involving the motor fibers, with a resultant loss of the intrinsic muscle mass of the foot.[9,24]

Important from a vascular standpoint is development of autonomic denervation, which can result in marked abnormalities of blood flow. Recent studies indicate a decreased forward flow in dilated inflexible arteries, as well as the absence of reverse flow (*i.e.*, a monophasic wave is seen instead of the usual triphasic wave on plethysmography) (Fig. 15-2).[9,24] An associated decrease in venous flow may also occur.[2] The change in both arterial and venous flow may result in arteriovenous shunts. The increase in venous pressure can result in peripheral edema secondary to impedence of outflow. Partsch reported the mean shunt value in neuropathies was 8.45% compared with 5% in controls.[41] The actual effect of the shunt is unknown in terms of metabolic effects, because measurement of the arteriovenous oxygen gradients between diabetics and nondiabetics does not show a significant difference. Nevertheless, the arteriovenous shunt probably contributes to the metabolic derangement noted in diabetic tissue. One possible explanation for the lack of an arteriovenous oxygen difference involves the effect of glucose elevation on hemoglobin. In diabetics, HbA_1C is a glycated hemoglobin that comprises 6% to 10% of the total hemoglobin; normally, this glycated hemoglobin comprises 3% to 5%. This type of hemoglobin is formed by the irreversible, post-translational, nonenzymatic glycation of hemoglobin A, and involves linkage of glucose to the N-terminal valine of the B-chain of hemoglobin. The actual mechanism involves the formation of a Schiff's base (Fig. 15-3). This hemoglo-

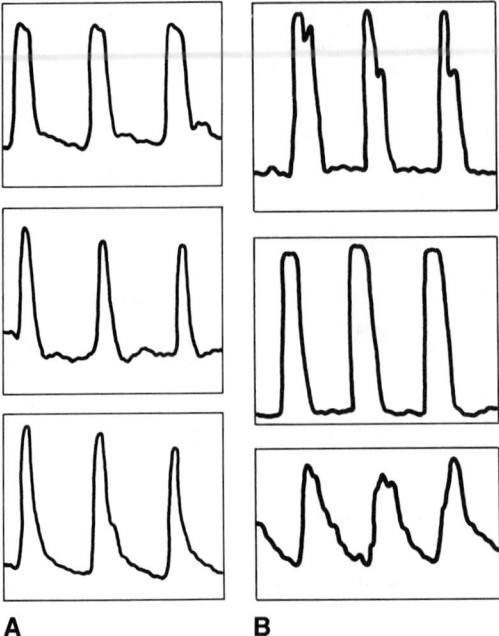

Figure 15-2. (A) The Doppler waveform of a normal vascular system—the waveform is triphasic with a normal forward flow, followed by a period of reverse flow and finally a return to forward flow. (B) The Doppler waveform of a diabetic vascular system—the waveform is monophasic. In the early diabetic patient, a marked increase occurs in the forward flow with loss of the period of reverse flow.

bin has less sensitivity to 2,3 diphosphoglycerate and, thus, decreased release of oxygen in the peripheral tissues. The mechanism could account for decreased delivery of oxygen to the peripheral tissue in the presence of a normal arteriovenous oxygen difference.[53]

Atherosclerosis in the diabetic involves two mechanisms. The first mechanism involves the cutaneous dysfunction mentioned above. The constant dilation of the arterial tree has been proposed as a predisposing factor in arterial medial wall calcification. This calcification has been suggested to play a role in the "lead-pipe" phenomenon seen in the Doppler evaluation of diabetic patients. The second mechanism of atherosclerosis in the diabetic patient is the disease of the larger vessels. No distinguishing feature exists to separate the diabetic from the nondiabetic. The disease begins classically as fatty streaks in the large vessels, which develop into

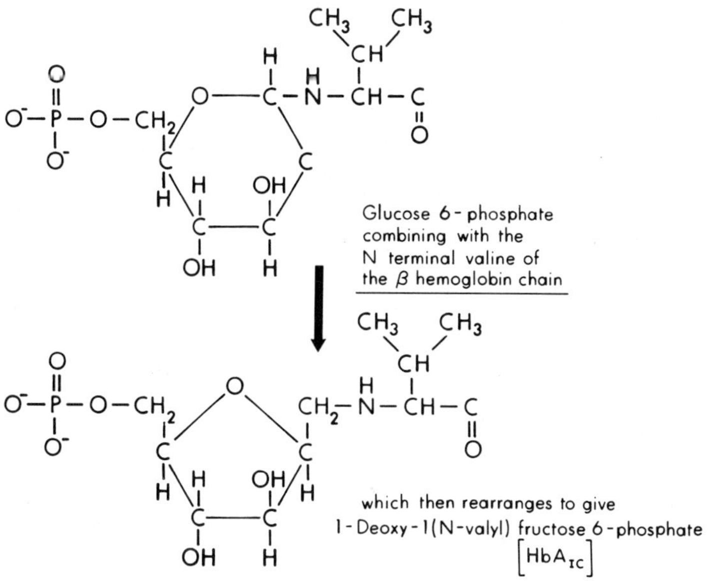

Figure 15-3. The formation of hemoglobin A₁C involves the glycation of the N-terminal valine of the β-chain. Glucose 6-phosphate appears to have an affinity for the binding site of 2.3 diphosphoglycerate, thus reducing hemoglobin affinity for the compound, resulting in decreased release of oxygen by hemoglobin at the tissue levels. The final step of this pathway, conversion to the fructose derivative, is irreversible.

atherosclerosis over time.[54] The result of progression of disease is ischemia of the extremity. As mentioned previously, the region of disease is usually distal, multisegmental, and bilateral when compared with that found in the nondiabetic. In type I insulin-dependent diabetes mellitus, the disease is small vessel: retinal, renal, and peripheral vascular. In type II non-insulin-dependent diabetes mellitus, the disease is similar to classic atherosclerosis or combined anatomic findings of small and large vessel disease. The type I patient dies of complications of multisystem disease. The type II patient lives longer and dies of cardiovascular disease, heart attack, and stroke. It must be emphasized that larger vessels are often involved and even smaller vessels can be revascularized. The areas involved are usually regions of high turbulence (*i.e.*, bifurcations—vessels of the lower extremity and foot are often significantly involved).[12,34]

DIAGNOSIS

Initial evaluation of the diabetic with peripheral vascular disease should begin with the history and physical examination. The initial history in the patient with peripheral vascular disease revolves around the five P's: pulselessness, pallor, paresthesia, pain, and paralysis. The important point in obtaining the history from a diabetic patient is to differentiate between the symptoms caused by vascular disease or diabetes, or a combination of both. Evaluation of the diabetic patient with peripheral vascular disease requires a complete understanding of the pathophysiology. Derangement at the cellular level helps to explain the alteration of symptoms. As discussed previously, defective glucose metabolism results in excessive sorbitol deposition in the nerve sheath, resulting in a subsequent neuropathy. These changes and symptomatology must be differentiated from ischemic changes. Even more difficult is when both vascular and diabetic components combine, making it difficult to determine the actual cause of the symptoms. The physician must elicit a careful, exact history to guide the evaluation in the proper direction.

Pain is the predominant reason both diabetics with peripheral neuropathy and patients with peripheral vascular disease appear for their initial evaluation. Pain associated with ischemic vascular disease is characterized by the syndrome of nocturnal foot pain, which occurs in the metatarsal location of the forefoot. This pain is often relieved by dependency.[27] The importance of the complaint of rest pain is that it is the predecessor to gangrene in the progression of peripheral vascular disease. Rest pain must be differentiated from diabetic neuropathy because rest pain and tissue breakdown are associated with limb loss. Diabetic neuropathy is most commonly a peripheral polyneuropathy and the presenting findings may be confusing. The syndrome is usually bilateral, characterized with numbness, paresthesias, severe hyperethesias, and pain. The pain, which can be severe, is deep-seated and usually worse at night. The pain syndromes are usually self-limiting and range from a few months' to a few years' duration.[15,21] It is obvious that the differentiation between the pain of vascular disease and that of diabetic neuropathy is not only difficult, but critical to the correct management of this patient population.

The presence of paresthesias or claudication requires an evaluation of hypoxia of the muscles of the lower extremity. Little distinction is noted in symptoms between the diabetic and nondiabetic patient. It is a reproducible physical finding in that a set level of activity produces symptoms relieved by a period of rest. Claudication is not associated with limb loss. The physiology involves anaerobic metabolism with the subsequent production of lactic acid, carbon dioxide accumulation, and hypoxia.[23] Although this can be an inconvenience to the patient, surgery is only recommended in unusual situations where significant limitation to lifestyle occurs. Only 1% to 3% of patients with claudication will progress to limb loss, and all will have further development of signs and symptoms of peripheral vascular disease leading to rest pain or tissue breakdown as the intermediate step. Patients who cannot work secondary to their claudication and have no other means of support need operative intervention. Evaluation of claudication is also important in long-term management of the patient with peripheral vascular disease. Progression of disease can be evaluated by worsening of the claudication (*i.e.*, less exercise, producing the same symptoms). Finally, in evaluation of claudication the symptoms must not be confused with intermittent cramps seen not only in diabetics, but also in certain electrolyte abnormalities.

The remaining three P's—pulselessness, pallor, and paralysis—in the evaluation of peripheral vascular disease involve physical assessment of the patient. Pulselessness reflects the ability to detect palpable pulses in the lower extremity. Measurement of the pressure associated with pulse, which will be discussed later, has become a major diagnostic tool in evaluation of peripheral vascular disease. Absence of a pulse, however, is not always indicative of associated vascular disease because 15% of all women and 5% of all men normally have the segmental absence of foot pulses.[46] In the diabetic patient, severe peripheral vascular disease may be present even with good palpable pulses. This disease syndrome has been described previously as "lead-pipe" disease.[12] Pallor appears with advanced arterial insufficiency. The characteristic vascular findings are a purplish rubor with dependency of the extremity, which changes to a pale foot with elevation. Again, this is not an absolute rule because pallor can also be associated with other disease states. Paralysis is more often associated with acute vascular occlusion, although it can be seen with chronic vascular insufficiency. It is a poor prognostic sign and amputation is often the only treatment left to the physician. In the patient with chronic vascular insufficiency changes, progression of claudication is rest pain to gangrene, but should be recognized and treated before the development of paralysis.

The physical evaluation of the diabetic patient with peripheral vascular disease would be incomplete without examination of the foot for ulcers. Important in the examination is to differentiate ulcers caused by diabetic neuropathy from those caused by vascular insufficiency. Figure 15-4 shows a classic neuropathic ulcer.[9] The location is usually the metatarsal heads, with other locations including the dorsum of the toes and heels; the pathology appears at points of initiation of pressure. The neuropathic ulcer is painless and usually surrounded by an elevated callus.[10] The ulcer often has a punched-out appearance, can involve the deeper tissue, and is usually superficially infected.[9] These ulcers are the result of noxious stimuli not perceived by the patient because of the loss of sensation of pain. The stimuli result in chemical, thermal, and mechanical injuries. Several additional mechanisms have been proposed to contribute to the formation of these ulcers, including the loss of sweating, loss of temperature and vibration sense, and arteriovenous shunting.[4,7,13,22] Arteriovenous shunting causes reduced nutrient delivery to the tissue by reduction of the capillary blood flow.[33] Injury is brought about by direct mechanical or repeated trauma to a callus formed previously. These ulcers have

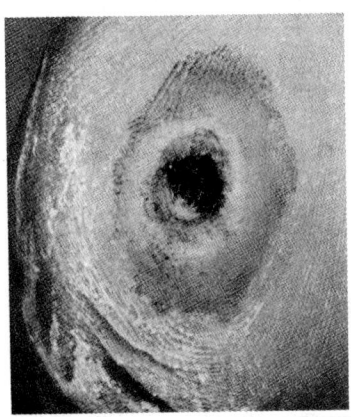 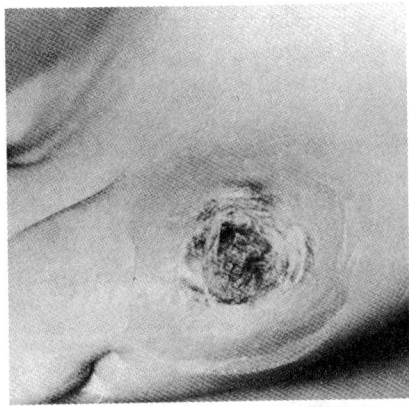

A   **B**

Figure 15-4. (A) Neuropathic ulcer of a diabetic patient. The neuropathic ulcer usually has a punched-out appearance surrounded by a callus. This ulcer is usually superficially infected and can involve the deep tissues. (B) Nondiabetic vascular ulcer. This ulcer is found in regions of poor vascular flow. Loss of hair, shiny skin, and muscle atrophy are characteristics of this region. In contrast to the diabetic ulcer, there is usually no callus, but a surrounding area of erythema does occur. These ulcers can also be superficially infected and, if allowed to progress, will proceed to gangrene. (Reproduced with permission from Edmonds ME: The diabetic foot: Pathophysiology and treatment. In Watkins PJ (ed): Clinics in Endocrinology and Metabolism. Vol 15, No 4, pp 889–916. Philadelphia, WB Saunders, 1986

been shown to occur at areas of maximal loading.[6,9,43] The diabetic ulcer must be contrasted to the ulcer associated with ischemic vascular disease. The nondiabetic vascular ulcer appears in a region of poor perfusion (Fig. 15-4,*B*). The more common sites include the great toe, medial surface of the head of the first metatarsal, lateral surface of the head of the fifth metatarsal, and heel. These ulcers can also be infected secondarily with both anaerobic and aerobic organisms. Atherosclerotic ulcers may be multiorganisms in character, but are predominantly *Staphylococcus aureus* (coagulase positive); diabetic ulcers have a variety of organisms including *Staphylococcus*. If allowed to progress, gangrene can develop in the region of ulceration. The ulcer usually has an area of necrosis; often the ulcer is surrounded by an area of erythema.[28] In contrast to the diabetic ulcer, no callus surrounds the vascular ulcer. The pathogenesis of the vascular ulcer is a loss of blood supply to the foot.[48] Histopathology is similar to that seen in nondiabetics with the development of extensive plaques, especially at points of bifurcation.[52] The initiating event of the vascular ulcer is usually perceived as minor trauma, which is then complicated by infection. Because of the poor blood supply, the patient cannot mount an adequate response; subsequently, the ulcer will develop. The ability to differentiate between neuropathic and vascular ulcers is extremely important because the treatment methods are markedly different. Furthermore, presence of neuropathy in the patient with peripheral vascular disease often causes the patient not to recognize the vascular ulcer until the disease is far advanced.

CLINICAL INVESTIGATION

After the initial examination (history and physical) indicates the presence of vascular disease, the next step in the evaluation is to determine the location and severity. The initial evaluation should begin with noninvasive studies that revolve around the blood flow laboratory. If the patient is found to have a surgically correctable lesion and is a candidate (appropriate cardiopulmonary and renal status) for reconstructive surgery, an arteriogram is performed.

NONINVASIVE BLOOD FLOW LABORATORY MEASUREMENTS

Although the physical examination can suggest the underlying problem initially, further techniques are needed to define more accurately the extent of the disease process. The role of a noninvasive vascular blood flow laboratory is to review the locations and severity of the disease and determine functional significance. Doppler ultrasonography measures blood pressure in a sophisticated fashion. The Doppler effect was first described in 1842. The basic concept is to evaluate the sound change produced by fluid in motion. It was popularized in 1969 by Yao when he compared the blood pressure in the upper extremity to that of the foot.[56] If a patient has a normal brachial blood pressure of 120, the posterior tibial and dorsalis pedis are exactly the same in the normal resting supine patient, which yields an ankle:brachial ratio of one. The device is based on the flow of blood through each vessel and because each vessel can be evaluated separately, the patency of each vessel can be determined. In this way, the vessels can be studied individually, and level of obstruction is suggested when a marked change in pressures is noted. Thus, a patient with a normal thigh pressure and a significantly decreased popliteal artery pressure will probably have superficial femoral artery disease.

Evaluation of ankle pressures is significant in determining the severity of peripheral vascular disease in the lower extremity. Table 15-1 indicates the various ranges and corresponding disease states. A ratio between 0.7 and 1.0 is usually considered normal; measurements in the range of 0.5 to 0.7 are usually associated with claudication; and measurements of 0.3 to 0.4 are compatible with rest pain. In the range of 0 to 0.2, the threat of imminent limb loss exists.[55] An additional pressure measurement is present in the diabetic patient, which occurs when the vessel cannot be occluded effectively by the blood pressure cuff and ankle pressures are higher than in the arm (*i.e.*, >1.0). This condition is seen with calcific vessels, described previously as the "lead-pipe" syndrome.[1]

Table 15-1

Ankle:Brachial Ratios and Corresponding Disease Stages

*Ankle:Brachial Ratio**	*Clinical Correlation*
0.7–1.0	Normal
0.6–0.7	Usually associated with claudication
0.3–0.5	Compatible with rest pain
0–0.3	Threat of imminent limb loss

*Values >1.0 can be obtained in diabetic patients, which is consistent with the phenomenon of "lead-pipe" disease.

Digital artery pressures are an extension of the Doppler pressure measurements. A digit cuff is applied, and photoplethysmography measurements are taken. The photoplethysmograph uses a transducer-emitting infrared light from a light-emitting diode into the underlying tissue.[55] The photoplethysmograph records instantaneous circulatory changes similar to those obtained from direct pressure measurements. Several studies have shown a strong correlation between blood flow and the ability to heal tissue.[3,11,44] In the diabetic patient, digit pressures >50 mmHg markedly enhance the potential to heal tissue.

The Doppler not only provides information by determining pressures, but also can provide significant data about the vessels by analysis of the waveform. Figure 15-5 shows the progression of disease as represented by the waveform. The normal waveform has a triphasic form, with a forward flow in systole, followed by a reversal of flow in diastole and a return to a short forward flow.[1] With the progression of disease, the triphasic wave will become monophasic with a decrease in amplitude, which must be differentiated from the monophasic form seen in the diabetic patient with neuropathy. In the diabetic patient, the monophasic wave shows a marked increase in the forward flow of systole (Fig. 15-2,B).[47] As the disease progresses, the waveform flattens. The significance of these changes is that the waveform is an early indication of peripheral vascular disease. The waveform will change first, followed by changes in the pressures.[16] Thus, in patients with minimal symp-

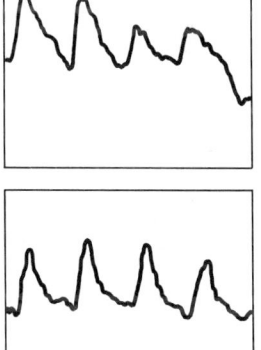
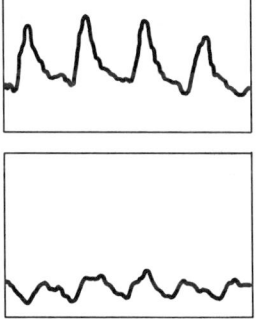

Figure 15-5. Doppler waveform of a diabetic patient with vascular disease. The waveform is initially the classical monophasic pattern in the femoral region. With the progression of disease down the extremity, however, a loss of amplitude and flattening of the waveform occur.

DIABETES AND VASCULAR DISEASE

toms, the waveform can indicate early disease. Changes in waveform and pressure will often allow the clinician to differentiate between neuropathy and vascular disease. Nevertheless, the two can co-exist, and often do.

Finally, noninvasive testing can also be used in association with treadmill testing. Patients may have normal pressures, palpable pulses, and waveforms in the presence of subcritical areas of stenosis. With the onset of ambulation at 1 mile per hour in the patient with a subcritical stenosis, the first changes are seen in the waveform. Figure 15-6 shows the progression of the waveform from triphasic to monophasic to flat in a patient who was otherwise normal on noninvasive evaluation. A decrease in pressure follows the changes in waveform. Patients who do not claudicate have normal pressures after 3 minutes. Patients who have changes in pressure have either a narrow, compressed, or inflexible vessel and they may be living off of their collaterals.

Noninvasive blood flow monitoring is a simple, effective, and relatively inexpensive way to evaluate the peripheral vascular system. It provides a rapid mechanism for determining the location of

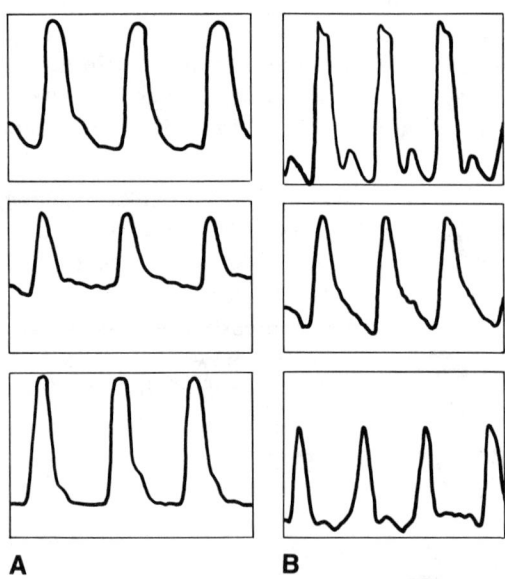

Figure 15-6. Doppler waveforms and treadmill testing. The patient initially had normal-appearing Doppler, as seen in A. After one minute on the treadmill, however, the Doppler exhibited a monophasic pattern, as seen in B. The patient's ankle:brachial ratio showed changes decreasing from .92 to .75 (dorsalis pedis).

significant disease and degree of compromise of flow. It also provides a mechanism to follow the patient over an extended period of time, evaluating for changes in waveform and pressure. Finally, noninvasive monitoring can be used to evaluate the immediate effect of medications on blood flow of the extremities.

ARTERIOGRAM

When the noninvasive evaluation suggests significant atherosclerotic disease, the next step in evaluation is the arteriogram. The critical question now becomes whether the patient is a likely surgical candidate. Patients who cannot tolerate a surgical procedure should not proceed to a dye study. The arteriogram is an invasive procedure and carries an inherent risk of complications (*i.e.*, anaphylaxis, hemorrhage, embolus, intimal flap, and acute renal or cardiac dysfunction). An arteriogram is the most accurate test to evaluate the peripheral vascular tree. It provides information not only on the suspected disease segment, but on the blood vessels both proximal and distal to the disease site. It is an anatomic study; the noninvasive laboratory is a physiologic assessment.

The arteriogram should be examined carefully to determine the full extent of the disease. Figure 15-7 is the arteriogram of a patient suspected of having bilateral superficial femoral artery disease on the basis of the noninvasive investigation. The arteriogram in this situation confirms the level of obstruction and shows little disease elsewhere. Furthermore, the distal vessel reconstitutes as the popliteal artery. The patient underwent bilateral femoral-popliteal artery bypass and subsequently did well. Often, significant disease occurs distal to the point of obstruction; this is seen in Figure 15-8 where the patient not only had superficial femoral artery disease, but did not reconstitute the popliteal artery. This patient did reconstitute at the more distal arteries, in this case the anterior tibial and peroneal arteries, and required a more extensive operation (femoral-anterior tibial bypass) to salvage the extremity. Subcritical disease more proximal to the obstruction can also be determined by arteriogram. Figure 15-9 is an arteriogram of a patient whose noninvasive studies suggested a left superficial femoral artery occlusion. This x-ray shows the patient had significant aortoiliac disease, as well as superficial femoral artery occlusion. The aortoiliac disease eventually required reconstruction. In the diabetic patient, atherosclerotic vascular disease is usually distal, multisegmental, and bilateral,[48] as seen in Figure 15-10.[42] The arteriogram demonstrates patent vessels with minimal disease to the level of the popliteal artery trifurcation. No major vessels can be

DIABETES AND VASCULAR DISEASE

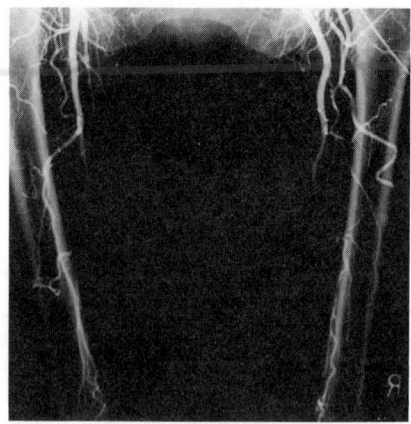

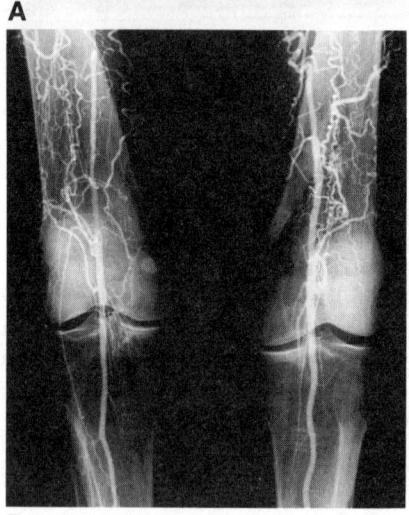

Figure 15-7. Arteriogram of a patient with bilateral superficial femoral artery occlusion. (A) Superficial femoral artery disease with mid-thigh occlusion; (B) reconstitution of popliteal arteries.

identified distal to the disease. This patient could not be bypassed and eventually required amputation. It is important to recognize that, while noninvasive methods can suggest levels of disease, the arteriogram is essential in preoperative patient evaluation to determine the correct management. The assessment will be, therefore, to reflect problems of inflow, outflow, or runoff.

The arteriogram carries a significant risk of complication. In addition to the technical problems of bleeding, embolus, and intimal flaps, a significant risk of acute renal dysfunction also exists. In the diabetic patient who has inherent microvascular renal disease, this risk is greatly amplified. Gomes and co-workers reported an overall incidence of acute renal dysfunction after arteriogram of

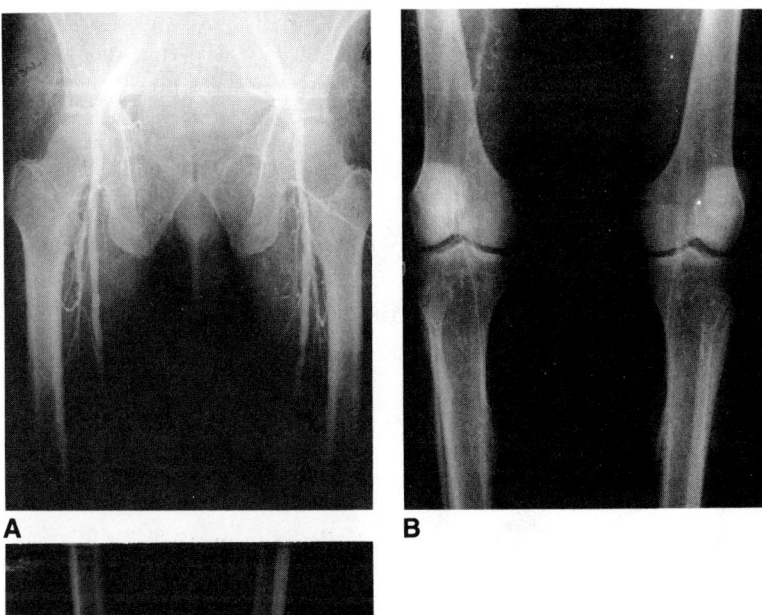

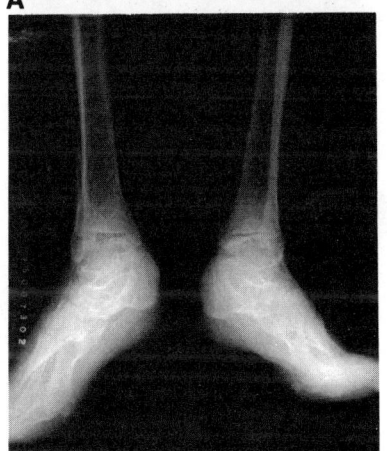

Figure 15-8. Arteriogram of a patient with vascular disease. (A) Normal aortogram with patent superficial femoral arteries; (B) occlusion of superficial femoral arteries with no reconstitution at level of popliteal artery of the trifurcation; (C) reconstitution of posterior tibial on left and anterior tibial on right.

7.1%.[20] Although most recovered, 1.4% eventually required dialysis. In patients with pre-existing renal disease, the incidence of acute renal dysfunction increased to 14.8%; 3.7% of these patients later required chronic dialysis. Several other authors have reported a significant renal risk associated with arteriogram.[25,37,38] In the diabetic patient who may have intrinsic renal disease, the risk of acute renal dysfunction with arteriogram is real. Pre-arteriogram preparation of the patient with mannitol, Lasix, and intravenous hydration has been shown to decrease the risk of complications; however, arteriogram should not be undertaken lightly.[30]

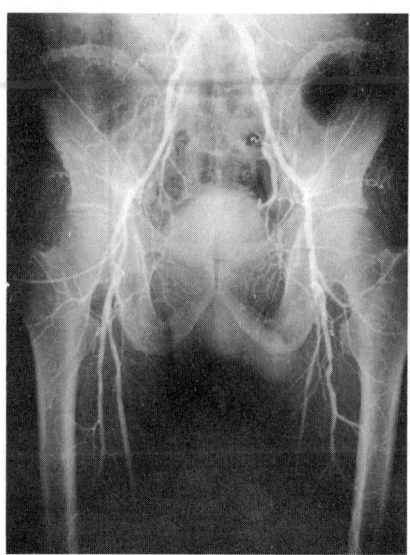

Figure 15-9. Arteriogram of a patient with a suspected left femoral artery stenosis. The arteriogram demonstrates a severe stenosis at the origin of the superficial femoral artery; however, the aortogram also exhibits significant aortic and iliac disease.

Over the last few years, several new nonionic contrast agents have been developed that reduce the osmotic load to the kidney and, thus, decrease renal tubular cell injury. Omnipaque-350® (Iohexol) is one of the commercially available nonionic agents. The iodine (radiopaque substance) is chemically bound, thus preventing disassociation and reducing osmotic load by 60%.[45] Reduction of the osmotic load has also been shown to reduce the pain associated with the arteriogram. Currently, the major problem with the new nonionic contrast agents is the prohibitive costs. The current price of Omnipaque-350® (Iohexol) is approximately $1000 per study, compared with $10 per study for dyes used currently. The cost, however, should not be a consideration in the patient with borderline renal function.

The value of the arteriogram in peripheral vascular disease cannot be overemphasized. Its role is essential in evaluation of the disease. It must also be emphasized that a high risk is associated with the procedure. Arteriogram, therefore, should only be performed in those situations in which surgical correction of the patient's peripheral vascular disease is contemplated.

MANAGEMENT

Management of peripheral vascular disease is dictated by the severity of the disease at the time of presentation. In the diabetic

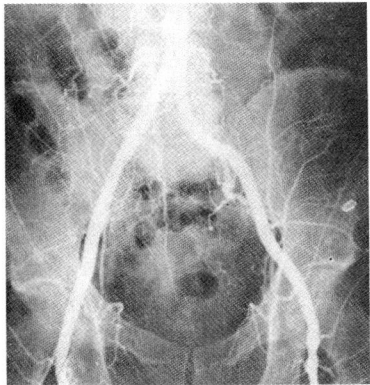
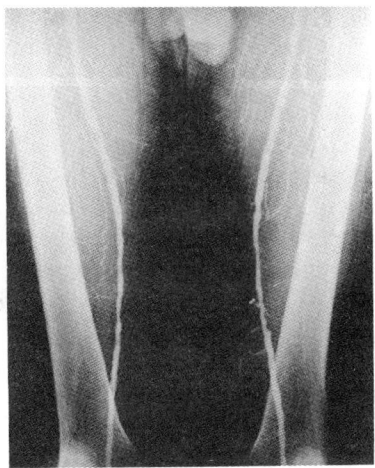
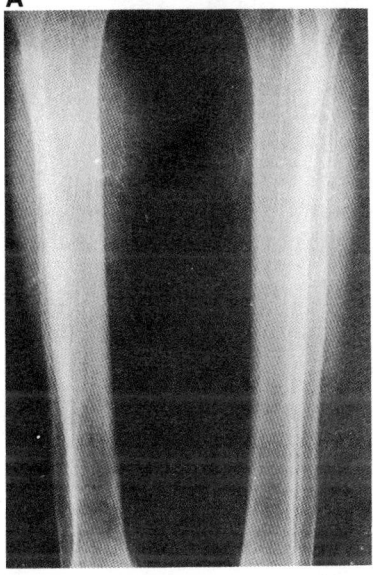

Figure 15-10. Arteriogram from patient with diabetic vascular disease. (A) Pelvic vessels show minimal atheromatous involvement. (B) Thigh vessels show moderate arteriosclerosis. (C) Branches of popliteal artery in same arteriogram show diffuse, severe occlusive vascular disease. (Reproduced with permission from Picus D, Staple TW, Gilula LA et al: Radiographic imaging and treatment of vascular disease in the diabetic patient. In Levin ME, O'Neal LW [eds]: The Diabetic Foot, 4th ed, pp 182–202. St. Louis, CV Mosby, 1988)

patient, management is further complicated by the associated underlying metabolic derangements. The dictum in management of any vascular patient is "life, then limb." All patients should be approached from this standpoint. The diagnosis of the severity of vascular disease has been described previously in this chapter. When the severity of the disease has been established, treatment should be instituted rapidly and aggressively.

When no immediate threat to life or limb is present, conservative therapy is the initial method of treatment of the diabetic patient with peripheral vascular disease. Control of the diabetes is an essential first step in any management plan. As discussed previously, elevated levels of glucose can cause serious metabolic derangement at the cellular level.[14,35,50] This will result in decreased tissue perfusion and reduction of the cellular delivery of nutrients. Elevated glucose levels also seriously inhibit the effectiveness of leukocytes.[15] The diabetic patient is also at risk because of the associated neuropathy that develops as a result of the elevated glucose.[35] This neuropathy can prevent the patient from recognizing significant signs and symptoms of advancing disease.

A second important aspect in the initial conservative management is to make the patient an integral part of the team. The patient must be made to recognize the seriousness of his condition and how he can help improve the situation. Instruction in proper examination and care of the foot is necessary to avoid serious complications. The foot should be examined daily for the effects of trauma or extremes of temperature. A podiatrist, if available, should be incorporated into the management team, to instruct the diabetic patient on care of the feet. Following is a list of information given to our residents, students, and patients regarding diabetic foot care.

- Feet should always be kept clean and dry.
- Nails should be trimmed regularly. The podiatry clinic is available if you are unable to trim your nails.
- Do not treat cuts, corns, or calluses yourself. See a doctor for advice.
- Wear comfortable shoes at all times.
- Never wear circular garters.
- Wear clean socks or stockings.
- Avoid garments that cause constriction around the thighs.
- Never go barefoot.
- Avoid positions that cause pressure on the legs (*e.g.*, crossing the legs, folding the legs under you).
- Avoid prolonged standing.
- Keep feet warm; avoid excessive heat.
- Sit with legs slightly elevated on something whenever possible.
- Avoid smoking—smoking causes the blood vessels to constrict, thereby causing a decrease in circulation of blood in the lower extremities.

In addition to patient education, the podiatrist or prosthetist can assist with obtaining proper footwear that redistributes the mechanical stresses away from areas of continued pressure.[5] Weight reduction, which should also be stressed to the diabetic patient, serves two functions: to reduce the trauma to the lower extremities, and to assist in better control of glucose levels in the adult onset diabetic. Patients should be encouraged to stop smoking because this can only worsen the situation. An aggressive exercise program should be established, especially in patients who have symptoms of claudication. Exercise does not increase patency of diseased vessels, but many function through improving collateral flow or improving oxygen extraction. In many instances, patient symptoms will improve with an aggressive exercise program. If conservative treatment is to be effective in management of peripheral vascular disease, the patient must adhere to each step in the treatment regimen. Should the patient have elevated triglycerides, particularly the low-density lipoprotein fraction, corrective action should be undertaken. If the patient is not overweight and lipid levels are normal, medication and inappropriate dieting have no place. One cannot make the well patient better!

All injuries and infections of the lower extremities in diabetic patients with peripheral vascular disease should be considered limb-threatening initially and treated rapidly and aggressively. If the patient initially has either an injury to the lower extremity or an infection, the primary evaluation should include a noninvasive evaluation to determine the presence and severity of the vascular disease. If the blood flow pattern suggests adequate perfusion for healing of the injury or infection, the patient should be treated with antibiotics and local wound care. In certain instances, the treatment may include operative debridement. In cases where the infection or injury is not severe enough to require hospitalization, the patient should maintain strict bedrest at home. Antibiotics should be administered. If there is any question concerning severity of the injury or infection, the patient should be hospitalized for aggressive wound care and intravenous antibiotics. All patients should receive frequent follow-up care as outpatients. If a nonhealing ulcer persists or a question of bone involvement arises, plain x-rays of the foot or a bone scan of the questionable area of osteomyelitis is required. The combination of vascular disease, diabetes, and digital osteomyelitis results in amputation—of the digit alone—if the blood supply is adequate.

When the patient suffers rest pain or is threatened with limb loss and the vascular evaluation suggests a significant disease process, a more aggressive surgical approach should be taken. If the arteriogram shows specific obstructed disease segment, revascularization can markedly improve tissue perfusion. The goal of all vascular reconstruction is to obtain maximal flow to the area of ischemia. As discussed previously, not only the specific disease site must be evaluated, but the entire vascular system both proximal and distal to the lesion must be examined.

Calcified aortoiliac disease is rarely the source of limb-threatening distal ischemia.[34] In the diabetic patient population, however, it is often a component of the multisegmental, bilateral nature of the disease process.[48] Reconstruction of the aortoiliac system by an aortobifemoral artery bypass is highly successful because it takes advantage of the high-flow states of these blood vessels. The distal portion of the bypass also allows evaluation and management of the profunda femoris, which is often the source of significant collateral circulation.[32] The purpose of aortobifemoral bypass is to establish adequate inflow into the vascular tree of the extremity. This procedure is highly successful and carries a 5-year patency rate of >85%.[49]

Femoral-popliteal and infrapopliteal bypasses are performed to establish maximal blood flow from the femoral region to the region of distal ischemia. A femoral-popliteal arterial graft can be performed to bypass an isolated superficial femoral artery occlusion, or in conjunction with an aortobifemoral bypass graft if more proximal disease is also present. The arteriogram must demonstrate good reconstitution of the popliteal artery with good run-off for this procedure to be successful. In the diabetic patient, however, usually multiple additional occlusions of the tibial and peroneal vessels are present. In these cases, infrapopliteal bypasses are necessary to establish maximal flow to ischemic tissue. Technical expertise and precision are absolutely essential in the infrapopliteal bypass to obtain optimal results.[39]

Long-term results have shown autogenous saphenous vein graft to be the most consistently reliable conduit. Veith and co-workers reported a significant advantage in maintaining patency in below-the-knee bypass grafts.[51] The site of the distal anastomosis should provide a direct channel to the pedal circulation. Intraoperative assessment with arteriogram is absolutely essential to determine that the best possible anastomosis has been performed. The 5-year patency rate for above-the-knee bypass is 75% to 85%. For a below-the-knee bypass, the patency rate at 5 years drops significantly from 30% to 40%, depending on the level of the distal bypass. Although many bypasses will subsequently thrombose, the procedure will significantly improve distal circulation in a number of patients, allowing the ischemic tissue to heal and collateral circulation to develop. Thus, femoral-popliteal and infrapopliteal vessel revascularization will produce a significantly higher increase in limb salvage.

Percutaneous transluminal angioplasty can also play a significant role in management of peripheral vascular disease. When the arteriogram suggests an isolated segment of disease, in many instances the segment will be amenable to angioplasty. The patency rate in many instances approaches that of surgery. The success rate of angioplasty of iliac arteries is 80% to 90% at 1 year and 70% to 85% at 2 to 3 years. In popliteal segments, the success rate is 70% to 80% at 1 year and 60% to 75% at 2 to 3 years.[1,8,29,54] These results are similar to those achieved with autogenous vein grafts and superior to those obtained with prosthetic material. It has been shown, however, that a poorer long-term result in patency does occur in the diabetic as opposed to the nondiabetic population.[19] The associated morbidity rate of the procedure is relatively small. In several series, the rate of complications has been reported at 10%, with major complications being groin hematoma.[18,36,40] Distal embolization has been reported to occur in 5% of the patients who undergo angioplasty; however, the majority of these are clinically insignificant.[26] Percutaneous transluminal angioplasty is an effective treatment method in management of isolated disease segments.

SUMMARY

Peripheral vascular disease alone is a significant disease process; in the presence of diabetes, diagnosis and management become much more complex. Diabetes also seriously worsens the patient's prognosis. Understanding the pathophysiology of the disease is essential to the physician who treats these patients; he must be able to interpret the clinical and laboratory findings. Treatment must be instituted rapidly and aggressively. It is apparent that the diabetic patient with peripheral vascular disease is extremely challenging in all aspects of management and treatment.

REFERENCES

1. Abbott WM: Percutaneous transluminal angioplasty: A surgeon's view. Am J Roentgenol 135:917–920, 1980
2. Archer AG, Roberts VC, Watkins PJ: Blood flow patterns in painful diabetic neuropathy. Diabetologia 27:563–567, 1984
3. Bone GE, Panajel MJ: Toe blood pressure by photoplethysmography: An index of healing in forefoot amputation. Surgery 5:569–574, 1981
4. Boulton AJM, Hardisty CA, Betts RP et al: Dynamic foot pres-

sure and other studies as diagnostic and management aids in diabetic neuropathy. Diabetes Care 6:26–33, 1983
5. Brand PW: The diabetic foot. In Ellenberg M, Rifkin H (eds): Diabetes Mellitus, pp 829–849. New York, New York Medical Examination Publishing, 1983
6. Ctereteko GC, Chanebhan M, Hutton WC et al: Vertical forces acting on the feet of diabetic patients with neuropathic ulceration. Br J Surg 68:608–614, 1981
7. Deenfield JE, Daggett PR, Harrison MJG: Role of autonomic neuropathy in diabetic foot ulceration. J Neurol Sci 47:203–210, 1980
8. Dotter CT: Transluminal angioplasty: A long view. Am J Roentgenol 135:561–564, 1980
9. Edmonds ME: The diabetic foot: Pathophysiology and treatment. In Watkins PJ (ed): Clinics in Endocrinology and Metabolism, Vol 15, No 4, pp 889–916, Philadelphia, WB Saunders, 1986
10. Edmonds ME, Blundell MP, Morris HE et al: Improved survival of the diabetic foot: The role of the special foot clinic. Q J Med (in press), 1989
11. Edmonds ME, Giley S, Walters HW et al: Improved survival of the diabetic ischemic foot. Diabetic Med 2:506A, 1985
12. Edmonds ME, Morrisson N, Laws JW et al: Medical arterial calcification and diabetic neuropathy. Br Med J 284:928–930, 1982
13. Edmonds ME, Nicolaides KH, Watkins PJ: Autonomic neuropathy in diabetic foot ulcerations. Diabetic Med 3:56–59, 1986
14. Edmonds ME, Roberts VC, Watkins PJ: Blood flow in the diabetic neuropathic foot. Diabetologia 22:9–15, 1982
15. Foster DW: Diabetes mellitus. In Petersdorf RG, Adams RD, Braunwald E et al (eds): Harrison's Principles of Internal Medicine, pp 621–629. New York, McGraw-Hill, 1983
16. Fulton TJ, Hamilton WAP, Graham JC et al: On-line analysis of the femoral artery flow velocity waveform and its application in the diagnosis of arterial disease. J Biomed Eng 5:151–156, 1983
17. Gabbay KH: The sorbitol pathway and the complications of diabetes. N Engl J Med 288:831–836, 1973
18. Glover TG, Rendick PJ, Dilly RS et al: Efficacy of balloon catheter dilation for lower extremity atherosclerosis. Surgery 91:560–565, 1982
19. Gollino A, Mahler F, Prolost P et al: Percutaneous transluminal angioplasty of the arteries of the lower limbs: A 5-year follow-up. Circulation 70:619–623, 1984

20. Gomes AS, Baker JD, Paredero MV et al: Acute renal dysfunction after major arteriography. Am J Roentgenol 3:1249–1253, 1985
21. Green DA, Brown MJ, Braunstein SN et al: Comparison of clinical course and sequential electrophysiological texts in diabetics with symptomatic polyneuropathy and its implications for clinical trials. Diabetes 30:139–147, 1981
22. Guy RJC, Clark CA, Malcolm PN et al: Evaluation of thermal and vibration sensation in diabetic neuropathy. Diabetologia 28:131–137, 1985
23. Guyton AC: Metabolism of carbohydrates and formation of adenosine triphosphate. In Guyton AC (ed): Textbook of Medical Physiology, 6th ed, pp 838–848. Philadelphia, WB Saunders, 1981
24. Harrison MJG, Farris IB: The neuropathic factor in the arteriology of diabetic foot ulcers. J Neurol Sci 28:217–223, 1976
25. Hass WK, Fields WS, North RR et al: Joint study of extracranial arterial occlusion. II. Arteriography, techniques, sites, and complications. JAMA 203:961–968, 1968
26. Health and Public Policy Committee, American College of Physicians: Percutaneous transluminal angioplasty. Ann Intern Med 99:864–869, 1953
27. Imparato AM, Riles TS: Peripheral arterial disease. In Schwartz SI, Shires TG, Spencer RC et al (eds): Principles of Surgery, 4th ed, pp 897–974. New York, McGraw-Hill, 1984
28. Kammel WB, Shurtloff D: The natural history of arteriosclerosis obliterans. Cardiovasc Clin 3:38–52, 1971
29. Katzen BT, Chang J, Knox WG: Percutaneous transluminal angioplasty with the Gruntzig balloon catheter: A review of 70 cases. Arch Surg 114:1389–1399, 1979
30. Kerstein MD, Puyau PA: Value of periangiography hydration. Surgery 96:919–922, 1984
31. Kilo C, Volger N, Williamson JR: Muscle capillary basement membrane changes related to aging and to diabetes mellitus. Diabetes 21:881–905, 1972
32. King TA, Depalma RG, Rhodes RS: Diabetes mellitus and atherosclerotic involvement of the profunda femoris artery. Surg Gynecol Obstet 159:553–556, 1984
33. Kozniewska F, Jung L, Skolasinska K et al: Changes in blood flow and permeability of vessels to protein preceding the development of cutaneous ulcers in the hind limb of the rabbit. Microvasc Res 19:189–196, 1980
34. Kwasnik RM: Limb salvage in diabetics: Challenges and solutions. Surg Clin North Am 66:305–318, 1986

CHAPTER SIXTEEN
Islet Transplantation in Animals and Humans

Kevin J. Lafferty
Lyndee Paris

INTRODUCTION

It is becoming widely acknowledged that type I diabetes has an autoimmune etiology. It is postulated that the diabetic initiates an immune response against his own islet tissue, thus destroying his source of insulin. The factor(s) that trigger this response are undefined, but may include abnormal antigen expression by the islet cell, an intrinsic defect in the immune system of the diabetic, or both. In our laboratories we have used both clinical and animal models to study the mechanism of the disease process, as well as to formulate treatments to prevent or correct diabetes. One corrective procedure we have used is the transplantation of normal adult islets of Langerhans to alleviate experimentally induced diabetes in mice.[9] This is the prototype experiment for the development of human islet transplantation. Before this procedure can be successful, however, two major obstacles must be overcome: the process of graft rejection and the underlying pathogenesis of the diabetic condition.

ALLOGRAFT RESPONSE

A major roadblock to achieving an understanding of the allograft response (*i.e.*, the immune response generated when tissue is grafted between histoincompatible patients) was the assumption that graft rejection was triggered solely by the graft antigens. Traditionally, the graft has been assumed to be composed of a relatively homogenous cell population, at least in terms of immunogenicity. It was believed that an immune response was generated against graft antigens that were shed and came into contact with the host lymphatic system (Fig. 16-1). According to this view, which dominates modern clinical transplantation, there are only two ways to prevent graft rejection. First, one may attempt to find a donor that is histocompatible with the recipient, which can only be accomplished in humans by using identical twins. The second option is immunosuppressive treatment of the recipient. Currently, clinicians depend almost entirely on immunosuppressive therapies, which leave the patient vulnerable to secondary infections and limit the widespread applicability of transplantation.

If one assumes that graft rejection is the result of an immune response toward shed antigens, then one encounters a "transplantation paradox." This paradox is composed of three propositions. The first is that allograft rejection is an immunologically mediated

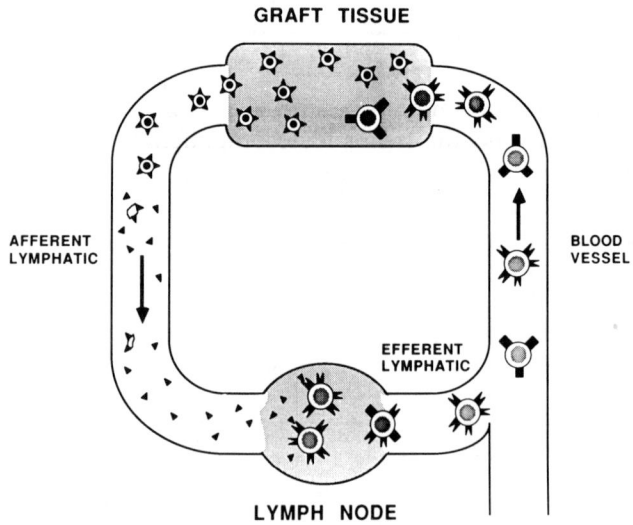

Figure 16-1. The classic view of graft sensitization. Graft cells bearing antigen enter the afferent lymphatic vessels. Here, the cells fragment as they move toward the lymph node, where peripheral T cells specific for graft antigens are activated. These cells leave the lymph node via the afferent lymphatic vessel, eventually finding their way into the bloodstream. Cells are carried by the blood to the graft, where they move through the vessel walls into the substance of the graft and trigger the series of events that culminate in destruction of the transplanted tissue.

process initiated by the recognition and response to transplantation antigens encoded by the genes of the major histocompatibility complex. Further, the allograft response is recognized as one of the most violent immune reactions known. When the major histocompatability complex antigens are isolated from the cell surface in soluble form, however, they serve as weak antigens.[2] Herein lies the paradox: how can such weak antigens trigger a vigorous response in the context of the allograft? Resolution of this paradox, essential for an understanding of transplantation, has resulted from a greater understanding of the signaling requirements necessary for generating an immune response.

The T cell needs two signals to become activated. Antigen provides one, and interaction with the major histocompatibility complex of the antigen-presenting cell causes it to release the second signal. In normal antigen recognition, a specialized lymphoid cell (probably a macrophage), the antigen-presenting cell, degrades or processes foreign antigen and presents it on its cell membrane (Fig. 16-2,A). The antigen-presenting cell has two markers that can be recognized by the T cell: processed antigen, and its own cell surface structures, its specific major histocompatibility complex. It is now thought that the major histocompatibility complex molecule on the surface of the antigen-presenting cell acts like a light switch. Interaction between the major histocompatibility complex and T cell receptor switches the antigen-presenting cell on and activates it to provide a second, inductive signal to the T cell.[1] Foreign antigen is recognized by the T cell in the context of the major histocompatibility complex of the antigen-presenting cell; therefore, the immune response is restricted by the major histocompatibility complex of the cell that presents antigen. When both signals are provided, the T cell can then become activated specifically against the control molecule/antigen complex, and proliferate.

When one applies this working model to antigen recognition in alloreactivity, it is evident that antigen alone on the graft cell surface cannot be strongly immunogenic (Fig. 16-2,B). The parenchymal cells of the graft are a source of antigen for the T cell, but they are not a source of second signal, which is required for T cell triggering. When these cells' antigens are processed by a host macrophage, they are recognized in context with the major histocompatibility complex of the host cell. Because those antigens do not appear on the graft cells in this context (*i.e.*, with the major histocompatibility complex of the host), the T cells produced cannot be specifically reactive to the graft cells. To produce a T cell that is activated against the major histocompatibility complex of the donor, antigen-presenting cells of the donor type must be present

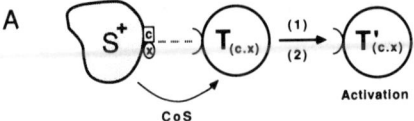

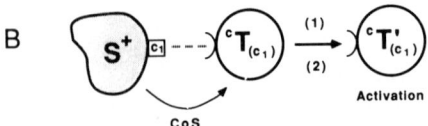

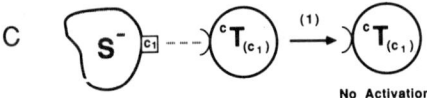

Figure 16-2. (A) The normal process of T cell activation. An antigen-presenting cell (S^+) degrades and processes foreign antigen (x) and presents it on its cell surface in association with the major histocompatibility complex (c). This complex is recognized by T cells of the specificity (c.x). The control structure (c) is engaged and the costimulator is released from the S^+ cell. The provision of these two signals results in T-cell activation. (B) T-cell activation by alloantigen. Allogeneic major histocompatibility complex (c_1) presented on the surface of S^+ cells is highly immunogenic for T cells of (c) genotype, which have a receptor for alloantigen (c_1). In this interaction, signals one and two are provided and the alloreactive T cell is activated. (C) Alloantigen on S^- cells is nonimmunogenic. Alloantigen (c_1) presented on the surface of an S^- cell can only provide signal one for the alloreactive T cell; S^- cells cannot provide a source of costimulator (CoS). As a result, those interactions do not lead to T cell activation.

in the grafted tissue mass (Fig. 16-2,C). The donor antigen-presenting cell is able to present its own major histocompatibility complex as foreign antigen to the host T cell as well as provide the second signal; therefore, the host T cell is both activated against the donor major histocompatibility complex and triggered, and can attack the graft cells.[7]

To obtain a nonimmunogenic graft, the stimulator (antigen-presenting) cells must be removed. There are a number of ways to eliminate a high percentage of lymphoid cells from a graft. Most of these techniques rely on the differential sensitivity between lymphoid cells and parenchymal cells to toxic agents. Much of the early work involving this treatment of tissue has been carried out with endocrine grafts. Islet tissue isolated by enzymatic digestion of the pancreas can be maintained in organ culture.[5] Islet tissue tends to be more hardy than lymphoid under adverse conditions. Lacy and co-workers in St. Louis have cultured islet tissue under low temperature conditions combined with a short period of immunosuppression with antilymphocyte serum after transplantation.[4] Hegre and co-workers in Minneapolis have used a clever technique using the selective growth of islet cells *in vitro* to eliminate passenger leukocytes.[3]

In our laboratories at the Barbara Davis Center, the islets of Langerhans are removed from the enzymatically digested pancreas, spun into clusters, and cultured in a 95% oxygen atmosphere for 1 week.[6] Because high oxygen concentrations are more toxic to lymphoid cells than to clusters of beta cells, a mass of graft tissue can be obtained that is relatively antigen-presenting cell-free. This technique has also been successful in the transplantation of thyroid tissue across major histocompatibility barriers.[8]

The removal of antigen-presenting cells from the donor tissue has a dramatic effect on rejection (Fig. 16-3). In Figure 16-3, CBA mice have been made diabetic with an injection of the diabetogenic drug, streptozotocin, and have received grafts of either cultured or uncultured Balb/c islet tissue. These two strains of mice have different major histocompatibility antigens, but the host was not immunosuppressed before or after transplantation. The mice who received cultured grafts free of antigen-presenting cells did not produce an immune response against the graft tissue. The islets they received began secreting insulin within a few days after transplant and their blood glucose fell into the normal range. The mice that received uncultured grafts were provided with both activation and triggering signals by the donor, and were able to reject their grafts. Graft rejection is indicated by the dramatic increase in blood glucose when the transplanted islets are destroyed. The rate of rejection in uncultured grafts is over 90%, but cultured allografts can remain indefinitely.

Grafts of this nature are in an immunologically precarious position. When the mice that accepted the grafts were challenged at day 30 after transplantation with donor spleen cells (capable of antigen-presenting cell function) they rejected their grafts. This finding points to the antigen-presenting cell as the primary element in graft rejection. The fact that these grafts can still be rejected many weeks after transplantation indicates that the graft is not in a stable state, although it can remain in a metastable state so long as the immune

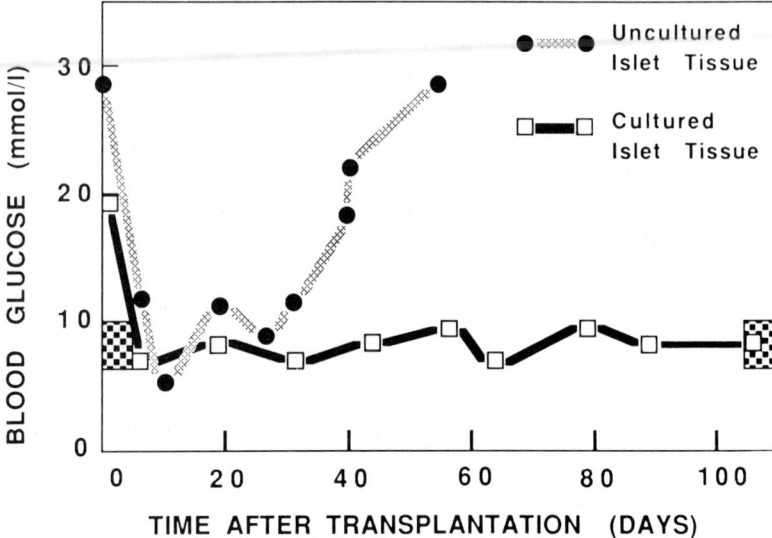

Figure 16-3. Blood glucose concentrations in diabetic mice following transplantation with either cultured or uncultured islet tissue. The normal blood sugar range is represented by the checkered area (5 to 10 mmol/liter). The solid line represents the prolonged decrease in blood glucose following transplantation of a cultured allograft. This reduction indicates that the graft is not rejected. The gray line represents the blood glucose level of a mouse transplanted with an uncultured allograft. The blood sugar decreased initially, but by 2 to 3 weeks the animal was hyperglycemic and eventually died on day 55.

system is not disrupted. With the passage of time, the graft shifts from a metastable configuration to a stable configuration. The stabilization of the graft is the result of tolerance induction in the adult animal.[6] We are still uncertain as to the detailed mechanism of this tolerance. We have evidence that it is a suppressive form of tolerance, which may be mediated by a humoral factor (unpublished data).

DISEASE RECURRENCE

Allograft response is the main concern when transplanting islets between animal or human major histocompatibility complex types. When confronted with type I diabetes, a complicating factor—autoimmune disease—comes into play. We have done many studies using the NOD mouse as a model for this type of diabetes. This particular strain of mouse develops an autoimmune response to its own islet tissue at about 120 days of age. The cause of this response is still unknown. Initially it was thought that an abnormal antigen was present on the surface of the islet and was recognized by the normal immune system of the animal as foreign. To test this hypothesis, a major histocompatibility complex-incompatible graft was transplanted into the NOD mouse after it had destroyed its own islets.[8] It was thought that if the major histocompatibility complex molecule on the cell surface of the graft islets was different, perhaps these islets could not be attacked by the immune system that was activated against self-aberrant antigen. Determining the cause of tissue damage in this case was problematic, because damage could be caused by either allograft rejection or disease recurrence in the transplanted tissue. To distinguish between these two, a graft of allogeneic pituitary and one of islet tissue from the same donor were transplanted under the kidney capsule of NOD mice to determine if inflammatory damage to the islets was tissue-specific and not an allograft response. The islet tissue in all mice was completely or almost completely destroyed, while the pituitary grafts showed little or no inflammation or lymphocytic infiltration. Selective destruction of islets demonstrated that islet damage in NOD mice is tissue-specific, and failure of the mouse to reject the pituitary graft ruled out the allograft response as the cause of islet damage. Disease recurrence, therefore, is a factor that must be kept in mind when considering clinical islet transplantation.

Human islet transplants were begun at St. Luke's Hospital in Denver, in coordination with the Barbara Davis Center in 1986.[10] When transplanting islet tissue into human patients, a problem arises immediately: Where will we obtain viable tissue? Five years of experimentation were required to develop a technique for the isolation, culture, and transplantation of islets in mice. It has proved to be a much more arduous process in humans. Isolating islets from the adult pancreas is extremely difficult because of its fibrous composition. Major advances in islet isolation from the adult pancreas have been made by Lacy in St. Louis. A few years ago, one was fortunate to recover 10% of the islets from an adult pancreas. Lacy and his colleagues are now able to obtain a 60% yield of reasonably pure islets. In Denver, fetal pancreas tissue from cadaveric donors has been used as material for transplantation into adult diabetics. At a gestational stage of about 3 months, the islet tissue is still undifferentiated. When transplanted, this tissue develops mainly into duct tissue from which islet tissue subsequently forms. For this reason, this tissue is slow to function.

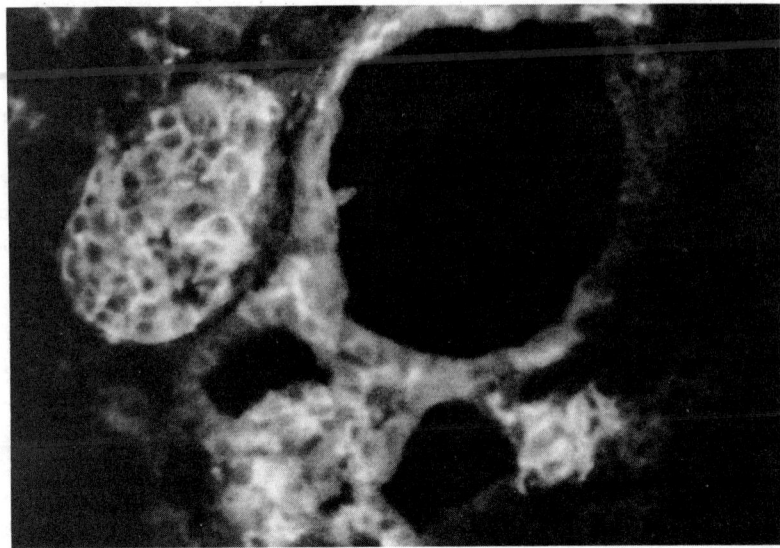

Figure 16-4. Pro-islets developing adjacent to ductal structures in the cultured fetal pancreas. The pro-islet material is stained with a fluoroscein-labelled monoclonal antibody specific for human islet β-cells and a subset of α-cells.

When using a monoclonal antibody specific for islet precursors to stain a histologic preparation of this seemingly undifferentiated tissue, tiny pearl-like pro-islets are visible (Fig. 16-4). By transplanting this tissue into athymic mice we have found that after a period of a few months the tissue begins to grow and differentiate, and eventually secretes hormones.

When attempting to transplant islet tissue into humans, allograft response must be considered, along with autoimmune disease. Diabetics may possess an aberrant T cell type capable of recognizing markers specific to the beta cell and attacking them directly. If this hypothesis were correct, the result would be the destruction of any islets transplanted into the diabetic after the destruction of their own islet tissue. This would make any attempt at islet transplantation after disease onset impossible without immunosuppressive therapy. For this reason, much more information concerning the disease process must be assembled. Also, early trials of clinical islet transplantation have been restricted to patients requiring immunosuppression for another reason (usually renal transplantation).

We have done two series of experiments to determine if islet tissue can survive in the human type I diabetic after disease onset. In the first series, cultured fetal tissue was transplanted into diabetic patients with end-stage renal disease at the same time they received a kidney transplant. Because of the immunosuppressive therapy, there was less chance of an immune reaction destroying the islets or affecting the development process. The optimal location for the graft tissue was not immediately apparent. At first the tissue was placed in the omentum. Of the five patients tested in this trial, none showed any detectable C-peptide production at the time of transplantation, or in the period from 1 month to 6 months after transplantation.

At this point in the investigation it was not certain if the tissue's failure to develop was the result of disease recurrence, problems with revascularization, or an unknown factor or factors. The only useful information gained from this particular series of investigations was that the treatment was not detrimental to the patients' health. They experienced no complications from the graft.

In our current investigations, islet tissue is transplanted under the capsule of the grafted kidney. At this site, blood vessels can grow into the graft from the healthy kidney parenchyma, which keeps the islet tissue in optimal condition and provides a means of entry for hormones from the graft into the systemic circulation. In coordination with Spees from St. Luke's Hospital in Denver, Colorado, the tissue is biopsied to determine if it is, in fact, differentiating in its adult host (Fig. 16-5). The biopsies provided evidence that the islet tissue could grow, differentiate and become integrated into the general circulation. A great deal of mitotic activity was noted in this tissue, and no evidence of rejection or disease recurrence. By 3 months post-transplantation we have seen evidence of islet differentiation with the accumulation of insulin somatostatin and glucagon within the alpha, beta, and delta cells of the maturing islets. Studies involving the grafting of human fetal pancreas in athymic mice have allowed us to follow development of glucose responsiveness in the grafted tissue. The function of human islet tissue in mice is easy to detect, because human C-peptide can be readily distinguished from mouse C-peptide in a radioimmunoassay. We and others have now shown that transplanted human islet tissue does not become glucose-responsive until about 4 months after grafting.

Studies in human patients are still in progress. We are conducting a clinial trial with 17 patients who have been transplanted with either low or high doses of pro-islet tissue. At this stage, a significant difference is seen between these two groups, with a

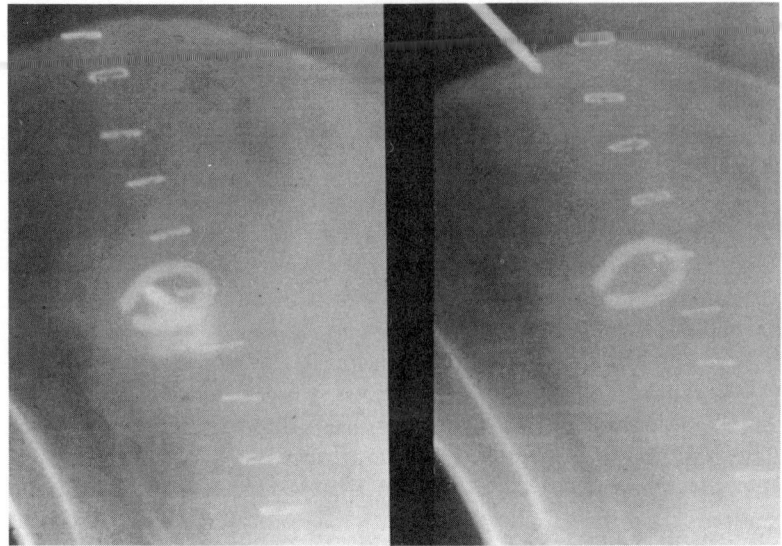

Figure 16-5. Needle biopsy technique. The grafted kidney is visualized radiographically. The location of the islet graft is marked by the radio-opaque horseshoe sutured to the kidney capsule at the time of transplantation. This technique allows percutaneous needle biopsy through the subcapsular region containing the grafted tissue.

large proportion of patients receiving high doses of pancreatic tissue showing a significant reduction in insulin requirement. While these studies are encouraging, no patients have as yet become completely insulin-independent. These studies are on-going, however, and each patient must be followed for at least 2 years before a statement of success or failure can be made concerning the procedure.

SUMMARY

Type I diabetes is most probably of autoimmune etiology with the diabetic developing an immune response against his own islet tissue. Clinical transplantation and animal models have been developed for islet transplantation in order to formulate treatment protocols. Graft rejections and the underlying pathogenesis are being explored.

REFERENCES

1. Babcock SK, Gill R, Bellgrau D et al: Studies on the 2 signal model for T cell activation in vivo. Transplant Proc 19:303–307, 1987
2. Batchelor JR, Welsh K, Burgos H: Transplantation antigens per se are poor immunogens within a species. Nature 273(5657):54–56, 1978
3. Hegre O, Marshall S, Schulte B et al: Nonenzymatic in vitro isolation of perinatal islets of Langerhans. In Vitro 19:661–691, 1983
4. Lacy P, Davie J, Finke E: Prolongation of islet allograft survival following in vitro culture (24 C) and a single injection of ALS. Science 204:312–313, 1979
5. Lacy PE, Kovstianovsky M: Method for isolation of intact islets of Langerhans from the rat pancreas. Diabetes 16:35–39, 1967
6. Lafferty KJ, Babcock SK, Gill R: Prevention of rejection by treatment of the graft. In Meryman H (ed): Transplantation: Approached to Graft Rejection, pp 87–117. New York, Alan R Liss, 1986
7. Lafferty KJ, Gill RG, Babcock SK et al: Activation and expression of allograft immunity. In Morris P, Tilney N (eds): Progress in Transplantation III, pp 55–84. New York, Churchill Livingston, 1986
8. Lafferty KJ, Prowse S, Simeonovic C: Immunobiology of tissue transplantation: A return to the passenger leukocyte concept. Annu Rev Immunol 1:143–173, 1983
9. Prowse S, Lafferty KJ, Simeonovic C: The reversal of diabetes by islet transplantation. Diabetes 31:30–37, 1982
10. Robertson RP, Lafferty KJ, Haug C, Weil R III: Effect of human fetal pancreas transplantation on secretion of C-peptide and glucose tolerance in type I diabetics. Transplant Proc 19:2354–2356, 1987

Index

Page numbers followed by *f* indicate figures, numbers followed by *t* indicate tabular material, and numbers followed by *n* indicate footnotes.

A

acetohexamide
  comparison of therapy with, 136*t*
  relationship among sulfonylureas, 135*t*
adenosine diphosphate, effect on platelet aggregation, 23, 25*f*
age, red blood cell filterability and, 19, 19*t*
allograft response, in islet transplantation, 267–72, 268*f*, 270*f*, 272*f*
alrestatin, in treatment of neuropathy, 174
aminophylline, effect on stiff red cell syndrome, 22
angioplasty
  laser, 237–38
  percutaneous transluminal, 235–36, 261
angioscopy, in arterial reconstruction, 237
ankle pressures, evaluation of, 250, 250*t*
antibiotic therapy, in infected foot ulcers, 207
anticoagulant(s)
  in intermittent claudication, 217
  in peripheral vascular disease, 234
antiplatelet agents
  in intermittent claudication, 217–18
  in peripheral vascular disease, 234
aortobifemoral artery bypass, in peripheral vascular disease, 260
ApoA$_1$/ApoB ratio, fructose and, 148, 149*f*
arachidonic acid metabolism, 30, 30*f*
arterial reconstructive techniques
  angioscopy, 237
  conventional bypass, 236
  in situ vein graft, 236–37
  laser angioplasty, 237–38
  local endarterectomy, 236

arterial reconstructive techniques (*continued*)
  percutaneous transluminal angioplasty, 235–36
arteriogram(s)
  in evaluation of peripheral vascular disease, 253–56, 254f, 255f, 256f, 257f
  of microvascular changes, 31, 32f
  of bilateral superficial femoral artery occlusion, 253, 254f
  of suspected left femoral artery stenosis, 253, 256f
arteriolar hyaline, incidence of lesions of, 62t
arteriole(s)
  description of, 2–3
  hemodynamic compensatory changes following dilatation of, 1–2
aspirin, treatment with
  of intermittent claudication, 218
  of peripheral vascular disease, 234
atherosclerosis
  pathophysiology of, 229–31, 244–45
  risk factors for, 230t
  smoking and, 230–31
autogenous saphenous vein graft, 260
autonomic denervation, pathophysiology of, 243–44

B

Belgian study on diabetic complications, 65, 66f
blood. *See also* whole blood
  filterability of, factors influencing, 11f
  fluidity
    critical reduction in, 3–4
    cyclo-oxygenase inhibitors as agents for improvement of, 30–31, 30f, 31f, 32f
    noninvasive monitoring of, 249–53, 250t, 251f, 252f
blood glucose
  concentrations of, following transplantation, 271, 272f
  postprandial, newer modes in normalizing of, 138–39
blood vessel, normal
  immediately after being injured by needle prick, 17, 17f
  one minute after, 17, 18f
  three minutes after, 22, 22f
  two minutes after, 17, 18f
  scanning electron microscopic view of, 16–17, 16f
bone marrow, of SS-genotype infant, 15f
British study on control of retinopathy, 71, 73f, 74f
Buerger's disease, red blood cell filterability in, 19, 20t
buffy coat elements, in normal spleen, 15f
buflomedil
  hemorrheologic effect of, 185
  mediator blockade by, 183t
bypass(es)
  conventional, in arterial reconstruction, 236

in management of peripheral vascular disease, 260

C

calcified aortoiliac disease, management of, 260–61
calcium channel blockers
 hemorrheologic effect of, 184–85
 in treatment of intermittent claudication, 225
capillary(ies)
 description of, 2
 small, red blood cell changes in, 9f
 types of, 2
capillary bed(s)
 draining of, 3
 flow of blood through, 1
Charcot's foot, 200, 201f, 202, 202f
chlorpropamide
 comparison of therapy with, 136t
 relationship among sulfonylureas, 135t
 in treatment of type II diabetes, 118
chronic occlusive atherosclerotic disease (COAD)
 platelet aggregate ratios in, 19, 21t
 red blood cell filterability in, 19, 20t
cigarette smoking
 atherosclerosis and, 230–31
 cessation of, intermittent claudication and, 216
 diabetes and, 43
 severe arteriosclerosis obliterans and, 44f

cinnarizine, mediator blockade by, 183t
circulation
 closed, successful function of, 2
 improvement of, 205–7
 cyclo-oxygenase inhibitors as agents for, 30–31, 30f, 31f, 32f
 primary function of, 3
claudication. See intermittent claudication
COAD. See chronic occlusive atherosclerotic disease
conventional bypass, in arterial reconstruction, 236
Coumadin, in treatment of peripheral vascular disease, 234
C-peptide
 responses in
  after glucagon stimulation, 158f
  after glucose tolerance test, 159f
 in treatment of diabetes, 156–58, 160
crenated red blood cell, 17, 18f
cyclo-oxygenase inhibitors, as agents to improve blood flow, 30–31, 30f, 31f, 32f

D

Dallas study on control of complications in diabetes, 76–78, 79f, 80f
dazadopine, in treatment of intermittent claudication, 225
denervation, autonomic, pathophysiology of, 243–44

281

dextrans, in treatment of intermittent claudication, 219–20
diabetes. *See also* diabetes mellitus; malnutrition diabetes
  cigarette smoking and, 43
  classification of, 114–16, 115*t*
  complications in
    alcohols and, 97–105
    animal model of, 100–1, 100*f*, 102*f*
    basic studies in, 98–99
    Belgian study on, 65, 66*f*
    British study on, 71, 73*f*, 74*f*
    classification of, 88, 88*t*
    clinical applications of, 102
    clinical trials on, 64–68
    controlled prospective trials on, 68–80
    Dallas study on control of, 76–78, 79*f*, 80*f*
    enzymatic activity in, 103
    genetic influences on, 53–54, 53*t*, 55*t*, 56*f*
    history of, 97–98
    hormonal influences on, 97–105
    increase in number of microaneurysms, 66, 67*t*
    influence of risk factors on, 104–5
    in vivo evidence about metabolic control and, 90–91
    Job study on, 65–66, 67*t*, 68
    Kroc study on control of, 74, 76, 76*f*, 77*f*, 78*f*
    macrovascular, 92–93
    Malmo study on, 64–65, 64*t*, 65*t*
    metabolic influences on, 56–59, 57*f*, 58*f*, 59*f*, 60*f*, 61*f*, 62*f*, 62*t*, 63, 63*f*
    microvascular, 88–90
    nephropathy, 50–51, 52*t*, 64*t*, 65*t*
    New Haven study on control of, 71, 73, 75*f*, 75*t*
    retinopathy, 51*f*, 65, 66*f*
    Steno study on, 68, 69*f*, 70*t*, 71, 72*t*
    strict glycemic control and, 91–92
    sugar and, 97–105
    vascular, after 40 years, 50*t*
  effect of, on l-albumin permeation, 100*f*, 101, 102*f*
  islet transplantation in, 267, 276
    allograft response, 267–72, 268*f*, 270*f*, 272*f*
    disease recurrence, 272–76, 274*f*, 276*f*
  microvascular changes in, 9–35, 9*f*, 10*f*
  natural history of, 49–51, 53
  prostaglandin E_1 combined with pentoxifylline in, 33, 34*f*
  red blood cell filterability in, 19, 20*t*
  trends in causes of death, 109, 110*t*, 111
  type I
    classification of, 115, 115*t*
    treatment of, 123–24
  type II
    choices of treatment of, 114
    classification of, 115, 115*t*
    combined insulin and glyburide therapy in, 139–40, 140*f*

INDEX

control of, 112–13
C-peptide responses to new treatment of, 156–58, 158f, 159f, 159t, 160
diet in, management of, 146–48, 147f, 148f, 149f, 150
diet in treatment of, 116–17, 126–29, 127f
exercise in, management of, 146–48, 147f, 148f, 149f, 150
exercise in treatment of, 129–30
impaired insulin secretion, treatment of, 143–44
increased hepatic production of glucose, treatment of, 145–46, 145f
insulin in treatment of, 117, 137–40, 140f
insulin resistance in, treatment of, 146
long-term control of, 112
management of, 111, 113, 116–20, 123–41, 146–56
metabolic control in, 125–26, 125f
metabolic defects leading to hyperglycemia in, 144f
modern treatment of, 109, 110t, 111, 120–21
noninsulin-dependent, pathophysiology of, 124–25, 125f
normalizing postprandial blood sugars in, 138–39
oral agents in treatment of, 117–19, 118t
oral agents combined with insulin in treatment of, 120

pancreatic functions and treatment of, 113–14
pharmacologic therapy, new strategies in, 150–55, 152t, 153f, 154f, 155t, 156f
receptor system and treatment of, 114
short-term control of, 111–12
sulfonylurea agents in, 130–34, 131f, 132f, 133f, 134f, 135t, 136t, 137
therapeutic modalities in, 125–30, 125f
weight control in, 126–29, 127f
type III, 115n, 116
Diabetes Control and Complications Trial, 79–80, 92
diabetes mellitus
classification of, 114–16, 115t
degenerative complications of
classification of, 88
glycemic control and, 87, 93–94
diabetic foot. See foot, diabetic
diabetic microangiopathy, genetic predisposition and severity of, 80–82, 81f
diabetic neuropathy. See neuropathy, diabetic
diabetic retinopathy. See retinopathy, diabetic
diagnosis
of intermittent claudication, 233
of peripheral vascular disease, 246–49, 248f
of peripheral vascular occlusive disease, 231–32, 233f

283

diet, treatment of type II diabetes with, 116–17
  newer modes of, 126–29, 127f
  new strategies in, 146–48, 147f, 148f, 149f, 150
diseases. *See specific diseases*
disorders. *See specific disorders*
Doppler waveforms
  of diabetic patient with vascular disease, 251, 251f
  and treadmill testing, 252, 252f
drug(s)
  that affect hemorrheology, 182, 183t, 187–88, 187f
  in treatment of peripheral vascular disease, 234–35

E

endarterectomy, local, in arterial reconstruction, 236
endothelial cells, in normal spleen, 15f
erythrocyte(s), 4–6. *See also* red blood cell(s)
exercise
  lack of, intermittent claudication and, 216
  treatment of type II diabetes with
    newer modes of, 129–30
    new strategies in, 146–48, 147f, 148f, 149f, 150

F

femoral-popliteal bypass, in management of peripheral vascular disease, 260
fish oil, hemorrheologic effect of, 186–87

flunarizine, mediator blockade by, 183t
foot, diabetic, 201f, 202f
  care of
    education of patient, 209–11
    infected ulcers, 207–9
    medical management of, 193–94, 211
    patient instructions, 210–11
    in peripheral vascular disease, 258
    team approach to, 209
  correction of vascular risk factors in, 204–5, 204t
  improved circulation in, 205–7
  with ischemic skin changes, 206f
  massive ulcer on plantar surface of, 202, 202f
  neuropathic ulcer, 248, 248f
  peripheral neuropathy in, 199–204
    causes of, 203
    signs and symptoms of, 199–200
  peripheral vascular disease, 194–98, 194t, 195f, 196f
    Doppler pressures in, 197–98, 199f
    Doppler waveforms in, 197, 198f
    signs and symptoms of, 196–97
  saving of, 204–11
foot ulcers, treatment of, 207–9
fructose
  ApoA$_1$/ApoB ratio and, 148, 149f

G

glipizide
  comparison of therapy with, 136*t*
  dosage of, 118*t*, 119
  relationship among sulfonylureas, 135*t*
  treatment with, 118–19, 118*t*
glucose
  blood concentrations of, following transplantation, 271, 272*f*
  increased hepatic production of, treatment of, 145–46, 145*f*
  response to glyburide, 152–54, 152*t*, 153*f*, 154*f*
  intolerance, insulin secretion and, 124, 125*f*
glyburide
  comparison of therapy with, 136*t*
  C-peptide levels and, 154–55, 154*f*, 156*f*
  dosage of, 118*t*, 119
  glucose response to, 152–54, 152*t*, 153*f*, 154*f*
  insulin combined with, 139–40, 140*f*
    glucose and C-peptide levels response to, 154–56, 155*t*, 156*f*
  relationship among sulfonylureas, 135*t*
  treatment of type II diabetes with, 118–19, 118*t*
glycation, nonenzymatic, diabetic neuropathy and, 171–72, 171*f*
graft(s)
  nonimmunogenic, obtaining of, 270–71
  rejection, in islet transplantation, 268–69
  sensitization, in islet transplantation, 268, 268*f*

H

hammer toe, 200
  progression of contractures leading to, 201*f*
hemoglobin A_1C, formation of, 243–44, 245*f*
hemoglobinopathy(ies), with relatively stiff red blood cells, 10
hemorrheologic drugs. *See also specific agents*
  mediator blockade by, 183*t*
  in treatment of peripheral vascular disease, 234, 234–35
hemorrheology, 181–82
  definition of, 2
  description of, 1
  drugs affecting, 182, 183*t*, 187–88, 187*f*
  microcirculation and, 1–7
hormonal hypothesis, of diabetic neuropathy, 172–73
hyperglycemia, metabolic defects leading to, 144*f*
hypertension, peripheral vascular disease and, 45

I

infections, management of, 259
infrapopliteal bypass, in management of peripheral vascular disease, 260
injuries, management of, 259
inositol hypothesis, of diabetic neuropathy, 168–70
in situ vein graft technique, in arterial reconstruction, 236–37

insulin
  glyburide combined with, 139–40, 140f
  glucose and C-peptide levels response to, 154–56, 155t, 156f
  newer modes of treatment with, 137–38
  normalizing postprandial blood sugars with, 138–39
  oral agents and, 120
  secretion
    glucose intolerance and, 124, 125f
    impaired, treatment of, 143–44
  treatment with, 117
  resistance, treatment of, 146
intermittent claudication, 215
  absolute claudication distance, 223f
  diagnosis of, 233
  improvement in, 224t
  initial claudication distance, 222f
  nonoperative treatment of, 215–25
  pharmacologic manipulation of, 216–25
    anticoagulants, 217
    antiplatelet agents, 217–18
    calcium channel blocking agents, 225
    prostaglandins, 218–19
    red blood cell deformability and, 220–22
    serotonin-related agents, 223, 225
    vasodilators, 217
islands of Langerhans, transplantation of, 267–76. *See also* islet transplantation

islet transplantation, 267, 276
  activation of T cells, 269–70, 270f
  allograft response in, 267–72, 268f
  in animals, 272–73
    blood glucose concentrations following, 271, 272f
  disease recurrence, 272–76, 274f, 276f
  graft rejection, 268–69
    in animals, 271–72, 272f
  graft sensitization, 268, 268f
  in humans, 273–76
  needle biopsy technique, 275, 276f
  obtaining nonimmunogenic graft, 270–71
  pro-islets developing adjacent to ductal structures, 273–74, 274f
  T-cell activation, 269, 270f

J

Job study on diabetic complications, 65–66, 67t, 68

K

ketanserin
  hemorrheologic effect of, 186
  mediator blockade by, 183t
  in treatment of intermittent claudication, 223, 225
Kroc study on control of retinopathy, 74, 76, 76f, 77f, 78f

L

laser angioplasty, in arterial reconstruction, 237–38

lidocaine infusion, in treatment of neuropathy, 175
lipoproteins, role of, in peripheral vascular disease, 43–45
liver-spleen scan, of SS-genotype infant, 14f
local endarterectomy, in arterial reconstruction, 236

M

Macaca arctoides, 23, 24f
macrovascular complications, metabolic control and, 92–93
macrovascular disease, risk factors for, 204–5, 204t. *See also* peripheral vascular disease
Malmo study on diabetic complications, 64–65, 64t, 65t
malnutrition diabetes, 115n, 116
membrane thickness, diabetes and, 53, 53t, 55t
mesenteric microcirculation, 9f
metabolic control, newer modes of treatment in, 125–26
microaneurysms
  increase of, in diabetes, 66, 67t
  Job study on, 65–66, 67t, 68
microcirculation
  description of, 2
  hemorrheology and, 1–7
  red blood cell in, 10f
microvascular complications
  metabolic control and, 90–91
  metabolic factors and, 88–90
  strict glycemic control and, 91–92
monkey, stump-tailed, stiff red cell syndrome and, 23, 24f

N

naftidrofuryl
  hemorrheologic effect of, 185–86
  mediator blockade by, 183t
  in treatment of intermittent claudication, 219
narcotic analgesics, in treatment of diabetic neuropathy, 175
needle biopsy technique, in islet transplantation, 275, 276f
nephropathy
  development of, 50–51, 52t
  incidence of, 65, 65t
  Malmo study on, 64–65, 64t, 65t
neuropathic ulcer, 248, 248f
neuropathy, diabetic
  classification of, 163
  clinical presentation of, 164–73
  development of, 242–43, 242f
  hormonal hypothesis of, 172–73
  inositol hypothesis of, 168–70
  nonenzymatic glycation and, 171–72, 171f
  painful, treatment for, 175
  pathophysiology of, 242–43, 242f
  polyol pathway and, 167–68, 167f
  postulated mechanisms of, 167–73
  prevalence of, 164
  treatment of, 173–75

neuropathy, diabetic (*continued*)
  types of, 163
  vascular hypothesis of, 170–71
neuropathy, peripheral, pathophysiology of, 243
New Haven study on control of retinopathy, 71, 73, 75f 75t
nondiabetic vascular ulcer, 248f, 249
nonenzymatic glycation, neuropathy and, 171–72, 171f
nonimmunogenic graft, obtaining of, 270–71

O

oral agents
  effectiveness of, 119
  insulin and, 120
  treatment with, 117–19, 118t
osteomyelitis, progression of contractures leading to, 201f

P

pain, in peripheral vascular disease, 259–60
  in diagnosis of, 246
pallor, in diagnosis of peripheral vascular disease, 247
pancreatic functions, treatment of diabetes and, 113–14
paralysis, in diagnosis of peripheral vascular disease, 247
patient education, in management of diabetic foot, 209–11

pentoxifylline
  biochemical mechanism of action of, 27–29, 29f
  combined with PGE_1, 33
  effect of
    on filtration rate of blood in sickle cell disease, 23, 24f
    hemorrheologic, 182, 184
    on *in vivo* platelet aggregation, 27, 27f
    in stiff red cell syndrome, 22–23, 22f, 23f, 24f, 27
    to facilitate perfusion, 31–35
  mediator blockade by, 183t
  metabolism of, 31–33, 32f
  red blood cell deformability and, 221–22, 222f, 223f, 224t
  reduction of aggregation index after pretreatment with, 27, 28f
  in treatment
    of intermittent claudication, 224t, 225
    of peripheral vascular disease, 235
peptide. *See* C-peptide
percutaneous transluminal angioplasty
  in arterial reconstruction, 235–36
  in management of peripheral vascular disease, 261
peripheral neuropathy
  causes of, 203
  pathophysiology of, 243
  signs and symptoms of, 199–200
  treatment of, 203–4
peripheral vascular disease, 194–98
  arterial reconstructive techniques in, 235–38

angioscopy, 237
conventional bypass, 236
laser angioplasty, 237–38
local endarterectomy, 236
percutaneous transluminal angioplasty, 235–36
in situ vein graft, 236–37
arteriogram from patient with, 195–96, 195f, 253–54, 255f, 257f
bilateral superficial femoral artery occlusion, 253, 254f
calcified aortoiliac disease and, 260
cigarette smoking and, 43, 44f
clinical evaluation of, 249–56
  ankle pressures, 250, 250t
  arteriogram, 253–56, 254f, 255f, 256f, 257f
  artery pressures, 251
  noninvasive blood flow laboratory measurements, 244f, 249–53, 250t, 251f, 252f
diagnosis of, 246–49, 248f
differences in, 194–95, 194t
Doppler pressures in, 197–98, 199f
Doppler waveforms in, 197, 198f, 251f
drug therapy in, 234–35
formation of hemoglobin A_1C and, 243–44, 245f
historical perspective of, 41–42
hypertension and, 45
lipoproteins and, 43–45
management of, 256–61
  aortobifemoral artery bypass, 260
  autogenous saphenous vein graft, 260

cessation of smoking, 259
diabetic foot care, 258
femoral-popliteal bypass, 260
foot care, 258
infections of lower extremities, 259
infrapopliteal bypass, 260
medical, 233–35
obtaining proper footwear, 259
percutaneous transluminal angioplasty, 261
occlusive, diagnosis of, 231–33, 233f
pathophysiology of, 241–45, 242f, 244f, 245f
physical evaluation of patient with, 247–49, 248f
prevalence of, 42–43
progression of, 45–46
red blood cell filterability in, 19, 19t
risk factors in, 43–45, 44f
signs and symptoms of, 196–97
sorbitol pathway, 242–43, 242f
surgical management of, 196f, 235
suspected left femoral artery stenosis, 253, 256f
PGE_1, combined with pentoxifylline, 33
pharmacologic agents
  red blood cell deformability and, 220–22, 222f, 223f, 224t
  in treatment of intermittent claudication, 216–25
pharmacologic therapy, new strategies in, 150–55, 152t, 153f, 154f, 155t, 156f

289

phenytoin, in treatment of neuropathy, 175
plasma viscosity, in normal circulation, 6
platelet(s), undergoing viscous metamorphosis, 23, 25f, 26f, 27
platelet aggregation
  effect of adenosine diphosphate on, 23, 25f
  in vivo
    effect of pentoxifylline on, 27, 27f
    measuring apparatus for, 23, 25f
    scanning electron microscopic view of, 23, 25f, 26f
polyol pathway, diabetic neuropathy and, 167–68, 167f
pores, occlusion of, by stiff red cells, 27, 28f
postprandial blood sugars, newer modes in normalizing of, 138–39
prostacyclin, in treatment of peripheral vascular disease, 235
prostaglandin E_1, combined with pentoxifylline, 33
prostaglandins, in treatment of intermittent claudication, 218–19
pulselessness, in diagnosis of peripheral vascular disease, 247

R

Raynaud's syndrome, red blood cell filterability in, 19, 20t
receptor system, treatment for diabetes and, 114
reconstruction, arterial, angioscopy, 237
  conventional bypass, 236
  in situ vein graft, 236–37
  laser angioplasty, 237–38
  local endarterectomy, 236
  percutaneous transluminal angioplasty, 235–36
red blood cell(s). *See also* stiff red cell syndrome
  aggregation of, 4–5
  concentration of, 4–5
  crenated, 17, 18f
  deformability of
    measurement of, 11, 12f
    measuring apparatus for, 11, 12f
    normal, 11, 13f
    normal circulation and, 5–6
    in sickle cell crisis, 11–12, 14f
    pharmacologic agents and, 220–22, 222f, 223f, 224t
  filterability of, 19, 19t, 20t
  in microcirculation, 10f
  microscopic view of, in sickle cell disease, 14
  normal, filtered, 13f
  parasitism, 10
  shape change by, in small capillaries, 9f
  SS-genotype, 15–16, 16f
red cell stiffness
  measuring apparatus for, 23, 25f
  occlusion of pores by, 25f, 27, 28f
renal function, Steno study on, 71, 72t
rest pain, in peripheral vascular disease, 259–60
retinopathy
  Belgian study on, 65, 66f

British study on control of, 71, 73f, 74f
classification of, 75t
as complication of diabetes, 65, 66f
Kroc study on control of, 74, 76, 76f, 77f, 78f
New Haven study on control of, 71, 73, 75f, 75t
prevalence of, in diabetes, 51f
Steno study on control of, 68, 69f, 70t, 71, 72t

S

saline, reduction of aggregation index after pretreatment with, 28f
saphenous vein graft, autogenous, in peripheral vascular disease, 260
serotonin-related agents, in treatment of intermittent claudication, 223, 225
sickle cell disease,
　effect of pentoxifylline in, 27, 28f
　prevention of, 34–35
　red blood cells in, 14f
smoking. See cigarette smoking
sorbinil, in treatment of neuropathy, 174
sorbitol pathway, 242f
spleen
　importance of circulation in, 14–15
　normal cortex of, 15f
　normal sinus of 15f
　in SS-genotype infant, 14f
SS-genotype
　infant
　　bone marrow of, 14, 15f
　　liver-spleen scan of, 12–14, 14f
　　red blood cells being deoxygenated before sickling, 15–16, 16f
Steno study
　on control of retinopathy, 68, 69f, 70t, 71, 72t
　on renal function, 71, 72t
stiff red cell syndrome
　adenosine diphosphate effect on platelet aggregation, 23, 25f
　blood vessel three minutes after needle prick injury, 22, 22f
　measuring apparatus
　　to determine *in vivo* platelet aggregation and, 23, 25f
　occlusion of pores in, 27, 28f
　pentoxifylline, effects of on
　　filtration rate of blood, 22–23, 23f, 24f
　　on animal model of vasoocclusive crisis, 27, 28f
　　on *in vivo* platelet aggregation, 27, 27f
　scanning electron microscopic view
　　of aggregating platelets, 23, 25f, 26f
　　of platelets undergoing viscous metamorphosis, 23, 26f
　significance of, 12–14, 14f, 15f
　stump-tailed monkey and, 23, 24f
　xanthine derivatives and, 22
stress, at microcirculatory level, 1
stump-tailed monkey, 23, 24f
sulfonylurea agents. *See also specific agents*
　comparison of, 136t

291

sulfonylurea agents (*continued*)
  newer modes of treatment with, in type II diabetes, 130–34, 131*f*, 132*f*, 133*f*, 134*f*, 137
  relationship among, 135*t*
surgery, in peripheral vascular disease, 235

T

T cell activation, in islet transplantation, 269–70, 270*f*
theophylline, effects on stiff red cell syndrome, 22
thromboembolism, red blood cell filterability in, 19, 20*t*
thromboxane synthetase inhibitors, in treatment of intermittent claudication, 219
tip-top-toe syndrome, 200, 201*f*
tolazamide
  comparison of therapy with, 136*t*,
  relationship among sulfonylureas, 135*t*
tolbutamide
  comparison of therapy with, 136*t*
  relationship among sulfonylureas, 135*t*
  in treatment of type II diabetes, 118
tolrestat, in treatment of neuropathy, 174–75
transplantation. *See* islet transplantation
treadmill testing, Doppler waveforms and, 252, 252*f*

Trental
  in stiff red cell syndrome, 22–23, 22*f*, 23*f*, 24*f*, 27
  in treatment of peripheral vascular disease, 235
tricyclic drugs, in treatment of neuropathy, 175. *See also* specific agents

U

ulcers, vascular. *See also* foot ulcers
  neuropathic, 248, 248*f*
  nondiabetic vascular, 248*f*, 249

V

vascular disease(s), risk factors for, 204–5, 204*t*. *See also* peripheral vascular disease
vascular hypothesis of diabetic neuropathy, 170–71
vascular system
  diabetic
    complications after 40 years, 49–50, 50*t*
    Doppler waveform of, 243, 244*f*
  normal, 243, 244*f*
vascular ulcer
  neuropathic, 248, 248*f*
  nondiabetic, 248*f*, 249
vasodilators
  in treatment of intermittent claudication, 217
  in treatment of peripheral vascular disease, 234
vein graft, *in situ*, in arterial reconstruction, 236–37
vessel wall disorders, with stiff red blood cells, 10

W

weight control, newer modes of treatment in, 126–29, 127f
whole blood, normal, 13f

X

xanthine derivatives, effect of, in stiff red cell syndrome, 22. *See also specific agents*